# Handbuch der Urologie
# Encyclopedia of Urology · Encyclopédie d'Urologie

*Gesamtdisposition · Outline · Disposition générale*

---

| Allgemeine Urologie | General Urology | Urologie générale |
|---|---|---|
| I   Anatomie und Embryologie | Anatomy and embryology | Anatomie et embryologie |
| II   Physiologie und pathologische Physiologie | Physiology and pathological physiology | Physiologie normale et pathologique |
| III   Symptomatologie und Untersuchung von Blut, Harn und Genitalsekreten | Symptomatology and examination of the blood, urine and genital secretions | Symptomatologie et examens du sang, de l'urine et des sécrétions annexielles |
| IV   Niereninsuffizienz | Renal insufficiency | L'insuffisance rénale |
| V/1   Radiologische Diagnostik | Diagnostic radiology | Radiologie diagnostique |
| V/2   Radiotherapie | Radiotherapy | Radiothérapie |
| VI   Endoskopie | Endoscopy | Endoscopie |

| Spezielle Urologie | Special Urology | Urologie spéciale |
|---|---|---|
| VII   Mißbildungen und Verletzungen. Urologische Begutachtung | Developmental anomalies and injuries. The urologist's expert opinion | Malformations et traumatismes. L'expertise en urologie |
| VIII   Entleerungsstörungen | Urinary stasis | La stase |
| IX/1   Unspezifische Entzündungen | Non-specific inflammations | Inflammations non-spécifiques |
| IX/2   Spezifische Entzündungen | Specific inflammations | Inflammations spécifiques |
| X   Die Steinerkrankungen | Calculous disease | La lithiase urinaire |
| XI   Tumoren | Tumours | Les tumeurs |
| XII   Funktionelle Störungen | Functional disturbances | Les troubles fonctionnels |
| XIII/1   Operative Urologie 1 | Operative urology 1 | L'urologie opératoire 1 |
| XIII/2   Operative Urologie 2 | Operative urology 2 | L'urologie opératoire 2 |
| XIV   Gynäkologische Urologie | Gynaecological urology | L'urologie de la femme |
| XV   Die Urologie des Kindes | Urology in childhood | L'urologie de l'enfant |
| XVI   General-Register und Schlußbetrachtungen | General-Index and Retrospect and outlook | Table de matières Conclusions |

# HANDBUCH DER UROLOGIE

# ENCYCLOPEDIA OF UROLOGY

# ENCYCLOPÉDIE D'UROLOGIE

HERAUSGEGEBEN VON · EDITED BY
PUBLIÉE SOUS LA DIRECTION DE

**C. E. ALKEN**   **V. W. DIX**   **H. M. WEYRAUCH**
HOMBURG (SAAR)   LONDON   SAN FRANCISCO

**E. WILDBOLZ**
BERN

XII

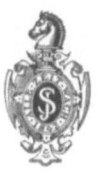

Springer-Verlag Berlin Heidelberg GmbH 1960

# FUNKTIONELLE STÖRUNGEN
# FUNCTIONAL DISTURBANCES

VON / BY

**ALFRED AUERBACK** · SAN FRANCISCO
**CARL E. BURKLAND** · SACRAMENTO
**GUSTAV-WILHELM PARADE** · NEUSTADT / WEINSTRASSE
**J. COSBIE ROSS** · LIVERPOOL - **DONALD R. SMITH** · SAN FRANCISCO
**WALTER W. WILLIAMS** · SPRINGFIELD

MIT 74 ABBILDUNGEN
WITH 74 FIGURES

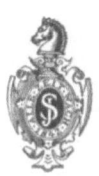

Springer-Verlag Berlin Heidelberg GmbH 1960

ISBN 978-3-662-21928-7    ISBN 978-3-662-21926-3 (eBook)
DOI 10.1007/978-3-662-21926-3

© by Springer-Verlag Berlin Heidelberg 1960
Originally published by Springer-Verlag OHG / Berlin · Göttigen · Heidelberg in 1960.
Softcover reprint of the hardcover 1st edition 1960

# Inhalt — Contents

**Neuromuscular Dysfunction and Paraplegia.** By J. Cosbie Ross. With 28 figures

**Male Sterility.** By Walter W. Williams. With 35 figures

## Mitarbeiter von Band XII — Contributors to volume XII

ALFRED AUERBACK, Professor Dr., University of California, San Francisco/USA.

CARL E. BURKLAND, M. D., Sacramento/USA.

GUSTAV-WILHELM PARADE, ord. Professor, Dr., Direktor des Städtischen Krankenhauses Neustadt a. d. Weinstraße.

J. COSBIE ROSS, Ch. M., F.R.C.S., Liverpool/Great Britain.

DONALD R. SMITH, M. D., Medical School, San Francisco/USA.

WALTER W. WILLIAMS, M. D., Springfield/USA.

# Functional Diseases

By

DONALD R. SMITH and ALFRED AUERBACK

With 7 figures

# A. The effect of the psyche on vesical function

## I. Introduction and review of the literature

Aberrations in vesical activity are very often caused by psychological disorders. Possibly 10% of patients with complaints consistent with "cystitis" are in this category. Emotional tension can act, through the autonomic nervous system, upon the posterior pituitary, adrenal cortex, smooth muscle, and blood vessels. Disturbances in their function or condition alter the amount of urine formed and the functioning of the neuromuscular mechanism of the bladder, thus causing urinary symptoms. What could cause a woman to urinate every 15 to 30 minutes during the first three hours after arising and yet have no further frequency during the day and no need to get up at night? Why would a 43-year-old man develop increasing nocturia such that he had to arise seven or eight times a night an yet had to void only three times a day? These two brief outlines of symptom complexes are typical of the psychosomatic urological disorder: Organic urological disease does not manifest itself in these ways—only nervous tension could account for such bizarre complaints.

The effect of acute anxiety upon bladder function is well known even to the layman. A typical example is the woman who felt she could not leave the bathroom on her wedding day because of severe urgency and frequency such as she had never before experienced and never suffered again.

It was early recognized (Guyon) that some patients suffered from urinary frequency because of emotional disturbance, yet in spite of many observations recorded in the literature this phenomenon has been little investigated by urologists. In 1890 one of Guyon's pupils, JULES JANET, published a monograph entitled, "Les troubles psychopathiques de la miction". He quoted Guyon as having said, "The bladder does not have an anatomical capacity; it has only a physiological capacity depending on its reaction to tension." Janet even discussed the habit of frequency which some men developed as a result of hearing other men urinate in the toilets on the avenues of Paris. He noted that male dogs wandering about the streets voided every time they sniffed a hydrant or a tree, but if confined to the house voided only three times a day. He knew how commonly medical students suffered acute urgency and frequency just before examinations.

JANET recognized that frequency was the most common symptom of the "nervous" bladder. He believed that the primary cause was an abnormal preoccupation with the act and organs of urination. Such preoccupation caused bladder contractions which were reflected in urgency. He noted that patients with this complaint nearly always had sexual difficulties as well.

Janet again quoted Guyon as follows: "It is easy to differentiate between psychic cystitis and true cystitis, for patients suffering from the former disease pass a large volume of clear urine." Janet observed that the nervous bladder would accept 300 ml of water by instillation, yet the patient might void only 100 ml every hour. On the other hand, in bacterial cystitis the capacity equalled the amount voided.

Janet recognized the fact that the patient with the irritable bladder caused by tension suffered day frequency but slept undisturbed all night. He cited the case of one patient who voided 16 to 24 times during the day but had no night frequency unless he had insomnia. If he was wakeful, his psyche remained active, according to Janet, so nocturia occurred as well. Janet recognized that even during the daytime frequency might cease as long as the patient was preoccupied.

In 1915 DÉJERINE and GLAUCKLER published a book, "The psychoneuroses and their treatment". They discussed frequency caused by nervousness, when frequency was periodic and associated with the voiding of large volumes of dilute urine. They attributed this type of frequency to acute emotional stress and thought it might become permanent through habit. They also discussed nervous polydipsia as a cause of frequency. They cited cases of urinary retention and incontinence caused by psychic disturbance. They thought frequency was often due to an obsession with urination, and they recognized that the pains of which their patients complained were not related to urination.

In 1929 MAYER described the case of a young woman who voided 40—60 times a day. She had desire for sexual experience, yet feared to allow it. She often dreamed of men and of voiding; urination became a substitute for her sexual drive. As a result of psychotherapy her frequency ceased.

In 1930 ALKAN discussed the polyuria and frequency which occurred secondary to emotional disturbance. He noted that frequency associated with external sphincter spasm led to hypertrophy of the detrusor, which can be recognized as trabeculation. The bladder then becomes contracted. When the patient undergoes psychotherapy, the bladder may slowly regain some of its capacity. This observation tends to corroborate our longstanding suspicion that interstitial cystitis represents the end stage of the bladder made irritable by emotional upset. We have reported a case of trabeculation of the bladder associated with emotional upset.

MENNINGER published a paper in 1941 which dealt with the vesical symptoms that develop secondary to psychological factors. He discussed the erotic and aggressive components in urination. He noted that urination produces a feeling of sexual excitement in the infant. Normally, with maturity, this type of sexual gratification yields to masturbation which in turn yields to the adult sexual attitude. In neuroses, regression toward the infantile state occurs; frequency may therefore develop, thus representing and replacing sexual activity. Many women enjoy the sexual act more if their bladders are partially distended. Some of these patients report dreams in which they are about to have sexual relations but the dream is interrupted by an urge to urinate.

MENNINGER believes that urination is also an aggressive act. Consider the phrase, "Piss on you!", which is often the strongest weapon at the disposal of the child. The child, knowing that this will irritate his parents, may urinate frequently at the time of bladder training in order to defy them.

In 1941 VAN DER HEIDE described in detail a case of pollakiuria nervosa in a patient whom he had analyzed.

In a series of articles on the psychosomatic perspective in urology, CHERTOK, ABOULKER et al. have given an excellent review of the problems of micturition and of hyperesthesia in the region of the female urinary bladder. In a study of cystalgia, or "unstable bladder," they cite MOMBAERTS for the following symptomatology:

1. Micturitional symptoms, including urgency, painful micturition, frequency, and inability to urinate.

2. Perineal symptoms, including shooting pains, twinges, throbbing, twitching tingling, burning, vulvar symptoms, and dyspareunia;

3. Feelings of heaviness and pain radiating to the iliac and lumbosacral regions,

Accompanying these complaints, which were reported mostly by women, MOMBAERTS noted emotional symptoms and generalized psychological disturbances. Despite these symptoms, however, he believed that endocrine dysfunction was the major cause of "cystalgia" because most of the patients were women past the age of the menopause. It is interesting to note that he found endocrine therapy rarely helpful. It is our belief that there are common underlying psychological causes for the "cystalgia" he discussed.

In their study, CHERTOK and his associates found that their patients had day rather than night frequency. Their symptoms were characterized by crises and remissions. The urine was clear; no pyuria was present, and the bladder capacity was normal. Urethroscopy occasionally revealed polypoid formations on the bladder neck. The authors studied 50 women with an age range of 22 to 64 years and with urinary complaints of from one month's to 15 years' duration. Most had had extensive urological treatment. In addition to a complete physical examination each patient had psychiatric interviews and psychological testing.

The nature of the patient's complaints was noted, particularly the description of the pain or discomfort suffered. In many cases the pain was poorly localized and hard to define. None of the patients had a satisfactory sexual life. Ninety per cent were frigid. The urinary complaints of most of the women had a sexual coloring; often, the patient commented spontaneously that the urinary symptoms arose in connection with a sexual trauma. In some patients, initial unpleasant sexual relations in marriage produced dyspareunia and urinary symptoms. Others developed symptoms following rape, divorce, menopause, marital conflict, or traumatic surgery. Separation from husband or children was interpreted as rejection and triggered symptoms. Since the patients had focused their attention upon the physical symptoms, it was only through psychiatric study or psychological testing that it became possible to elicit the underlying neurotic problems. Some of the patients had phobias or other hysterical or psychosomatic symptoms.

The authors found that their female patients with cystalgia fell into two major categories. One group consisted of women possessing essentially masochistic personality traits. These patients were passive and somewhat depressed; aggressiveness was strongly repressed. Their prevailing attitude was a feeling of resignation in the face of misfortune. They had a "need for atonement," being the women who "gave all they had" or were "too good" and permitted themselves to be "used." The second group consisted of women with strongly aggressive, assertive personalities. Their behavior might be considered masculine in that they were outgoing and explosive. Some patients fell into an intermediate group showing mixed patterns of the two more clear-cut categories. Control subjects did not show these two categories of personality traits.

In conclusion, CHERTOK et al. summarized the factors and symptoms which they found in their cases:

1. Frequent absence of any organic illness (where illness existed, it did not explain the severity of the symptoms);

2. A coincidence between the onset of the complaint and the presence of a crisis or conflict situation in the patient's life;

3. Psychosexual disturbances in all patients;

4. Aggravation of the symptoms when treated locally and by surgical intervention;

5. Pain of an unusual character and a unique expressive (symbolic) value.

Our findings, previously reported, are in accord with the observations of CHERTOK and his co-workers. The majority of women we studied were frigid or had feelings of guilt about sexual activity which precluded complete satisfaction. Many had noted that prolonged love-making without coitus produced lower abdominal pain and urinary symptoms, most often frequency. The symptoms of "cystitis", or cystalgia were usually worse on the day following unsatisfactory intercourse. Marital strife often acted as a trigger. Feelings of "burning anger" or of "wanting to explode" were frequently expressed.

The initial urinary symptoms often appeared abruptly after a sexually stimulating situation which, for physical or psychological reasons, proved unsatisfactory. Many times the patient was not consciously aware of erotic feelings. The sexually inexperienced or prudish young woman may interpret the pelvic tumescence resulting from sexual stimulation as a need to urinate. By denying to herself that she has any arousal, she displaces all sexual feelings to the urinary system and establishes this pattern for tension discharge. It must be emphasized that this is an unconscious process, entirely beyond the patient's control and awareness. Once this mechanism is operative, sexual stimuli are responded to by urinary symptoms.

A study of patients with cystalgia shows a profound degree of sexual misidentification. The passive woman as described by CHERTOK considered the sexual act a function for the husband's pleasure and herself the exploited person. The aggressive woman felt "burning anger" at being used. Once these pathways for tension discharge had become established, the patients responded to any situation of anger, frustration, anxiety, or emotional distress by urgency and a sensation of burning. These symptoms then occurred as an automatic reaction with no conscious relationship to the emotional crisis setting off the response.

### Illustrative Cases

Case 1. A 45-year-old divorcee, eager for marriage, became engaged to a man whom she considered socially her inferior. Her fiance persuaded her to engage in premarital coitus. Torn between her desire to satisfy her fiance and a feeling of exploitation, she submitted. The following day she had intense burning, urgency, and frequency of urination. Cystoscopic examination was negative, and no pus or bacteria were found in the urine. Despite the use of various antibiotic and sedative drugs her symptoms became worse and continued intense until she left for a protracted vacation. It appeared that she unconsciously sought to avoid any further sexual contact by the continuation of her urinary symptoms.

Case 2. A 35-year-old married woman had been brought up in a strict religious home where sexual expression in any form was considered sinful. The initial episode of cystitis in this patient occurred following a physical examination by her physician when during the examination she had become aware of intense sexual feelings toward the physician, feelings she sought to repress.

One Sunday her husband insisted on intercourse at a time when she believed they should be in church. She was sexually aroused but because of her guilt feelings could not reach orgasm. She was angry with her husband and herself and was aware of a need for punishment. The next morning she awoke suffering from extreme urgency and burning.

Case 3. A 32-year-old woman who had been deserted by her husband became aware one evening of an intense sexual urge which was not relieved by masturbation. "I felt so full, as though I was going to burst." In a short time she developed frequency which continued for several hours, with a gradual diminution of her erotic feeling.

Case 4. A 49-year-old unmarried woman executive had had complaints of burning, frequency, and perineal pain for 14 years. Extensive urological treatment had achieved variable results: her condition had intermittent remissions and recurrences. The pain was severe enough to lead to consideration of possible nerve-block surgery. The patient's mother had died when she was born, and she had been raised by a maiden aunt who had impressed on her that she was superior to men and had no need for marriage. When the patient was 10 years old and the aunt 35, the latter began an affair with a suitor which lasted many years. The patient was perplexed and angered by this behavior but never dared speak about it. During this time she developed a "crush" on a female teacher whom she visited daily after school. Being with the teacher aroused her sexually and gave her a feeling of bladder fullness. She refrained from using the toilet in the teacher's home. However, in her own home it was necessary to pass through the aunt's bedroom to reach the bathroom; but when the aunt's lover was in the room she was refused admission despite her urgent appeals. She retaliated by urinating in the aunt's flower box.

The patient avoided male contacts and embarked upon an active homosexual life. She entered a field of endeavor normally reserved for men and won equal status with them because of her drive and ability. Her symptoms began at the age of 35, the same age at which her aunt had become involved with her lover. Psychiatric study revealed a struggle between the patient's wishes to be accepted as equal to men and her equally strong desire to be a fragile woman courted by men. The unusual perineal pain was relieved by using a cold or hot compress wedged between her legs and pushing on the perineum. When the patient understood that this represented a symbolic penis, the pain disappeared, although it had given her many years of almost constant distress. As she understood her identification with and hostility toward her aunt, the urgency and frequency also ceased.

This patient presented the syndrome described by CHERTOK: urinary symptoms, unusual pain, and a masculine aggressive personality.

Interstitial cystitis (Hunner's ulcer of the bladder) is an uncommon disease of unknown etiology characterized by progressive submucosal fibrosis with a reduction in vesical capacity and with cystoscopic evidence of ischemia and linear ulceration of the bladder dome. It is most prevalent in middle-aged females of neurotic temperament and is rarely found in men. The urine is clear. The reduced bladder capacity results in frequency of urination. Some writers have noted the relationship of this disease to emotional disorders; a recent report by BOWERS, SCHWARZ and LEON describes a psychiatric study of a case:

A 29-year-old unmarried woman had had an incapacitating bladder dysfunction of many years' duration. The disease had been diagnosed as interstitial cystitis by a number of urologists. The patient's bladder capacity was 175 cc. Frequent, uncontrollable bladder spasms resulted in virtual incontinence, with voiding of 1-ounce amounts day and night. A urethral catheter could not be tolerated; cystotomy drainage was unsuccessful. Cystoscopy revealed severe ischemia of the bladder neck. Transurethral resection of the bladder neck proved useless. Biopsy of the bladder dome showed chronic cystitis. Cystograms showed reflux up the left ureter. Transplanting the ureters into an ileal loop did not relieve the bladder spasms. Finally a transvaginal cystectomy was done. The pathological report was extreme fibrosis of the bladder wall with squamous cell metaplasia of the lining.

Psychiatric study of the patient revealed that after early successful toilet training, enuresis set in at the time of the birth of a baby sister and the post-partum death of the mother. A maiden aunt raised the patient. Whereas cruel punishments were meted out to her for bed-wetting, the rewards she was promised for keeping dry were never received by her. She could never express anger and soon began to wet herself during the day at school or at home when she was angry. Joking comments that "her wetting would wash her husband out of bed" if she married and other unfortunate episodes with men led to avoidance of male contact. Practically the only men in her life were the many urologists she consulted, who performed over 200 cystoscopies upon her.

The authors concluded that the bladder served as a pathway for the discharge of unconscious hatreds. The psychological factor, together with a bladder infection during puberty, started a vicious cycle of hate, repression, enuresis, superimposed infection, inflammation, and iatrogenic traumas which apparently culminated in the chronic interstitial cystitis.

A study of the emotional factors in a case of recurrent urinary retention has been reported by WILLIAMS and JOHNSON. Their patient, a 28-year-old woman, complained of vague abdominal and pelvic pains and recurrent episodes of urinary retention lasting up to 36 hours. Urological examination was negative. Psychiatric study revealed that the patient had gone through a severe toilet training with shaming and physical punishment for "accidents" or for touching her genitals. However, her aunt and uncle, who were raising her, paid excessive attention to her genitals and toilet habits. Her uncle repeatedly manipulated her genitals while forbidding her to do so or to permit other men to do as he did. Her initial episode of retention occurred at the age 17 following rape by her uncle.

In the patient's life outside the home, contacts with men in a superior position such as employers were disturbing to her because she unconsciously anticipated exploitation. The tension associated with contact with any employer mounted, and retention developed. However, as the patient learned to express her anger verbally, the episodes of retention occurred less often.

Study of patients with acute psychogenic retention reveals that they feel themselves in an overwhelming situation with which they are unable to cope. They have no resources with which to handle the crisis and feel swamped, hopeless and depressed. Many men are unable to void lying down because of their previous toilet training and the fact that this passive position mobilizes unconscious anxieties. Some men cannot urinate in the presence of other men. They experience feelings of shame about making a noise in urinating, of concern about the size of the penis, and they often have accompanying unconscious homosexual fears.

An excellent study of incontinence was made by SCHWARTZ and STANTON in a mental hospital. They studied a group of patients who were repeatedly incontinent and the situations in which the incontinence occurred. They found that the following situations tended to produce incontinence: those which made the patient feel abandoned and isolated, those in which the patient's self-esteem was severely hurt, and those in which a conflict was present which the patient felt unable to handle.

The recent *urological* literature on the relation of the emotions to bladder function is sparse indeed. In 1933 Clancy discussed psychosomatic bladder dysfunction briefly; CONE (1946) recognized that the patient with the psychosomatic bladder suffered from day but not night frequency. We recorded a summary of our experiences with the urological manifestations of emotional disturbance in 1952, and in 1953 one of us (D.R.S.) published a paper on a similar subject written in a non-psychiatric vein. In 1954, GREEN and DEAN also briefly discussed the genito-urinary symptoms caused by emotional difficulties. In the textbook, "General Urology", published by one of us (D.R.S.), one chapter is devoted to urological syndromes of psychosomatic origin.

# II. Experimental studies of the psychodynamics of vesical function

## 1. The influence of the emotions on vesical activity

MOSSO and PELLACANI in 1881 were the first to study the effects of the emotions upon vesical function by means of cystometry in dogs and in the human female. They found that a tactile sensation, a loud noise, the sound of running water, a strong emotion, or intellectual work caused vesical contraction. They observed that the mere thought of urination led to contraction of the detrusor muscle.

In 1949, STRAUB, RIPLEY, and WOLF studied a group of neurotic patients, who complained of vesical dysfunction, by means of cystometry. A catheter was placed in the bladder and 50–200 ml of water, depending upon the amount the patient could comfortably hold, were instilled. The catheter was then connected to a recording cystometer. Fig. 1 shows the small rises in intravesical pressure which obtained with physical straining and mental stress. The bladder gradually filled with urine as the experiment progressed. As much as 700 ml were drained from the bladder at the end of the experiment, in spite of the fact that most of these patients were complaining of frequency. After a period of non-conflictual conversation, the interviewer began discussion of a subject to which the patient was psychologically sensitive. This was followed by inconsequential discussion or intravenous sodium amytal. Two types of response were noted:

### a) Hypermotility of the bladder

This was the most common reaction. A 35-year-old single woman developed frequency and urgency when she was in a state of conflict over her relations with a suitor. She was undecided about marrying him. From early childhood, she had been closely attached to her father; she had gone out to dinner and to the theater or movies with him. Her mother was never invited. Her father died when she was 23 years old, but even at the time of the examination, twelve years later, she cried at the mention of his name. She compared other men unfavorably with him and was therefore unable to become closely attached to another man.

Her episodes of urgency and frequency were related to feelings of resentment. Arguments with her employer set off attacks of severe vesical irritability. Fig. 2 shows the cystometric tracing which was obtained during an interview. It will be seen that initially the bladder would accept only 50 ml of water and that even when it contained so little, transient severe urgency occurred until the patient was reassured. During a discussion of her new job, the patient's intravesical pressure remained at 7 ml of water, but when her old job was mentioned, it rose to 75 ml of water. Many uninhibited contractions occurred because of

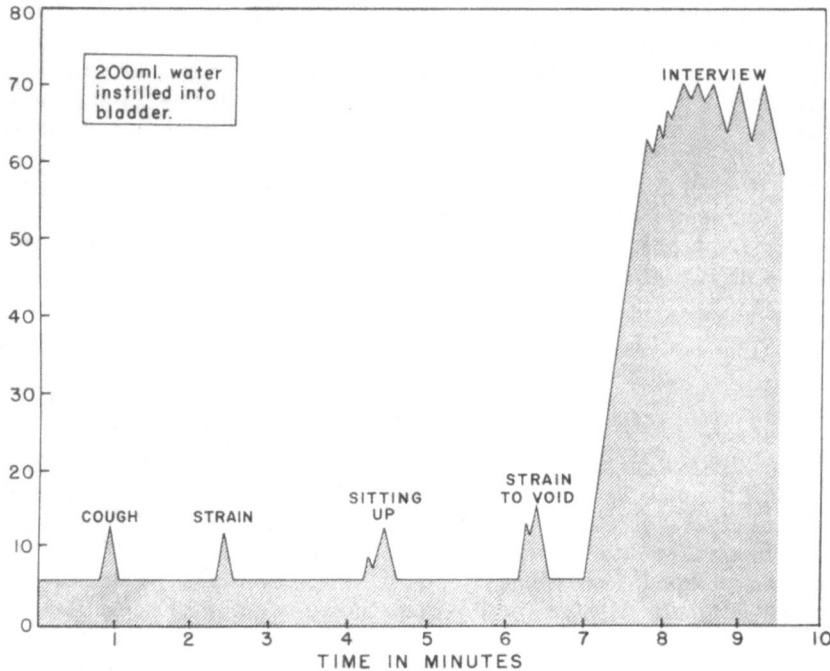

Fig. 1. Cystometrogram showing that only relatively small rises in intravesical pressure occur with voluntary strain whereas intracystic pressures rise sharply when psychic stimuli are present. [Modified, with permission, from L. R. Staub, H. S. Ripley and S. Wolf: J. Amer. med. Ass. **141**, 1139—1143 (1949)]

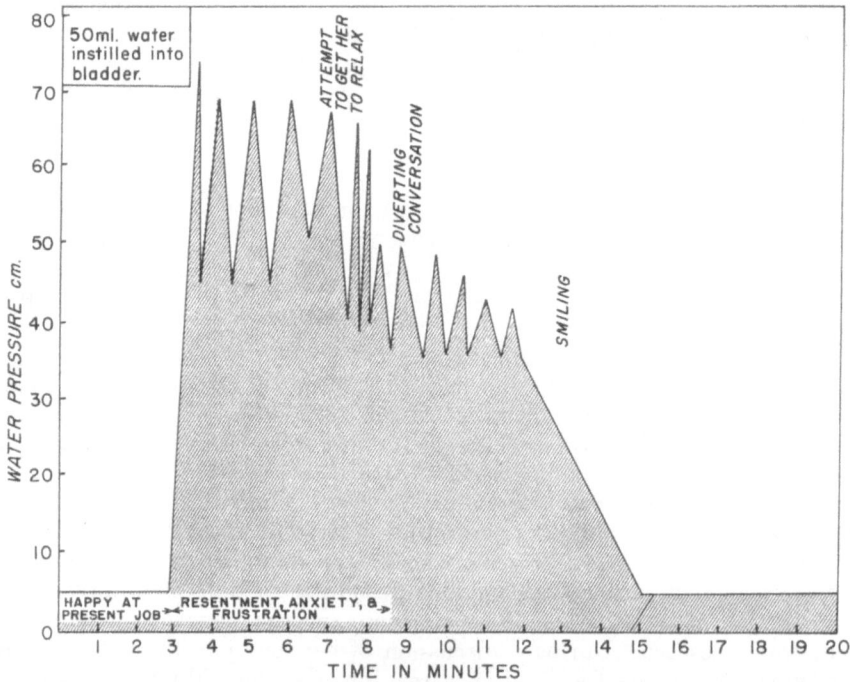

Fig. 2. Cystometrogram showing spasticity of the bladder developing with emotional stress. [Modified, with permission, from L. R. Staub, H. S. Ripley and S. Wolf: J. Amer. med. Ass. **141**, 1139—1143 (1949)]

feelings of resentment, frustration, and anxiety. When an attempt was made to
change to diverting conversation, she persisted in discussing distasteful aspects
of her old job. Finally, however, she relaxed and smiled; intravesical pressure
returned to normal.

A few months after the patient's discharge from the hospital, she was threatened with rape. She reacted with urinary retention. After being periodically
catheterized for a few days, she returned to the hospital. One thousand milliliters
of urine were drained from her bladder. The cystometrogram was typical of an
atonic bladder. Thus, whereas the patient's usual response to stress was frequency
and urgency, she suffered urinary retention when the situation became perilous

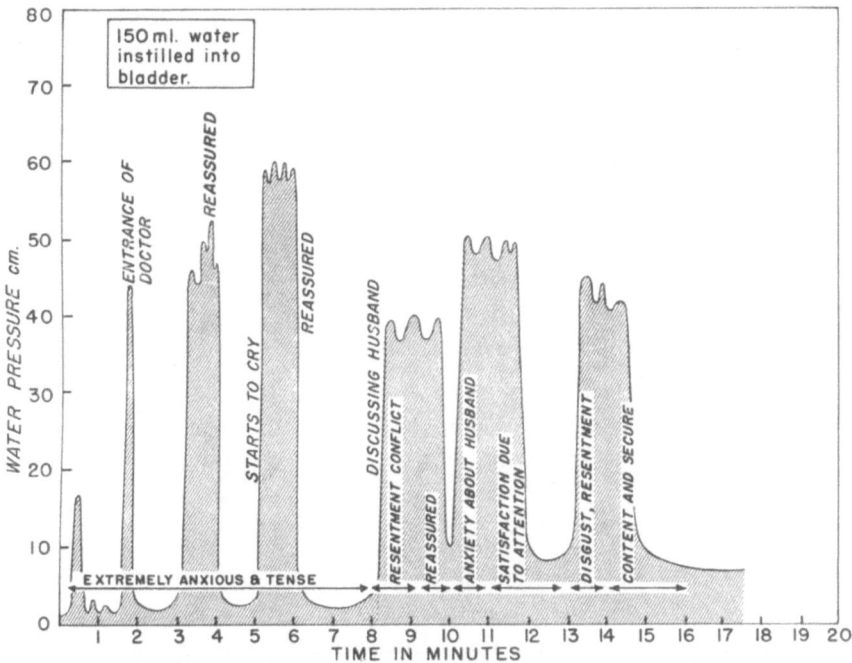

Fig. 3. Cystometrogram showing changes in intravesical pressure paralleling the condition of the psyche. [Modi-
fied, with permission, from L. R. STAUB, H. S. RIPLEY and S. WOLF: J. Amer. med. Ass. 141, 1139—1143 (1949)]

and out of hand. Her inability to have strong feelings for a man, probably
because of her earlier relationship to her father, led to repression of normal
sexuality.

Another example of the hypermotile bladder, also abstracted from the paper
by STRAUB et al., follows.

A 40-year-old woman was very tense and anxious about her marriage. A separation had occurred, but her husband desired a reconciliation. The woman was
physically attracted to him yet felt she could not be happy with him. During
this emotionally trying time she had bouts of urinary frequency.

Fifty milliliters of water were instilled into her bladder; marked but temporary
contractions occurred (Fig. 3). Following reassurance, she was finally able to
accept 150 ml. When the doctor entered the room, intravesical pressure rose
to 45 ml of water. She complained bitterly about the whole procedure; the
pressure rose to 50 ml of water. Her anger persisted; the pressure rose to 60 ml.

The cystometrogram reflects the response of the patient's bladder to discussions about her husband; vesical contractions were initiated which were not quieted until she was reassured.

This type of reaction (vesical hypermotility) was associated with general tension, anxiety, and resentment. Frequency, urgency, dysuria, and small bladder capacity were the rule.

### b) Hypomotility of the bladder

This was a less common response of the bladder to emotional factors. The hypomotility culminated in urinary retention, which was, for example, the

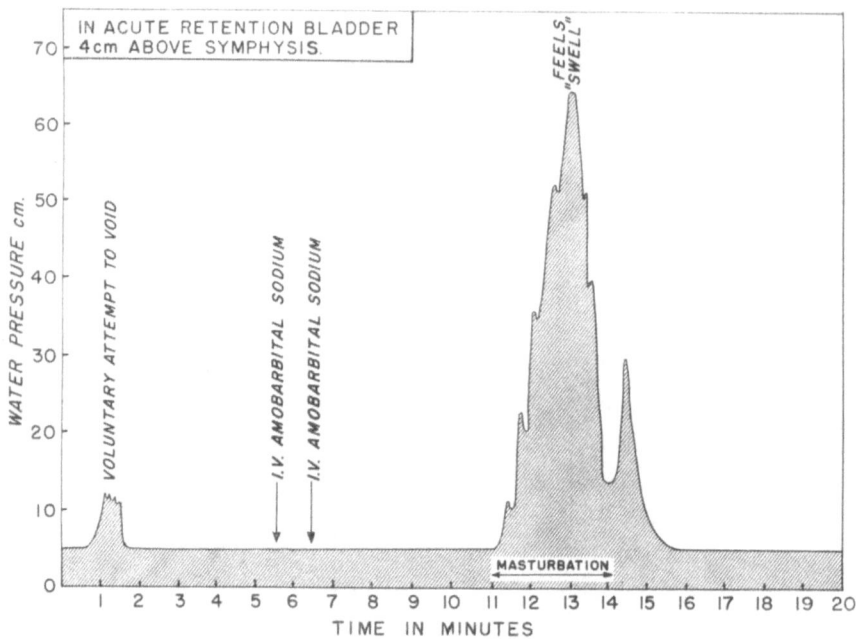

Fig. 4. Cystometric pattern of a woman who developed urinary retention due to psychic stress. [Modified, with permission, from L. R. Staub, H. S. Ripley and S. Wolf: J. Amer. med. Ass. **141**, 1139—1143 (1949)]

presenting symptom of a 25-year-old single woman patient. The patient's father had died when she was three years old. Her mother was an alcoholic who alternately indulged and threatened her children. The patient became withdrawn, cried often, and felt unwanted. She was shy and had few friends. She started to masturbate in adolescence and continued twice a week up to the time of the investigation. If, however, she was interested in a man, she gave up masturbation. She had dreams of intercourse culminating in orgasm. Often she planned to have intercourse, but always retreated if her partner made advances. On one of these occasions, though she wanted to cooperate, she rebuffed her partner. This made her feel humiliated and ashamed, and as a result unworthy, hopeless, and dejected. She reacted with urinary retention. Since bladder function failed to return, she was hospitalized.

Examination revealed that her bladder was 4 cm above the symphysis pubis. The bladder was not drained; the catheter was connected to a manometer. The intravesical pressure was low (Fig. 4). Two intravenous injections of sodium amytal were given. The patient finally closed her eyes and began to masturbate.

The bladder pressure rose to 65 cm of water, and she said she "felt swell". She voided spontaneously that night, but on the next day, since she again felt depressed, urinary retention recurred. She underwent psychotherapy; after 10 days spontaneous voiding started again.

Patients of this type have atonic bladders. This aberration in vesical function is accompanied by feelings of being overwhelmed and by hysterical reactions.

TAUBER, LEWIS, and LANGWORTHY (1938) noted that catatonic patients had cystometrograms which showed a rather rapid increase in intravesical pressure associated with many uninhibited contractions. However, even when the intravesical pressure reached 60 ml of water, no voiding occurred around the catheter.

### c) Discussion

Many normal persons develop acute vesical irritability under stress. We may cite the urinary frequency of the medical student facing his final examinations. The psychiatrist sees some patients who must leave his office one or more times during the hour. Even the female dog, excited when her family returns home after a vacation, may wet the floor.

A cystometrogram obtained from a patient with psychosomatic frequency is usually typical of an uninhibited neurogenic bladder. It must be remembered that a similar tracing may be the earliest sign of multiple sclerosis. However, the latter often responds to methantheline bromide (Banthine); the psychogenically irritable bladder usually does not.

Thus, STRAUB et al. have clearly shown the effect of the emotions on vesical function and have confirmed the cystometric findings of MOSSO and PELLACANI.

## 2. The influence of the emotions on the renal excretion of water and salt

### a) Animal experiments

Another mechanism which may cause frequency has to do with aberrations in renal function. BLOMSTRAND and LÖFGREN have recently discussed the influence of emotional stress on the renal circulation. They had observed that emotional stress could cause both diuresis and antidiuresis. They had also noted that stimulation of the pressor area of the cortex of cats produced ischemia of the kidneys. This reaction appeared to be similar to that of a patient described by Charcot in 1877 who developed anuria during a hysterical attack. BLOMSTRAND and LÖFGREN noted that Homer Smith had seen altered diuretic reactions which he thought were dependent upon psychogenic renal vasoconstriction. They cited the work of Bykow and Alexejew-Berkman, who had dogs drink water under certain constant conditions, thus establishing certain conditioned reflexes. Later, the same conditions were capable of causing diuresis without the administration of water.

BLOMSTRAND and LÖFGREN performed the following experiment; They passed 4 F. catheters into the right common carotid arteries of cats. The ends of the catheters were placed just proximal to the renal arteries. Seventeen of these cats were then confronted with barking dogs. While the cats were in a state of rage, india ink was quickly injected into the catheters, and immediate nephrectomy was performed. The kidneys of these cats were compared with those of three cats not subjected to stress. The kidneys of the control group were uniformly tinged with ink. The cortex was darker than the medulla (Figs. 5, 1). The kidneys from the frightened, enraged cats showed mottled (Figs. 5, 2) or completely blanched surfaces. Section showed the cortex to be pale, while the medulla was deeply stained (Figs. 5, 3). Microscopic examination showed no engorgement of the glomeruli. The mechanism for the glomerular ischemia was, therefore, afferent arteriolar spasm which, of course, causes oliguria, even anuria. We have seen a case of psychogenic anuria in clinical practice.

BLOMSTRAND and LÖFGREN believed that the stress reaction caused the liberation of epinephrine in accordance with Cannon's "emergency" theory. VERNEY has demonstrated that emotional stress leads to an increase in the amount

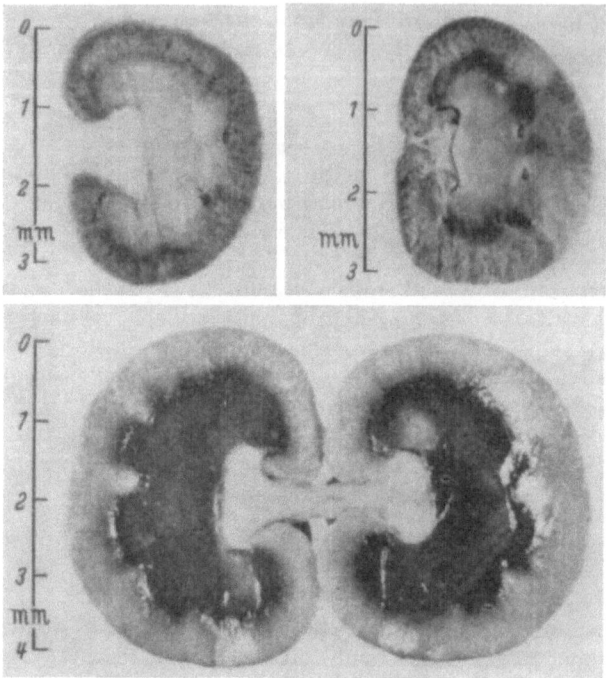

Fig. 5. *1* Kidney section from cat at rest (intravital India ink injection). *2* Kidney section from a cat in a state of emotional stress. Alternating blanched and ink-filled areas in cortex (intravital injection). *3* Kidney section from a cat in a state of emotional stress. Medulla saturated with India ink but cortex uniformly ink free (intravital injection). [Reproduced, with permission, from R. BLOMSTRAND and F. LÖFGREN: Psychosom. Med. 18, 420—426 (1956)]

of antidiuretic hormone from the posterior pituitary gland. He believes, therefore, that the diuresis is not caused by changes in renal blood flow or hormonal output from the adrenal glands.

## b) Observations in human subjects

The proof that this reaction occurs in man has recently been adduced by SCHOTTSTAEDT, GRACE, and WOLFF. They studied the rates of water, sodium, potassium, and creatinine excretion in five subjects in normal and stressful situations. They first established the normal excretion rates for these subjects; they found such factors as diet and exercise changed these values in only minor ways. Gross alterations in excretion of water and certain electrolytes were, however, observed when the subjects were subjected to severe emotional upset.

The findings in one woman were typical of the group (Table 1). She was a research worker who was unusually sensitive to implied or actual rejection by others. She had been adopted by wealthy parents in order to bolster their faltering marriage, but the adoption only increased the parents' tensions. The patient

Table 1. *Showing various rates of excretion of water and salt depending on the type of emotional stress. It demonstrates the oliguria-diuresis cycle which is dependent upon acute changes in renal blood flow or upon the amount of antidiuretic hormone liberated by the pituitary gland.* [Reproduced, with permission, from W. W. SCHOTTSTAEDT, W. J. GRACE and H. G. WOLFF: J. Amer. med. Ass. **157**, 1485—1488 (1955)]

Renal excretion rates associated with various life situations

| Situations | Urine volume | | Sodium excretion | |
|---|---|---|---|---|
| | ml/min | ml/4 hr. | mEq./min. | mEq./4 hr. |
| Tranquil state . . . . . . . . . . . . . . . | 0.83 | 199 | 85 | 340 |
| Alert behavior, confidence, feeling of tension | 0.66 | 158 | 55 | 220 |
| Return toward tranquility, freedom from tension . . . . . . . . . . . . . . . . | 1.35 | 324 | 68 | 272 |
| Reactions provoking retaliation, anger . . . | 2.47 | 592 | 201 | 808 |

openly preferred her father, and he reciprocated. The mother was jealous and disapproved of the child. The patient developed temper tantrums and was referred to the clinic because of uncontrollable bursts of anger. Her relations with her fellow workers were tempestuous; she was usually not on speaking terms with them.

Day after day, when in a tranquil state, she excreted an average of 0.83 ml of water and 85 mEq of sodium per minute. Over a four-hour period urine output was then about 200 ml. When she felt alert, confident, and tense, urine output decreased by 20 per cent and sodium by 35 per cent. As she became more tranquil a marked water and sodium diuresis occurred. If, however, situations developed which evoked retaliation and anger, a sharp increase in water and sodium excretion followed. Fluid output rose 300 per cent and sodium excretion increased 237 per cent above the norms for the tranquil state.

When situations evoking listlessness, hopelessness, and depression developed, the 5 subjects uniformly excreted about 30 per cent less water and 33 per cent less salt than when in a tranquil state. This condition was of course followed by diuresis.

These beautiful clinical experiments demonstrate that different emotional states can cause either diuresis or fluid retention and oliguria followed by diuresis. The degree depends upon the emotional reactions of the person. The mechanism for water retention or diuresis is activated by changes in renal blood flow or excretion of posterior pituitary hormone.

## c) Discussion

This knowledge can be used to explain the vesical habits of some emotionally disturbed patients such as the one who voids large volumes of pale urine frequently for a few hours each morning. We may postulate that as the day wears on, fluid and salt are retained because of feelings of tension. By morning, due to a return to the tranquil state, marked diuresis occurs. This phenomenon could also be explained by the development of anger or by a feeling of retaliation against the spouse following an incomplete sexual experience or other psychological traumata on the previous evening.

We have observed one patient who noted that under stress (depressed feelings) he gained as much as 11 pounds (5 liters of water) in 24 hours. Naturally, during these periods, he had oliguria and developed temporal headache, a feeling of fullness behind the eyes, and some peripheral edema especially about the face.

He developed a sense of overpowering restlessness and of dissatisfaction; he became irritable and wanted to be left alone.

Usually by the next day the sense of depression lifted and a marked diuresis (with physiological frequency) occurred. This caused relief from all the somatic symptoms which had been present on the preceding day. The patient's weight rapidly returned to normal.

The patient found that when the premonitory symptoms of fluid retention became noticeable, he could limit their severity by avoiding salt, limiting fluid intake, taking a high protein diet, and getting plenty of exercise.

Another patient, an 18-year-old boy who was exceedingly tense during the period preceding final examinations at college, was essentially anuric for 48 hours before his last examination. As he left the classroom he experienced a strong desire to void. He passed a large quantity of pale urine. During the next six hours he voided unusually large volumes of urine every half hour.

### 3. Polydipsia

Another cause for frequency of urination is a large intake of fluid which may not be consciously recognized by the patient; hence the need to ask the patient if, with his frequency, he voids large amounts. If he does, he may be drinking excessively. A patient of this type may complain of a tight feeling or dryness of the throat which is interpreted as thirst demanding to be quenched.

Many patients, thinking urine is dirty, have a fetish for "flushing out" the kidneys or bladder and therefore drink water incessantly. Frequency in this instance is physiological, but the cause of the polydipsia is not.

### 4. Comment

These animal experiments and clinical observations explain the abnormal vesical reactions which are seen in emotionally disturbed patients. A woman intensely angry with her husband experiences marked diuresis as part of an alarm reaction and at the same time develops the psychogenic uninhibited neurogenic-bladder response with extreme frequency. If she has an obsession leading to polydipsia as well, her frequency may become unbearable.

## III. The clinical picture
### 1. The history

The mere recording of the presence of day frequency, nocturia, urgency, burning, pain, and the size and force of the urinary stream is not enough if "nervous bladders" are to be correctly diagnosed. Let us take each symptom in turn and point out the important information to be gleaned.

#### a) Frequency during the day

1. Does the frequency persist all day, or does it occur only for a few hours ?
2. Does the frequency occur every day, or is it periodic ?
3. With the frequency, are the urine volumes large or small ?

Frequency due to organic disease is consistent and persistent; that caused by emotional upset is not. Typically, the nervous patient suffers frequency for only a few hours a day, particularly in the morning. Frequency may be severe on one day, yet absent the next.

Organic frequency is accompanied by small urine volumes. The same may be true of psychosomatic frequency, but at times the patient will admit that though frequency is present, the volume of each urination is about normal. This can only mean that the bladder has suddenly been presented with a large urine volume; frequency in this instance may be physiological.

### b) Nocturia

Is nocturia associated with the frequency?

The outstanding clue to the unstable bladder of psychic origin is *day frequency without nocturia*. On rare occasions a patient may have severe nocturia without diurnal frequency.

### c) Urgency

Is urgency associated with the frequency?

Urgency is usually present in cases of both organic and psychogenic vesical irritability.

### d) Burning on urination

Does the patient experience a feeling of burning in the urethral region during urination?

Despite great frequency and urgency, burning felt in the urethra during urination may be absent in patients with vesical dysfunction of psychogenic origin.

### e) Pain

Is there a complaint of pain? Where is the pain located?

Many women complain of pains which are atypical both in type and in location. They may feel "a knife in the urethra", "a twisting sensation in the vaginal area", "a pressure feeling in the lower abdomen as though something were pressing on the bladder". Men may complain of aching in the perineum or scrotal contents, or of sharp lancinating pains in the penis.

These aberrant pains, it should be pointed out, are not related to the act of urination. That in itself should arouse the suspicions of the clinician.

### f) The urinary stream

1. Is there hesitancy in initiating urination?
2. Is there impairment of the size and force of the stream?
3. Are these changes consistent?

In nervous pollakiuria, it is common to find that at some times urination is difficult while at other times it is perfectly free. This suggests the presence of periodic sphincter spasm.

### g) Fluid intake

1. Does the patient drink fluid excessively?
2. Is most of the fluid intake crowded into a few hours?

One woman drank two glasses of water at bedtime and another glassful every time she got up to urinate. Naturally she had severe nocturia.

Many patients who have frequency will volunteer that they void large amounts each time, yet they will deny polydipsia. Have them time and measure the volume of liquid intake and of each voiding for a few days. This will usually prove that they are unconsciously imbibing a large amount of fluid.

Some people drink large amounts of water as a "healthy" habit, others because of a need to "flush out" the kidneys and bladder and remove the dirty urine.

### h) Recurrent edema

Is edema ever observed ? Where does it occur ?

Many women who suffer from psychosomatic cystitis note periodic edema of the ankles, hands, and face. In the absence of cardiorenovascular disease the edema must be secondary to retention of water (and salt). These patients, of course, develop frequency when the inevitable diuresis sets in.

### i) The effect of the menses upon the bladder

Psychogenic urinary frequency may occur at the time of the menses. The accompanying pelvic congestion may become confused with sexual feelings. In these patients, whose sexual expression has been transferred to the bladder, vesical frequency may tend to afford them some sexual satisfaction.

### j) The effect of intercourse on bladder function

Does the patient observe exacerbation of symptoms following sexual intercourse ?

In the psychosomatically ill woman, the bladder is at its worst on the day after intercourse, for almost without exception a patient with this symptom complex is sexually frustrated. *This is the common denominator.*

It is important to ask the patient why the sexual act does not afford her satisfaction. The answer is usually that the patient no longer loves her spouse or that the spouse no longer loves the patient. The anger or hurt from rejection is great and gives rise to tension which results in frequency.

### k) The events preceding the first attack

What events preceded the first attack of frequency ?

Often women report that frequency was first noticed after some form of sexual trauma or the threat of a feared sexual act. Attempt or actual rape, disharmonious or unsatisfactory intercourse, forbidden sexual activity, sexual temptation, or the worry of an impending marriage have triggered the appearance of urinary symptoms.

### l) History of enuresis as a child

Is there a history of childhood enuresis ?

Patients having irritable bladders often admit a history of enuresis in childhood; the reasons for this will be discussed in the section dealing with enuresis.

### m) The patient's own theory as to the cause of bladder dysfunction

What does the patient believe to be the etiology of his complaint ?

It is most important to ask the patient his or her theory of the cause for the vesical dysfunction. Women often ask the physician if he thinks "nerves" could be the cause. Women appear to be more willing than men to admit that emotions and feelings govern their lives *and* organic functions.

## 2. The examination of the patient with psychogenic bladder dysfunction

### a) General appearance

Two types of women develop psychogenic bladder dysfunction. One is the aggressive, seemingly confident, yet tense and anxious type; the other is subdued and repressed. Men with this complaint are usually also meek and mild. They appear to have a poorly developed sense of masculinity.

## b) Urinalysis

The urine is normal microscopically. The stained smear and culture reveal no bacteria.

## c) Rectal examination

The anal sphincter may be hypertonic. The prostate may be unusually tender; the patient may faint after the lightest massage; he is apprehensive and has a low threshold to pain. The gland may be congested due to lack of intercourse.

## d) Vaginal examination

Though no organic pathology can be found, undue tenderness of the urethra may be noted; movement of the cervix may be unusually painful.

## e) Residual urine

Residual urine is usually absent except in the relatively rare depressed patient with an atonic bladder.

## f) Urethral exploration

A moderate-sized catheter may be inserted with difficulty yet can be withdrawn with ease. This observation suggests urethral spasm rather than organic stenosis.

## g) Cystoscopy

Trabeculation may be noted. This is not necessarily pathognomonic of organic obstruction; sphincter spasm can also cause detrusor hypertrophy. In women, polyps on the bladder neck may be seen, but their destruction has seldom dramatically relieved symptoms in our patients.

The trigone and urethra may be hypersensitive and reddened. These changes are caused by the patient's psychosexual difficulties and are due to pelvic congestion. Treatment of the "trigonitis" and "urethritis", therefore, usually fails to afford relief.

Even though the patient complains of frequent small voidings, the capacity of the bladder may be normal. If this is the case, a psychological cause for the frequency may be suspected.

# IV. Management

## 1. The effect of organic (empirical) treatment

Organic treatment for patients with psychogenic bladder dysfunction usually affords them little relief. Women are often subjected to bladder irrigations and instillations of various chemicals, fulguration of vesical-neck polyps, urethral and bladder-neck dilatations, and even transurethral resection of the bladder neck. Men are given frequent prostatic massages, urethral dilatation, and, at times, transurethral resection of the prostate, though no convincing evidence of obstruction is adduced. Both sexes may undergo endoscopic applications of noxious chemicals to the reddened trigone and urethra. This treatment obviously causes these areas to blanch! The administration of bladder sedatives, including methantheline bromide (Banthine), seems logical but usually fails to help.

Some patients may improve following organic treatment, but it is a question whether this is not merely because painful manipulations plus the receipt of a medical bill punish them sufficiently to relieve their guilt feelings temporarily. The masochist is happy for a while. The physician who has most success with this mode of therapy is unconsciously a good psychotherapist. He is sympathetic, listens to the complaints of his patients, and, with his manipulation of the erotically sensitive lower urinary tract, affords them some unconscious sexual satisfaction.

## 2. Psychotherapy as treatment for psychosomatic bladder dysfunction

Toilet training of the infant usually begins during the second year. During infancy, when sufficient urine or fecal matter has accumulated in the bladder or bowel, the muscles of these organs contract suddenly and the waste matter is expelled. The child wets and has bowel movements in accordance with his physiological needs and finds pleasure and relaxation in these releases of physical tension. When he soils, he gains his mother's attention: she wipes, changes, and holds him. However, both the mother and the other persons in the environment find this uncontrolled elimination disturbing and seek to change the child's habits. The infant is trained to signal his need to eliminate; gradually, he learns to perform in a designated manner and place. This learning process necessitates adequate neurophysiological and psychological maturation and the development of an awareness of bladder and bowel sensations. Too early training imposes a strain on the child, since his capacity for delay is limited. Many a child who is trained early may lose his training at a later age when stressful situations arise.

The desire to please the parent is the stimulus for learning control of bladder function. If too much pressure is put on the child, together with over-concern by the parent, he may also lose his learned control and revert to infantile habits of elimination. Frequently shaming is used as a means of "socializing" the child. When the mother over-stresses the dirtiness of the eliminative functions, the child's attitudes to elimination will reflect this attitude. Taboos regarding sex enter the picture, since elimination requires exposure of the genitals. Excessive modesty may develop, with a need to urinate in private. It may become impossible for the man to use public toilets in later years.

From all this it is obvious that toilet function is not an activity that develops spontaneously, like learning to crawl or walk, but rather necessitates a prolonged conditioning period with much trial and error. During this training period there is some degree of conflict between the child and the environment, particularly between the child and the mother. The social setting will demand that the child's eliminative reflexes conform to the mores, taboos, and toilet rituals already established. If the child can successfully negotiate this difficult transition, achieving it in large degree by virtue of the mother's love, support, and understanding, he wins social approval and status and runs little risk that this will become an area of conflict in his life. However, if the training period is stormy, if there is frequent loss of nocturnal control, if feelings of shame and disgust with overtones of "sexual wrongness" develop, the stage is set for potential future problems involving the elimination processes.

In urinating, the boy must handle his penis. His mother, reacting to this situation with mixed emotions, stresses that the penis should be handled only for urination and not at other times and that the hands should be washed after handling the penis. The boy, however, becomes aware of a pleasurable sensation; thus, masturbation becomes associated with feelings of greater or less guilt, depending upon the environmental attitude. At about the same time, boys and girls become interested in the anatomical differences between the sexes. Frequently little girls attempt to urinate standing up. They may feel resentful of the anatomical difference, so that a feeling of competitiveness with boys may ensue. In females there are two basic reactions to the absence of the penis and the necessity to urinate in a different manner. Some women, as mentioned above, are resentful and competitive and go through life fighting back, in an attempt to prove their own worth. Others accept the anatomical difference and its many implications with a feeling of defeat and helplessness. The majority of women have an admixture of both feelings with a greater or lesser acceptance of their role as women. The conflict engendered in women by the lack of a penis has been called "penis envy" or the "masculine protest".

The little boy, too, is aware of the sex difference associated with his pattern of urination. The thought of possibly losing his penis and with it his masculinity occasions him great concern. This "castration anxiety" is heightened by guilt feelings over masturbation and the parent-child conflict during what has been called the "oedipal phase". The young boy competes with his father for the mother's love and attention. The fear of physical punishment by the father includes conscious and unconscious concern regarding the penis. Many little boys learn to urinate mechanically to avoid any pleasurable sensations from the penis.

It is apparent that the achievement of bladder control is a highly complex learning process colored by feelings of shame, guilt, and anxiety. Both sexual and aggressive components are present in the urinary act. Some boys find pride in achieving control. Others, feeling overwhelmed by environmental pressure, adopt a passive attitude. Similarly, some girls develop a passive, helpless, "just let go" attitude, while others react with aggressive, explosive behavior.

Urination, a physiological process for relieving bladder tension, also serves as a means of expressing psychological tensions and attitudes. The intimate anatomical, embryological, and especially neurological connection between the urinary and genital systems permits physiological and psychological stimuli in one system to flow over and find discharge in the other.

In the child, urination produces a feeling of pride and of physical satisfaction. Under stress, the adult may revert to this act as a source of physical pleasure. Some persons substitute urinary symptoms for sexual satisfaction when the latter is unobtainable. Some may retain large amounts of urine in the bladder because they experience a pleasurable sensation on voiding. Others consciously or unconsciously enjoy the frequent passage of urine, even in small amounts. When sexual arousal first takes place in the child or adolescent, the unfamiliar feelings of tumescence and pelvic fullness are often interpreted as stimuli from the bladder with a feeling of the need to urinate. Some adults have found that partial distention of the bladder increases their erotic feelings in sexual activity. Some individuals, particularly women, may, as a result of various conditioning experiences in their lives, have no conscious sexual feelings; they have displaced them entirely to the urinary system.

It is important for the physician to recognize that individuals with urogenital dysfunction, whether it is the result of organic or functional conditions, have some degree of anxiety, consciously or unconsciously, that their previous sexual activity has some connection with the presenting difficulty. Feelings of guilt about masturbation, pre-marital or extra-marital sexual temptations or activities, or worry about the normalcy of their sex life, are common concerns. Long-forgotten threats of punishment for masturbation are revived when symptoms develop in the bladder or lower genito-urinary tract. The urologist should be cognizant of this fact and tell his patient that the presenting disorder is not the result of "sexual abuse" or venereal disease. Since most patients are afraid to ask because of feelings of guilt or shame, the physician can alleviate much anxiety by this direct reassurance.

However, patients whose condition, after careful examination and evaluation, appears to stem from functional causes need more than just reassurance. It is imperative that they receive psychotherapy in addition to whatever treatment the organic manifestations of the disease may require.

It is our impression that cystalgia, the "irritable bladder" and interstitial cystitis (Hunner's ulcer), are all manifestations of a urinary syndrome intimately associated with the personality problems of the individual. The pattern of toilet training which the child has experienced, especially if it involved the use of shame and punishment and a conscious or unconscious linking with sexual functions, may set the stage for later urological troubles. In many patients, stress may result in a need to void immediately and recurrently, even in minute amounts. In a lesser number, voiding is accompanied by strong guilt feelings resulting in a tendency to retain urine, with the possibility of secondary anatomical changes.

# B. Functional enuresis

## I. Introduction

### 1. Definition

The term enuresis refers to a periodic unconscious loss of urine. Through usage, it has come generally to mean "bedwetting" during sleep. Though most enuretic persons wet the bed only at night, a few may also lose urine involuntarily during the day, and in rare cases, only during the day.

It is generally agreed that a normal child should acquire diurnal control of the bladder by the age of two and one-half years and control during sleep by the age of three years. Despert cites the average ages as 21.4 months and 27.3 months, respectively.

Enuresis by itself is rarely a symptom of organic disease, since organic diseases of the genito-urinary tract usually excite symptoms more severe and more constant than enuresis. For instance, urgency, burning on urination, frequency, and nocturia are common complaints of the patient with cystitis; and frequent losses of urine day and night are often secondary to neurovesical disease (e.g., myelo-meningocele).

### 2. Historical references

Glicklich has written a scholarly paper dealing with historical descriptions of enuresis. She notes that enuresis was discussed in the Papyrus Ebers, dated 1550 B.C., and that many references to enuresis appeared in the Middle Ages. References to enuresis in the medical literature of the nineteenth century are impressively extensive, and many theories concerning the etiology of enuresis were propounded during this period. Glicklich also states that in primitive tribes enuresis has been considered a problem.

### 3. Incidence

Bakwin, studying 1000 children between the ages of 4 and 12 years, found that 26 per cent were enuretic. Crosby constructed a graph showing the incidence of enuresis by age (Fig. 6). He found that 50 per cent of children at the age of four years have enuresis, but by the age of 10 years only 8 per cent wet the bed. By the age of 20 years, only 1 to 2 per cent have enuresis. Thorne found that of 1000 draftees, 16 per cent were enuretic after the age of five years, but only 2.5 per cent were enuretic after the age of 17 years.

Many children do not acquire voluntary control of the bladder, which empties automatically from birth through infancy, and therefore fail to become toilet trained at the usual time. Others attain voluntary control at the usual time only to regress at a later date. STOCKWELL and SMITH found that 59 per cent of a group of bedwetters studied by them once had normal control, while both ANDERSON and PINCK noted only 20 per cent of their patients regressed after control had been established.

BAKWIN thought that the incidence of enuresis was lower in negro children than in white children. He attributed this to the fact that the negro children received better care from their parents and developed fewer psychological troubles. ANDERSON, however, did not find any racial differences.

SHLIONSKY, SARRACINO, and BISCHOF studied 100 enuretic men who were in the U.S. Army during World War II. These writers were surprised to find that enuresis appeared to be common in enlistedmen but rare in officers. They also noted a high incidence of bedwetting among soldiers as compared to that of civilians. It should be appreciated, however, that the allegedly high incidence of enuresis among enlisted personnel may have resulted from the fact that enuresis cannot be hidden in barracks, whereas officers and civilians in private quarters can hide their affliction more easily.

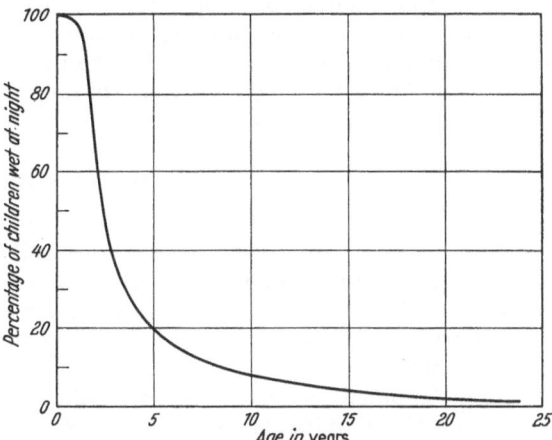

Fig. 6. The incidence of enuresis by age. This graph demonstrate the high incidence of spontaneous acquisition of nocturnal urinary control. [Reproduced, with permission, from N. D. CROSBY: Med. J. Aust. 2, 533—543 (1950)]

# II. Etiology

The causes of enuresis remain obscure; undoubtedly there are many factors which may produce this condition. A review of the literature quickly reveals the confusion in ascribing causes to enuresis.

## 1. Maturational factors

The bladder of an infant operates as an uninhibited neurogenic organ. Its motor activity (expulsion of urine) is governed by its sacral reflex arc when capacity is reached; it lacks cerebral control. Along with maturation of the central and peripheral nervous systems, maturation of the bladder progresses, and finally urination is controlled by the child. Early toilet training (i.e., before the age of 18 months) is usually fruitless. McGRAW studied two sets of twins from the time of their birth in the following manner: One twin from each set was subjected to training technics a few months after birth. The other two were not. Interestingly enough, all four became toilet trained at the same age.

It is conceivable that maturation progresses more slowly in some children than in others. The persistence of enuresis beyond the age of three years may be a concomitant of a slow rate of maturation.

THORNE believes that enuresis may be caused by a developmental defect which disappears when maturation within the central nervous system is completed. Certainly it is true that the majority of enuretic children overcome this affliction spontaneously by the age of 10 years.

BOSTICK and SHACKLETON warn against beginning toilet training at too early an age. They fear that beginning training too soon interferes with the natural rate of development, thereby delaying the accomplishment of bladder control.

CROSBY thinks that enuresis is a true disease entity and that it is not usually caused by psychological difficulties. He states that in order to gain nocturnal continence a child must develop a degree of cerebral inhibition such that dispersion of sleep occurs, allowing him to urinate voluntarily. He states further that cerebral inhibition is encouraged by the discomfort the child experiences when he is wet. Thus, he concludes that the infant, needing to void, first awakens, urinates, then cries because he is wet.

## 2. Hereditary factors

Many observers have noted a high incidence of enuresis in the families of enuretic children. SHLIONSKY, SARRACINO, and BISCHOF, in a study of 100 soldiers with enuresis, found 15 enuretic parents and 40 enuretic siblings in the families of 36 of these men. STOCKWELL and SMITH noted that 63 per cent of the parents and 21 per cent of the siblings of the 100 enuretic children whom they studied also had enuresis.

FRARY studied 59 "clans", which included 221 families, and 787 individuals. He found 239 individuals who were known to be enuretic, and postulated that enuresis was caused by a "single recessive gene substitution". HUBERT noted that 40 per cent of the parents of his enuretic patients had had enuresis, while ADDIS cited parental enuresis in 26.6 per cent of his enuretic patients. Most authors, however, believe that enuresis is not truly hereditary. They attribute the high incidence of enuresis in families to a basic psychoneurotic behavior trait common to the parents which their offspring acquire through environmental influences.

## 3. Mentality

Though it is true that in some cases it is impossible to toilet train children who have low intelligence quotients, studies of groups of enuretic children have provided evidence that this factor has little influence upon the incidence of enuresis (STOCKWELL and SMITH).

MICHAELS and SECUNDA found abnormal (immature) curves in electroencephalograms recorded from enuretic patients.

## 4. Anomalies

### a) Spina bifida

Spina bifida has been considered as a possible cause of enuresis, if paresis of the sacral nerves, causing neurogenic vesical dysfunction, is associated with it. Enuresis in this instance probably would be associated with other urinary symptoms and signs including slow urinary stream, frequency or dribbling, and pyuria.

KARLIN found that 21 of 25 patients (84 per cent) with enuresis had spina bifida, whereas in a control group of 50 randomly selected subjects, 27 (54 per cent) had spina bifida. He pointed out, however, that the enuretic patients with spina bifida had more extensive bony defects than subjects in the control group and also often had cutaneous sensory changes.

SANFORD and KLIMAN studied a group of enuretic and nonenuretic soldiers and found no significant difference in the incidence of spina bifida occulta in comparing the two groups (62 per cent and 64 per cent, respectively). STOCKWELL and SMITH, in a survey of 100 enuretic children, found that 46 per cent had spina bifida.

It is clear that the presence of spina bifida should be sought in all enuretic patients. If it is present, and particularly if it is extensive, a careful neurological examination with particular reference to perianal sensation, tone of the anal sphincter, estimation of residual urine, and cystometry should be done.

### b) Myelomeningocele and meningocele

Myelomeningocele, and often meningocele, are associated with lesions of the sacral roots of the cauda equina; neurogenic dysfunction of the bladder is present in these cases. The vesical reaction may be spastic, atonic, or a mixture of these two. In almost every instance, children with these conditions have many complaints in addition to bedwetting and, therefore, obviously do not suffer from simple or functional enuresis. These complaints include weakness or contractures of the lower extremities, constant dribbling of urine, involuntary urination, distended bladder, deficiencies in bowel control, and obvious peripheral neurologic disturbances. Residual urine is present and one may expect to find evidence of infection in the urine. A plain x-ray film of the abdomen may reveal spina bifida, which, if present, is often extensive; and the cystometrogram will have pathognomonic manometric curves.

## 5. Organic disease

Estimates of the percentage of children who have enuresis which is caused by organic disease vary. CAMPBELL states that 90 to 95 per cent of enuretic children wet the bed as a result of functional problems, whereas only 5 to 10 per cent have organic disease. He also states, however, that of those who do not respond to medical therapy within four months, more than 50 per cent have organic disease, usually involving the lower tract, which is detected at the time of complete urologic examination.

PINCK, in a study of 100 children and adults with enuresis, found that 18 per cent had organic disease. In the remainder the cause was functional. STOCKWELL and SMITH found organic causes for enuresis in 13 per cent of 100 children studied by them.

## 6. Neurological factors

Some enuretic patients have a myoneurovesical dysfunction that causes no related symptoms or obvious signs. PINCK has demonstrated both uninhibited and atonic neurogenic vesical responses in cystometry of enuretic patients who have no other neurologic abnormality. STOCKWELL and SMITH obtained 37 cystometrograms with abnormal tracings from 90 of 100 enuretic patients; some had spastic bladders with small capacities while the remainder had atonic bladders with increased capacities. NASH's findings were similar.

HALLMAN measured the volume of voided urine from a group of enuretic children and from a group of normal children. He observed that normal children four years of age and older have bladder capacities of at least 300 ml, whereas most enuretic children have capacities of less than this amount.

## 7. Psychological factors

Though many urologists still believe that enuresis is organically caused, present day knowledge indicates quite clearly that bed-wetting is usually a neurotic disorder occurring in a physically healthy child with no evidence of urinary-tract disease. In a socio-cultural setting in which toilet training is ignored and it is assumed a child will achieve control by himself, only a few children do not achieve control and continue to be enuretic.

GERARD, in a study of 72 enuretic children, found that organic factors were responsible in only seven. Of these seven cases which were organically caused, three were associated with epileptic states, three were caused by bladder infections, and one by spina bifida. Of the remaining 65 cases, four could be ascribed to faulty training, and were corrected in 1 to 2 weeks by establishing regular toilet habits—these children showed no evidence of neurotic traits or behavior disorders and in 61 of the 72 children emotional problems were the causes of enuresis.

Gerard's study showed that the majority of enuretic children had definite neurotic behavior patterns such as nail biting, temper tantrums, thumb sucking, or eating problems, in addition to their urinary problems. For some the onset of wetting coincided with the birth of a baby in the family. Enuresis at this time is part of a general regression to a more infantile mode of behavior in order to compete with the baby for the mother's attention, along with whining, clinging to the mother, refusing to eat, and even physical attacks on the sibling.

In a few instances the mothers had rejected the children, sometimes openly, considering them unwanted. Resenting the children, these mothers were nagging, punitive, and demanding in their rearing. The children responded with varying degrees of open hostility, stubbornness, and aggressive behavior. Most of these children had never achieved toilet control and often deliberately soiled to anger and punish their mothers. Sometimes, even though the mothers were accepting parents, harsh, punitive, rejecting fathers evoked the same rebellious pattern. The family settings were so turbulent and these children were so disturbed that often placement in foster-homes was necessary, and in most cases this placement effected improvement in behavior and cessation of wetting. In a situation in which a child is aware of parental hostility and is able to respond by being hostile, the neurotic disability is not severe, and a rapid response to environmental changes may be expected.

However, 46 of the 65 patients described above had complex clinical syndromes, of which enuresis was only one symptom; and study of the attitudes of these patients' parents showed similar patterns. In the cases of enuretic girls, the important parental figures were fathers, some alternating extremely affectionate behavior with episodes of physical punishment. The maternal figure was sometimes affectionate and sometimes rejecting, but rejecting to a much lesser degree than the mother of an openly rebellious child, as described above. A few of the fathers were openly seductive to their daughters. The enuretic girls were active, outgoing, independent children, usually doing well in school work and in their associations with other children. In play, they were strongly competitive in their attitudes towards boys and generally verbally depreciative of males. While fearless in daytime activities, they had night-time fears, usually nightmares of physical attack, which deeper psychological study revealed as unconscious fears of sexual attack.

Enuretic boys had different character structures. Within the family, the mother's personality was dominant; she usually unconsciously rejected the boy and over-compensated by excessive concern and protectiveness, and had many fears of injury to the child. The father played a secondary role, although he generally urged the boy to be more outgoing and expressed his displeasure and irritation at his son's fearfulness and generally passive behavior. These children were poor students; they avoided physical-contact sports; they tended to be passive, retiring, and self-depreciatory. They were slow and dawdling in dressing, eating, or doing assigned chores, demanding an unusual amount of help and encouragement from parents and teachers. While enuretic girls behaved in ways as though equal or superior to boys and girls generally, enuretic boys behaved as though they were inferior to their fellows. The boys as well as girls had night fears; however, those of the boys were associated with injury at the hands of a woman. Because of this fear of women they avoided the active role of the male, and sought refuge in general non-activity.

Most enuretic children of both sexes had suffered sexual traumata. Many had been exposed to their parent's sexual life through sleeping in the same room or in an immediately adjacent room, and had observed or heard their parent's sexual activity. A few had experienced sexual seduction or attack, or had engaged in disturbing sex play with other children. Because sexual activity had a disturbing quality these children masturbated less than other children and unconsciously substituted urination as a sexual outlet. After puberty, the physical need to masturbate, despite feelings of anxiety and guilt, led to resumption of this act, coincident with which enuresis usually ceased.

SEARS, MACCOBY, and LEVIN studied child-rearing patterns by observing 379 American mothers and their children. They found three factors related to the late persistence of bedwetting: severity of toilet training, lack of warmth in the mother's attitude toward the baby, and intensity of the mother's personal sexual anxiety. The combination of severe toilet training, a relatively cold and undemonstrative attitude toward the child, and great sexual anxiety were very likely to produce enuresis. If the mother was affectionate and gentle in toilet training, the child usually remained dry all night by the age of two. SEARS, MACCOBY, and LEVIN also found that if a child had an eating problem, he was less likely to be enuretic. Refusing to eat or wetting the bed are two possible reactions to severe parental discipline, and a child who uses one response does not ordinarily require the other. They did not find that bed-wetting was consistently related to the general level of infant frustration, to the birth of a sibling, or to the demands and restrictions of the environment.

## III. Symptoms

Though bed-wetting may be the chief problem with which a patient comes to a physician, other symptoms of concurrent urinary disorders are common. STOCKWELL and SMITH, in their study of enuretic children, found that 41 had only enuresis, 47 suffered urgency and frequency during the day, as well as enuresis, while 10 had occasional diurnal incontinence but no enuresis. SHLIONSKY, SARRACINO, and BISCHOF noted that the majority of 100 enuretic soldiers suffered from frequency and urgency also. BAKWIN observed that the victims of enuresis have increased frequency with excitement or cold; and, as a rule, all enuretic patients have "sensitive" bladders throughout life. In other words, as adults they are likely to develop periodic or persistent urgency and frequency when under emotional stress. Nocturia without day frequency may be the adult counterpart of enuresis.

Pinck observed that 27 per cent of enuretic patients had diurnal incontinence, while Bakwin noted that 40 per cent of an enuretic group he studied also had diurnal incontinence.

It is important that a physician learn whether a patient's enuresis has persisted since birth, or whether it recurred after a period of complete control, since reverting to incontinence after having gained bladder control suggests psychologically caused regression to an infantile attitude. Stockwell and Smith noted that 59 per cent of their enuretic patients once had bladder control, while Anderson and Pinck each reported that 20 per cent of their patients had become enuretic after having been continent.

The presence of abnormal gait, impaired force of the urinary stream, undue constipation, or bowel incontinence should suggest the possibility of abnormalities affecting the sacral nerve roots. Burning on urination, hematuria, or cloudy urine may be present if there is infection of the urinary tract.

The emotional background of the patient should be explored. As described above, Gerard has observed that enuretic girls tend to be aggressive and confident, whereas enuretic boys are reserved, repressed, and unsure of themselves. It will usually be observed that parents are overly anxious about their child's enuresis and may reveal exasperation and impatience with him; these attitudes only add to the child's anxiety and insecurity.

## IV. Physical examination

The physical examination should include the following procedures in order to determine whether signs of organic disease are present:

1. Palpation of the kidneys. Enlarged kidneys suggest hydronephrosis secondary to obstruction of the lower urinary tract.

2. Palpation and percussion of the suprapubic area. This procedure may reveal a distended atonic bladder, which may be secondary to neurogenic disease or obstruction of the urethra or bladder neck.

3. Observation of the size and force of the urinary stream. If the urinary stream is normal, neurogenic dysfunction or obstruction is, for all practical purposes, ruled out.

4. Examination of the penis. Meatal stenosis or phimosis with secondary balanitis should be sought for, though it is questionable that these lesions play a part in causing enuresis.

5. Examination of the rectum. Diminished tone of the anal sphincter is strong evidence of a defect of the sacral nerve roots and suggests neurovesical disease.

The bulbocavernosus reflex should be elicited. With the finger in the rectum, the glans penis or clitoris is squeezed. This maneuver should cause an involuntary contracture of the anal sphincter. If it does not, a lesion of the sacral roots (lower neuron) is present.

6. Examination of the lower spine. Evidence of myelomeningocele or meningocele should be sought for. A dimple or a group of hairs growing over the midline of the sacral area may indicate the existence of spina bifida.

7. Examination of the nervous system. Abnormalities in the patient's gait may suggest defects of the sacral nerves. Reflex and sensory changes may also be discovered. Perianal sensory losses are of particular significance because they suggest interruption of the sacral reflex arc.

## V. Laboratory tests

### 1. Complete blood count

A complete blood count is not useful unless chronic infection of the urinary tract or uremia is present.

### 2. Urinalysis

Urinalysis is of the greatest importance. A midstream specimen from either sex, or a catheter specimen from the female, must be immediately examined microscopically. The unstained sediment must be studied in order to detect the possible presence of pus and red blood cells; whether pus cells are present or not, the sediment must then be stained with methylene blue so that the presence or absence of bacteria can be established. In the urine specimens of many patients, particularly those with residual urine in the kidneys, ureters, or bladder, even though infected, few or no pus cells will be observed; but bacteria will be present. Their presence establishes the diagnosis of infection of the urinary tract, for it means that at least 10,000 organisms per ml of urine are present. If the urine has not been stained, it has not been completely examined. The stained smear is the simplest, least expensive, and best screening test for the presence of urinary infection. In some cases, quantitative cultures of the urine may be necessary. The discovery of infection places the patient in the "organic enuretic" class.

### 3. Renal function tests

Of all the tests for renal function, the phenolsulfonphthalein test gives the most accurate information most quickly. It not only measures renal function, but it also rules out or implies the presence of vesical or ureterorenal residual urine. Since the accuracy of this test does not depend upon the volume of urine flow, it is not necessary for the patient to force fluids beforehand. In fact, the test is most valuable when small volumes are voided. In most instances, a specimen obtained one-half hour after the injection of phenolsulfonphthalein is all that is needed; small children normally excrete 60 to 80 per cent of the dye at this time, and older patients 50 to 60 per cent. If the volume of urine is 50 ml or less and the amount of dye recovered is normal, there is no appreciable residual urine.

If the specific gravity of the morning urine is 1.024 or higher, and if the amount of PSP excreted one-half hour after its injection is subnormal, the presence of residual urine and its approximate amount can usually be established by collecting a second specimen 30 minutes later. If the percentage of PSP in the second specimen is only a little less or a little more than that found in the first specimen, residual urine is usually the cause. For example,

| Time after injection of PSP minutes | Quantity of urine voided ml | Amount of PSP present % |
|---|---|---|
| 30 | 25 | 25 |
| 60 | 50 | 20 |
| Total | 75 | 45 |

In this instance, the results of the PSP test can be diagrammed as a "flat" curve (25 per cent — 20 per cent) which signifies that residual urine (vesical or ureterorenal) is present and that renal function is about normal. Also in this example, the amount of residual urine does not exceed 25 ml, which is the amount that would contain another 25 per cent of the dye; consequently, a total 50 per cent of the dye was excreted in 30 minutes. If there is reason to question the results of the PSP test, the patient should be catheterized immediately after the specimen has been voided. A post-voiding film taken in conjunction with excretory urograms will also reveal residual urine, if it is present.

In functional enuresis there is no residual urine and no depression of renal function. If the PSP excretion is not normal, a thorough urological examination is indicated.

# VI. Special diagnostic procedures
## 1. Excretory urograms

Excretory urograms should be obtained and then the patient should void. After the patient voids, a film of the bladder area should be taken so that the presence or absence of residual urine can be ascertained. Evidence of obstruction in the urinary tract indicates that enuresis is not caused by a functional disorder. A film of the bladder area may also reveal spina bifida. Such a finding, if the lesion is extensive, strongly suggests damage to the sacral nerves.

## 2. Cystometric study

Stockwell and Smith recorded cystometrograms from 90 enuretic patients; 37 tracings showed abnormal responses. They felt that this procedure was definitely a help in the diagnosis of 80 of these patients. Pinck also stressed the importance of this procedure in the diagnosis of neurogenic or instrinsic neuromuscular dysfunction of the bladder.

Hodges and Keizur employed cystometry in their studies. Cystometrograms of 4 of their 13 patients contained curves characteristic of an uninhibited neurogenic bladder.

Nash noted abnormalities in the cystometrograms of many enuretic subjects. Some indicated highly tense bladders with small capacities, with or without uninhibited contractions, while others indicated bladders of low tension and large capacity, also with or without uninhibited contractions.

Abnormalities in cystometric tracings may suggest delay in maturation or may represent evidence of a psychosomatic response to unfavorable early sexual adjustments or harsh toilet training, as discussed in the chapter "The Effect of the Psyche on Vesical Function". Cystometry should prove helpful in discovering the uninhibited type of bladder, and this type of bladder should respond well to parasympathetic blocking agents.

## 3. Urethrography and cystography

Cystograms and urethrograms are not indicated if no infection is present, if intravenous urograms are normal, and if no residual urine is revealed by the post-voiding film. If there is evidence of infection or obstruction, a trabeculated bladder with small capacity or a large smoothwall bladder caused by neurovesical disease or obstruction may be seen in cystograms. Reflux of radiopaque material into the ureters may occur, defining hydroureteronephrosis.

## 4. Cystoscopy and panendoscopy

These procedures are not indicated if all previous examinations have indicated that the patient is normal (normal urinary stream, normal neurological examination, normal urinalysis, normal PSP test, normal excretory urograms, and no evidence of residual urine); they are reserved for examining patients who show evidence of organic disease. SPOCK has pointed out that from the psychologic standpoint, enuretic children, particularly boys, already have a dread of genital injury, and cystoscopy may only accentuate this fear (castration complex).

## 5. Electroencephalography

MICHAELS and SECUNDA studied the electroencephalograms of adolescents with enuresis. Though many of the tracings were normal, some showed border-line immature reactions and others showed definite abnormal immature tracings; a wave of slow rate was the most common recording. It is not clear, however, how this test may be useful in the diagnosis or treatment of enuresis.

## VII. Differential diagnosis

If the physical examination, urinalysis, PSP test, excretory urograms, and cystometrogram have indicated that the patient is normal, there is very little probability that enuresis is caused by any of the common organic diseases.

1. Ectopic ureteral orifice in the female. Patients with this anomaly, though they dribble urine constantly or intermittently, also urinate regularly with normal control. Upon examination of the vulval and vaginal areas the abnormal orifice will usually be discovered. If possible, a ureteral catheter should be passed up this ureter; the urine from it will almost always contain evidence of infection. A pyelogram can then be obtained, and it will give evidence of hydro-ureteronephrosis.

If the ectopic orifice cannot be found, excretory urograms will usually afford the evidence from which this diagnosis can be inferred. The ectopic ureter usually drains a duplicated renal pelvis. This pelvis may be hydronephrotic and may even fail to excrete the radiopaque material. Such a finding, in addition to cystoscopic evidence of a single ureteral orifice on one side, is typical of this congenital anomaly.

2. Neurogenic vesical disease. Patients with neurogenic vesical disease are usually incontinent during the day as well as at night. They dribble urine, often have a slow flow, cloudy, odorous urine, and have difficulty with bowel control. Physical examination may reveal a distended bladder, impaired tone of the anal sphincter, and absence of the bulbocavernosus reflex (lower motor lesion — atonic bladder). Evidence of myelomeningocele or meningocele and other abnormalities may be found in the course of the neurological examination.

Urinalysis usually reveals infection. PSP excretion is reduced because of the presence of residual urine or renal damage, or both; excretory urograms may demonstrate hydronephrosis and either a dilated, smooth-walled bladder (atonic bladder), a small, heavily trabeculated bladder, or a distorted bladder (spastic bladder). The post-voiding film will show residual urine.

The cystometrogram will contain evidence of a flaccid, spastic, or "mixed" type of neurogenic bladder; cystograms and cystoscopy will confirm this diagnosis.

3. Obstructive uropathy. Patients with obstructive uropathy complain of more than enuresis. They usually suffer from frequency, both day and night, burning on urination, urgency to the point of incontinence, recurrent fever, renal pain, and poor force and caliber of the urinary stream.

Physical examination may reveal renal enlargement (caused by hydro-nephrosis), distention of the bladder (caused by urethral or bladder neck obstruction), or stenosis of the urethral orifice. Urinalysis usually shows infection, the PSP excretion is depressed because of residual ureterorenal or vesical urine or impairment of kidney function, and excretory urograms will demonstrate obstruction or vesical residual urine.

Cystography and cystoscopy will help in outlining more completely the pathologic changes caused by obstructive uropathy.

## VIII. Treatment

Treatment of enuresis should be based upon knowledge of its cause; however, as has been shown, many theories as to its etiology have been propounded. Some theories appear to be more reasonable than others, but there is no unanimity of opinion in behalf of any one of them.

It is difficult to judge the efficacy of treatment because, as CROSBY has shown, in almost half the children who are enuretic at the age of three years spontaneous cure occurs during the two subsequent years. Furthermore, BROWNE and FORD-SMITH, in a study of 13 enuretic boys, observed that they obtained results with placebos that were as good as those obtained with drugs such as ephedrine and belladonna.

Before beginning treatment, some attempt should be made to diagnose the cause of the enuresis in each patient. The following principles should prove helpful:

1. If a child is continent for a number of months or years and then experiences enuresis again, the cause must almost certainly be psychological. The fact that complete continence was gained even for a short time rules out neurovesical disease, delayed maturation, and other organic causes.

2. If a patient suffers from diurnal incontinence in addition to enuresis, as well as urgency or frequency or both, a neurogenic type of vesical disease or a psychologic cause is suggested.

3. If a patient has never had nocturnal continence he may have some type of intrinsic neurovesical dysfunction or his maturation may be delayed. The cause could also be psychogenic.

### 1. Symptomatic measures
#### a) Limitation of fluids

This is the most time-honored treatment of enuresis. Fluid intake is restricted late in the afternoon and forbidden after a dry supper. These restrictions are employed to decrease nocturnal urinary output and thus decrease the chances of bedwetting. Unfortunately, nocturnal incontinence usually occurs when the bladder is only partially filled. Certainly the effect of this type of therapy is not dramatic.

#### b) Measures to increase vesical capacity and to increase acuity of inhibitory response

BAKWIN recommends that enuretic children be encouraged to put off urination during the day in order to increase the degree of afferent impulses from the bladder; cerebral consciousness of the urge to urinate as well as the capacity of the bladder are thus increased. NICHOLS also stresses this aspect of treatment. Most writers believe that an enuretic child should be thoroughly wakened once or twice a night and caused to urinate. This is also meant to develop the inhibitory reflex. If wakening by an adult proves efficacious, the child should be wakened by an alarm clock for many weeks so that he can assume the responsibility of voiding himself.

## c) Drugs

Various types of drugs have been used in the symptomatic treatment of enuresis.

### α) Parasympatholytic drugs

Since the bladder of the enuretic patient undergoes involuntary spasm in unconscious voiding, the administration of atropine-like drugs seems to be a logical means of attempting to interrupt impulses of the parasympathetic nerves to the bladder.

Tincture of belladonna. Tincture of belladonna has been the most widely used drug in the treatment of enuresis. The initial dose may be five or ten drops at bedtime, and the continuing dose should be increased to the maximum which can be tolerated or until the desired result has been obtained. This usually requires a dose of 20 to 30 drops. If diurnal incontinence, urgency, or frequency accompany enuresis, the drug may be taken before mealtimes as well as at bedtime.

Parasympathetic blocking agents. Parasympathetic blocking agents block the transmission of impulses in the postganglionic fibers of the parasympathetic nerves, and if a large enough dose is given bladder function may be completely paralyzed. Propantheline bromide (Probanthine), methantheline bromide (Banthine), or similar drugs are particularly useful in treating a patient in whom cystometry reveals an uninhibited neurogenic bladder. Patients with uninhibited neurogenic bladders are likely to have urgency, frequency, and occasional diurnal incontinence, as well as enuresis. For enuresis in children, the initial dose at bedtime is 25 mg, and the dose may be increased to 75 mg. For adolescents, larger doses may be prescribed. If there are symptoms of vesical irritability, the drug may be given in doses of 25 to 50 mg every six hours with the largest amount given at bedtime (HODGES and KEIZUR).

### β) Sympathomimetic drugs

Ephedrine. Ephedrine-like compounds are administered in order to increase resistance at the bladder neck by increasing the muscle tone of the internal sphincter. The initial dose for a child is 0.03 gm at bedtime. This may be gradually increased by 0.03 gm increments, depending upon result and side effects, to a possible total of 0.3 gm (BROOKFIELD). This drug may also help in the control of enuresis by causing some degree of wakefulness.

Dextro-amphetamine sulfate. Dextro-amphetamine sulfate is a central nervous system stimulant which, when administered at bedtime, decreases the depth of sleep. Some writers believe that one cause of enuresis is an unusually deep plane of sleep. The usefulness of this drug in the treatment of enuresis lies in the hope that it will cause wakefulness, thus allowing the patient to waken promptly when the urge to void is perceived.

The dose for children is 5 mg at bedtime, and it may be increased to 10 mg or even 15 mg if necessary.

### γ) Parasympathomimetic drugs

In a few enuretic patients, the cystometrogram may reveal vesical atony. Drugs such as bethanecol chloride (urecholine chloride) may decrease vesical capacity and increase the contractile power of the bladder. In children, the initial dose may be as low as 5 mg given three or four times a day. It may be increased to as much as 20 to 30 mg in adolescents. It is also advisable to insist that patients with vesical atony void every two hours whether or not they have the urge, and also strain abdominally as much as possible.

### δ) Antidiuretic hormone

Posterior pituitary snuff has been administered at bedtime in order to limit the formation of urine during the night. Mason thought it had particular usefulness if vesical capacity was smaller than normal. HALLMAN found that the capacity of the bladders of children suffering from enuresis was smaller than that of a control group.

MARSON treated four enuretic adolescents with posterior pituitary snuff, at times substituting a placebo for the hormone without the patient's knowledge. The results were superior when posterior pituitary hormone was administered. He suggested the use of 50 mg in each nostril at bedtime; it is effective for five to ten hours.

### ε) Sodium chloride

ROSENSON and LISWOOD treated 28 enuretic children between the ages of four and ten years by giving them sandwiches at bedtime containing five grams of salt. They claimed 27 were cured. This form of therapy, first suggested in 1927 by Kranogorski, who reported 78 per cent of 125 enuretics cured, is based upon the fact that the ingestion of about five grams of salt at bedtime causes the retention of fluid in the extracellular space, thus limiting urinary output during the night. This form of treatment has met with little enthusiasm.

## d) Reenforcement of conditioned reflex

Various machines for the treatment of enuresis have been used in the past without great success; however, MOWRER and MOWRER wrote of gratifying results obtained with a conditioning apparatus which was constructed so that an electrical circuit closed when voiding began. Closing of the circuit gave the patient an electrical shock which woke him. DAVIDSON and DOUGLAS claimed cure in 15 of 20 enuretic patients with the MOWRER device. They noted that it was necessary to use it for periods ranging from one to three months, and occasionally even longer.

SEIGER uses an apparatus which sets off an audible signal (a bell) when the circuit is closed, thus awakening the patient; and a nearby floor lamp lights up simultaneously! He treated 106 enuretic patients after which almost 90 per cent of them were dry for periods ranging from two months to many years. Ten per cent either suffered relapse or never ceased to wet the bed occasionally.

BEHRLE, ELKIN, and LAYBOURNE made an interesting study of 20 enuretic children who were treated with the type of apparatus used by SEIGER. Though these writers felt that the cause of enuresis in these patients was psychological, not incomplete maturation, they noted cure or marked improvement in 15 of 20. They questioned the danger of this type of treatment for a psychosomatic complaint, and were able to show that these children not only did not develop symptoms referred to other organs, but, in fact, were psychologically much improved after cure. They attributed this improvement to the fact that the patients were now socially acceptable, their anxieties and those of their parents were relieved; and they had thereby increased their self-confidence.

CROSBY believes that enuresis is a disease entity and not a symptom. Though he concedes that many cases of enuresis are due to psychological causes, he believes that the majority arise from a physiological abnormality. He thinks that during normal development a child acquires a degree of inhibitory tone such that, even though he sleeps deeply, he is awakened by the urge to void, and is therefore completely continent. If, however, this maturation is incomplete, and if the child becomes inured to the physical discomfort of being wet, enuresis persists.

CROSBY also believes that the use of a machine, similar to those used by others which shocks the patient when involuntary urination occurs, increases his somatic discomfort, which he resents, and develops the cerebral inhibitory reflex as well. The parents are also automatically wakened so that the child is escorted, wide-awake, to the bathroom. CROSBY found that it was often necessary to use the machine only on five successive nights, though a few children required its use for 15 to 40 nights. He also prescribed drugs (described above) as he thought indicated.

### e) Empirical organic therapy

The passage of sounds and the injection or instillation of chemical solutions into the urethra are mentioned only to be condemned. Children with enuresis are overly anxious and many of the boys have a definite fear of castration based upon threats of punishment for the bedwetting. These fears are only emphasized by procedures such as those mentioned above.

## 2. Psychotherapy

Successful psychotherapeutic treatment of enuresis necessitates realization by parents and physician that enuresis is a symptom of emotional unrest in a child. Parents must realize that punishment and disparagement of a child increase his feelings of inferiority and unworthiness. The physician must give the child a feeling of support, of being on his side. He helps the child think of his enuresis as a symptom, not as a disease or a "badness", thus relieving his feelings of guilt. The physician who can communicate in a "man to man" relationship with the child, treating him as a worthwhile individual, will achieve the best results in therapy. Strong suggestion and reassurance, made either directly or through the use of hypnosis, will bring about a remarkable degree of improvement. Instrumental manipulation should be avoided.

In addition to treating the child, the physician should provide guidance for the child's parents. They should understand their role in the child's difficulties without being made to feel guilty or to feel that they have failed as parents. They should be helped to realize that a home atmosphere of consistent good will and understanding will help the child attain self-confidence and, eventually, bladder control.

## IX. Prognosis

Fifty to 75 per cent of enuretic patients will probably respond well to symptomatic therapy; and many of the remainder may be helped by psychotherapy. A few of the remainder will not respond to any treatment, and some seem to overcome this difficulty spontaneously, since the incidence of enuresis at the age of twenty is only 1 to 2 per cent.

Many authors have observed that a number of previously enuretic patients continue to have nocturia, urinating once or twice during a night, and diurnal urgency and frequency at times; these are symptoms of an uninhibited neurogenic bladder and they may persist throughout life. A significant number of patients who were enuretic as children may notice as adults periodic or even persistent vesical irritability when under psychic stress. (This type of vesical irritability is described in "The Effect of the Psyche on Vesical Function"). This is further evidence of the psychological cause of enuresis.

# C. Impotence in the male

## I. Introduction

Among the commonest maladies affecting mankind one is still cloaked in shame and secrecy—sexual maladjustment. In men it appears as impotence; in women as frigidity. Many marriages are touched by it in some degree. ENGLISH and PEARSON have said; "When the sexual adjustment in a marriage is good it constitutes about 10% of the positive side of marriage but when it is bad it constitutes 90% of what is wrong in a marriage". Its repercussions may appear in extramarital affairs, marital friction, or divorce. It may cause nervous symptoms, chronic ill-health, depression, melancholia, or even suicide. It prevents some men and women from marriage; in others it impels frantic sexual activity with many partners.

The cultural reaction to sexual matters is mixed. On one hand sexual activity is surrounded by taboos and restrictions, considered dirty and indecent, something to joke and deride; and yet we talk of it as a wonderful, spiritual experience. The degree of misunderstanding and misinformation about this primary biological drive is truly astounding. To many, masturbation is still unnatural and disgusting. Every young man is disturbed by masturbation or nocturnal emissions until he somehow learns they are normal. The sexual impulse in the male is strongest between the ages of 15 and 19 years, at a time when society frowns on sexual activity. The prohibitions against and the misconceptions about this biologically normal function set the stage for greater or lesser difficulties in later years.

Impotence, the inability to perform the sexual act, is the commonest sexual difficulty in the male. It may occur as inability to achieve erection, to sustain erection, or to ejaculate; as premature ejaculation; or as loss of sexual desire.

There is much misunderstanding about the causes of impotence. It has been ascribed to neurological or urological disease (both are rarely etiological factors); hormonal deficiency; homosexuality, masturbation or sexual excesses; business or other real worries; fears of having children; frigidity in the wife or living with a wife who has lost her attractiveness; a natural occurrence with advancing age or after years of marriage to the same wife; ignorance of sexual technique; a reaction against the "bestiality" of sex or a belief in the "purity" of women. It is generally agreed among urologists that most impotence is of psychological or behavioral origin.

Although impotence is seldom due to physical causes (perhaps in only 1 to 5% of the cases that the urologist sees), medicine has always focused upon possible organic causes. The view to be taken in this chapter is that, although the presence of organic reason for impotence (known anatomicophysiologic defect, disease or influence) should first be ruled out, the possible psychological or psychiatric reasons for impotence (herein called *behavioral*) then require thorough consideration.

## II. Anatomy and physiology of the male genital organs

In order to understand the organic causes of sexual difficulties in the male, a knowledge of the anatomy (blood and nerve supply) and physiology of the genital organs is necessary.

### 1. Nerve supply (see Fig. 7)

The male sexual apparatus has parasympathetic, sympathetic, and somatic innervation. Sensory neurons which complete the reflex arcs course with motor neurons. The nerves that govern the sex act are essentially the same ones that regulate the act of micturition.

### a) Parasympathetic (visceral motor)

Parasympathetic fibers from the second, third, and fourth sacral segments of the spinal cord (S2—4) form the pelvic nerves, or nervi erigentes, which mingle with the sympathetic nerves in the inferior hypogastric plexus. Some

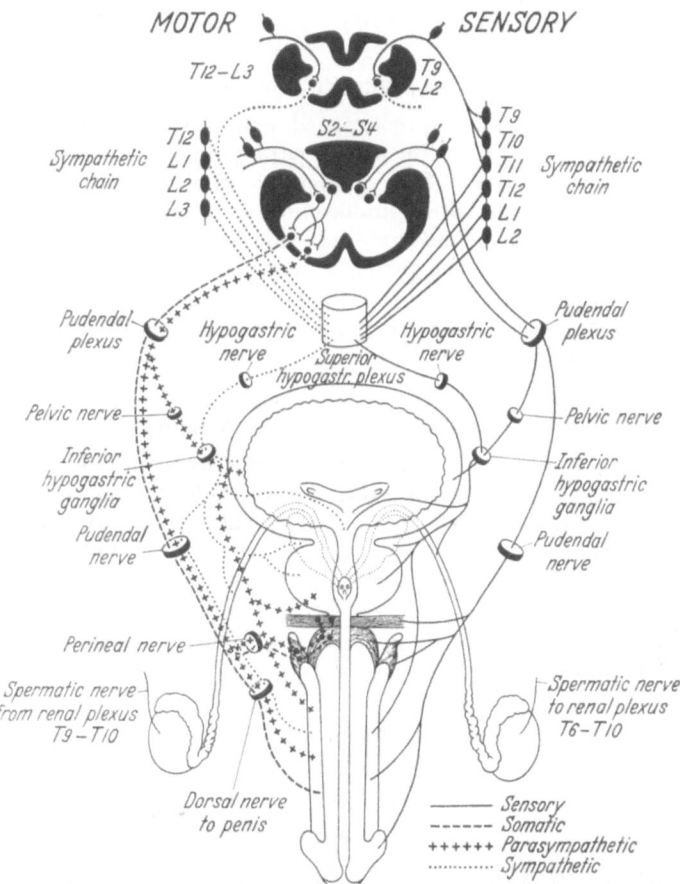

Fig. 7. Motor and sensory nerve supply of the bladder and internal and external genitalia of the male with particular reference to the phenomenon of sexual function. [Modified, with permission, from E. BORS: J. Nerv. Ment. Dis. **116**, 572—8 (1952)]

of the parasympathetic fibers of these nerves pass to the bladder wall (controlling its entire motor function) and to the prostate gland. Others continue distally through the urogenital diaphragm to the accessory muscles of ejaculation. Some parasympathetic fibers also join the pudendal nerve and are distributed to the arteries of the penis.

### b) Sympathetic (visceral motor)

Though some of the sympathetic nerves which contribute to the hypogastric (presacral) nerves descend along the aorta from the renal-aortic plexuses (T5 to T12), the nerves most vitally concerned with sexual function arise from T12—L3.

Their preganglionic fibers pass through the inferior mesenteric plexus to the superior hypogastric plexus. Their postganglionic fibers descend as the hypogastric nerves to the inferior hypogastric plexus, where they become associated with the sacral parasympathetic nerves arising from S2—4. From here, sympathetic nerves are distributed to blood vessels of the bladder, and to smooth muscles of the bladder neck, prostate, vasa, and seminal vesicles. Some sympathetic nerve fibers join the pudendal nerve with which they descend to innervate the arteries (constrictors) and the veins (dilators) of the penis and the musculature of the corpora cavernosa (constrictors).

### c) Somatic motor

The somatic fibers intimately concerned with sexual function are carried in the pudendal nerve and, like the sacral parasympathetic outflow, arise from S2—4. The perineal branch of the pudendal innervates the external urinary sphincter, ischiocavernosus, and bulbocavernosus muscles in addition to the transverse perinei, levator, and external anal sphincter muscles. The other branch, the dorsal nerve of the penis, is distributed to the body of the penis, the glans, and the corpora.

As noted above, the pudendal nerves carry parasympathetic and sympathetic fibers to the penis as well as somatic fibers.

### d) Somatic and visceral sensory

The sensory nerve-fibers involved in sexual function are in the pudendal (S2—4) and the hypogastric (T9—L2) nerves. The former carries sensations from the glans, skin, and deep structures of the penis and from the striated muscles of the perineum, including the ischiocavernosus, bulbocavernosus, and external urinary sphincter.

The sensory nerves that accompany the sympathetic fibers transmit impulses from the blood vessels of the penis, prostate, seminal vesicles, vasa deferentia, bladder, and bladder neck.

## 2. Blood supply

Only those blood vessels concerned with erection will be discussed.

### a) Arterial

The arterial blood which causes engorgement of the corpora of the penis comes from the internal pudendal, a branch of the hypogastric artery. The internal pudendal artery has three paired branches that are concerned with erection.

#### α) Artery to the corporus cavernosum

These are the main arteries to the corpora cavernosa. They anastomose freely with each other, the artery to the bulb, and the dorsal arteries of the penis.

#### β) Artery to the bulb

These arteries supply the corpus spongiosum.

#### γ) Dorsal artery of the penis

These arteries supply the penile integument and the erectile tissues of the glans.

## b) Venous

DEYSACH, from careful morphologic studies, has described the penile venous system as follows:

### α) Venae profundae

There are three or four of these "sluice valves" in each corpus spongiosum. They are of large caliber and have very thick muscular walls. They therefore resemble arteries more than veins. Through their walls course both small and large veins. The latter drain into the plexus of Santorini and thence to the prostatovesical venous plexus which joins the hypogastric veins.

### β) Superficial dorsal vein

These veins drain blood from the penile integument, anastomosing freely with the deep dorsal veins.

### γ) Deep dorsal vein

These veins carry blood from the glans and prepuce into the prostaticovesical plexus. They anastomose with the veins of the corpus spongiosum.

## 3. Physiological mechanisms

The sexual apparatus in the male is largely under the control of the autonomic nervous system. The total reaction of the penis to the complete sexual act can be divided into four phases: erection, emission, ejaculation, and subsidence of erection. The integrating site of sexual activity in the male is in the region of the upper lumbar cord (T12—L3).

### a) Erection (largely parasympathetic)

Normally erection is initiated by stimulation of the glans penis or psychic stimuli (or a combination thereof).

Afferent impulses arising from the glans pass, via the dorsal nerves of the penis, through the pudendal nerves to the posterior roots of S2—4 and through the hypogastric nerves to the upper lumbar portion of the spinal cord. Descending nerves from the cerebral cortex also communicate with the sacral portion of the cord (S2—4).

These sensory impulses set up a reflex arc through the sacral parasympathetic outflow (S2—4) with motor impulses reaching the arterioles of the penis over the pudendal (and vesicoprostatic) nerves. Such stimulation causes relaxation of these arterioles which are therefore able to deliver an augmented supply of blood to the corpora cavernosa.

The venae profundae contract (sympathetic nerve effect?) thus lessening the outflow of blood from the corpora through the small venous sluice channels. By this mechanism the blood pressure in the corpora approaches that of the carotid arteries, and erection is thus attained.

### b) Emission (largely sympathetic)

Afferent impulses from the moist and stimulated glans reach the sacral cord and the integrating center in the upper lumbar cord (T12—L3) via the dorsal nerves of the penis and the hypogastric nerves. A moment before actual orgasm occurs, a massive stimulus is sent out through the thoracolumbar sympathetic outflow, causing contracture of the smooth muscle of the prostate, seminal vesicles, and the vasa deferentia and thereby forcing the contents of these structures into the posterior urethra. At the same time, the bladder neck is tightly closed, thus preventing retrograde ejaculation.

### c) Ejaculation (largely parasympathetic)

Immediately after emission, the rhythmic reaction of ejaculation ensues. This consists of spasmodic contractions of the bulbocavernosus and the ischiocavernosus muscles accompanied by contractions of the external urinary sphincter, the pelvic floor, and the external anal sphincter (parasympathetic fibers in the pudendal nerves). Often, there are also spasmodic contractions of the extensor muscles of the thighs. These strong rhythmic muscular spasms force jets of semen down the urethra. Accompanying the motor activity of ejaculation is a strong sensory component (orgasm) which correlates well with the muscular spasms described above.

### d) Subsidence of erection (largely sympathetic)

At the time of emission-ejaculation-orgasm, sympathetic stimulation causes contraction of the arterioles leading to the corpora cavernosa and dilatation of the venae profundae which leads to subsidence of the erection; the smooth muscle of the corpora contracts, and the penis may, therefore, temporarily become smaller than normal.

# III. Organic etiology of impotence

## 1. Interference with arterial blood supply to the penis

Interruption or diminution of blood flow through the hypogastric arteries will of necessity have a deleterious effect upon erection. In the aging male, atherosclerotic or thrombotic processes affecting the hypogastric arteries or the aortic bifurcation will cause impairment of erection or premature loss of erection.

If thrombosis complicates surgical procedures on the aorta, or if retrograde occlusion of the hypogastric arteries ensues, loss of erection may develop from diminution of the arterial supply to the corpora of the penis.

Leriche has described a syndrome which arises from thrombotic obliteration of the bifurcation of the aorta. Such a condition can afflict young men as well as older men. These symptoms include an inability to sustain an erection, fatigue of the extremities on exertion (without claudication), atrophy of the muscles of the extremities without trophic changes, and pallor of the legs and feet. Physical examination reveals diminution or absence of pulses in the legs and iliac arteries, and thrill or bruit may be noted over the femoral arteries. The blood pressure is higher in the arms than in the legs.

## 2. Interference with nerve supply

Disease or injury affecting the sacral or upper lumbar and lower thoracic portions of the cord, the cauda equina, the sympathetic outflow from the sexual integrating centers of the cord (T12—L3), or the pudendal nerves may have an adverse effect upon one or more of the sexual reactions (erection, emission, etc.). A proper neurological examination will reveal changes reflecting injury to the nerves or centers which control sexual activity.

## a) Anomalies

Serious defects of the cauda equina, which include both efferent and afferent sacral roots, result in sexual malfunction. Most of the patients afflicted with myelodysplasia and extensive spina bifida will be completely impotent.

## b) Acquired diseases

Diseases of the peripheral nerves (sensory, motor, or both) or the spinal cord may cause deleterious effects upon the power of erection, emission or ejaculation. They include tabes dorsalis, tumors, and the toxic or degenerative lesions (i.e., as may occur in multiple sclerosis, diabetes mellitus, Parkinsonism, etc.).

## c) Traumatic injuries

Trauma to the nervous system is probably most common organic cause of aberrations of sexual power in the male. This trauma is usually due to external injury involving damage to the spinal cord.

### α) Affecting erection

Injuries to the spinal cord often impair or abolish erection but even more often abolish the ejaculation of semen. Of 408 paraplegic patients reported by TALBOT, 33.5% had no erections, 46% could get erections secondary to local stimulations, while only 20.5% experienced erections from either local or psychic stimuli. He reported that one third of those who could get an erection had had intercourse and one half of this group experienced some gratification.

MUNRO surveyed a group of 84 paraplegics of whom 74% had erections. He noted that the higher the lesion in the cord the more likely the patient was to have erections. Thus, of 54 patients with lesions above the sacral cord, 48 obtained erections. His 12 patients with lesions affecting the parasympathetic and somatic outflow (S2—4) had no erections.

ZEITLIN, COTTRELL, and LLOYD analyzed 100 patients with traumatic lesions of the spinal cord. Thirty-three of their patients had cervical lesions. Of these, 27 had normal erections. In 4 they were incomplete, while 2 had none. Twenty-one patients had upper thoracic injuries. In this group, 15 had good erections, 4 noted impaired erections, while 2 had none. Of those 39 patients who suffered damage to the lower half of the thoracic cord, 18 experienced normal erections, 12 noted some difficulty, while 9 were impotent. Seven of their group had sustained injury to the lumbar and sacral cord; 4 had good erections, 2 experienced some difficulty, and one patient was impotent.

Summarizing their series, 64% could develop normal erections. This compares fairly well with the figures of MUNRO (74%) and TALBOT (66.5%).

### β) Affecting ejaculation

The power to ejaculate is destroyed in most men who have suffered injury to the spinal cord at whatever level. MUNRO found that only 7% of his 84 paraplegic patients produced semen. ZEITLIN, COTTRELL, and LLOYD reported that only three of their 100 patients ejaculated semen.

Damage to the lower thoracic and upper lumbar segments of the cord interferes with the sympathetic outflow which controls the emission of semen into the posterior urethra by stimulating the contraction of the smooth muscle of the prostate, vasa deferentia, and seminal vesicles. The trigone also contracts, thus occluding the bladder neck. Lack of ejaculation of semen can be caused either by lack of emission of semen or by failure of the bladder neck to close though semen is forced into the urethra. In the latter instance, retrograde ejaculation into the bladder occurs.

### γ) Affecting orgasm

Possibly half of these men who have successful intercourse report sexual gratification, but few experience an orgasm (TALBOT). ZEITLIN, COTTRELL, and LLOYD stated that only 10% of their men who could gain an erection had orgasm, which the authors described as an "uninhibited spastic reaction" of the legs and perineum. Such a reaction, however, proved psychologically beneficial to h ese men.

### d) Neurosurgical interventions

Certain neurosurgical procedures may have damaging effects upon sexual functions.

### α) Sympathectomy, ganglionectomy, and splanchnicectomy

These procedures, used in the treatment of hypertension and certain peripheral vascular diseases, are often complicated by changes in sexual power. Furthermore, the type of difficulty which arises after these procedures throws further light upon the neurophysiology of the sexual apparatus in men.

Table 2. *Impairment in sexual power following sympathectomy* (WHITELAW and SMITHWICK)

| Extent of sympathectomy | Number of patients | Impairment of erection | Permanent loss of ejaculation of semen |
|---|---|---|---|
| T1—T12 . . . . . | 19 | 11 (57%) | 0 |
| T7—L3 . . . . . . | 116 | 26 (23%) | 24 (21%) |
| L1—L5 (unilateral) | 12 | 2 (17%) | 0 |
| L1—L5 (bilateral) . | 11 | 7 (63%) | 6 (54%) |

WHITELAW and SMITHWICK aalyzed the effectson sexual power in a group of 158 patients upon whom limited and more extensive operations were performed. Their observations are summarized in Table 2.

Since erection is activated by the sacral parasympathetic outflow, the above incidence of impairment of erection may seem surprising. WHITELAW and SMITHWICK offered three hypotheses to account for this in the groups subjected to extensive thoracic sympathectomy:

1. Increased peripheral sympathetic activity distal to the point of interruption of sympathetic nerves may lead to constriction of the arterioles of the penis, thus counteracting the dilator effect of the parasympathetic nerves.

2. Extensive thoracic sympathectomy causes vasodilatation of the blood vessels in the abdominal viscera thereby decreasing the supply to the penis.

3. After degeneration of preganglionic and postganglionic sympathetic fibers, sensitization to circulating epinephrine occurs and causes vasoconstriction of the penile arterioles. This hypothesis, however, does not seem to account for the weakened potency observed in those men subjected to a limited bilateral lumbar sympathectomy.

Another factor would appear to be the existence of a "sexual integrating center" in the lower dorsal and upper lumbar region of spinal cord which exercises some control over erection as well as emission and ejaculation. From the data formulated from the work of WHITELAW and SMITHWICK above, it seems clear that when the nerves emanating from that center are divided bilaterally, changes in erection and ejaculation of semen are common.

Fortunately, though erection is affected to some degree in many patients subjected to sympathectomy, this aspect seldom is sexually disabling. On the other hand, lack of ejaculation means infertility which may be a tragedy for a young man.

In order to preserve the power of ejaculation, WHITELAW and SMITHWICK suggested that thoracolumbar sympathectomy extend down to L1 on one side and T12 on the other. They further stated that bilateral lumbar sympathectomy would not harm the ejaculatory function if L1 were left intact bilaterally.

ROSE analyzed the effect of sympathectomy upon the ejaculation of semen. Of 30 patients subjected to bilateral lumbar sympathectomy, including L1, 27, or 90%, of the patients noted no impairment. When, however, a more complete sympathectomy was performed (T9—L3) each of eight patients failed to ejaculate semen. Of these eight, five failed to force any semen into the posterior urethra. The other three patients refluxed their semen into the bladder whose neck had not contracted.

### β) Operations to improve function of the neurogenic bladder

1. Pudendal neurectomy, if done on both sides, usually causes loss or weakening of erectile power (BORS). This is because the pudendal nerves contain both parasympathetic fibers to the arterioles of the penis and the sensory fibers from the penis; cutting them abolishes the reflex arc. Unilateral nerve severance has a much better chance of preserving this function.

2. Subarachnoid alcohol block, by destroying the sacral cord and cauda equina, destroys the center for erection.

3. Sacral neurectomy, if complete, has the same effect as subarachnoid alcohol. Differential sacral neurectomy may preserve erection.

4. Pelvic neurectomy (sacral parasympathetic outflow) must of necessity cause impotence.

5. Rhizotomies (either anterior, posterior, or both) will destroy the power of erection if the operations include the sacral nerves. Rhizotomies above S1 rarely have an adverse effect on erections.

6. Cordectomy causes loss of erection.

Ejaculation of semen may cease after these destructive neurosurgical procedures for improvement of bladder function. Since most of these patients, however, have already lost the power of ejaculation and are undergoing such interventions for serious disabilities, this threat can be ignored.

### γ) Prostatectomy, cystectomy, and abdominoperineal resection of the rectum

1. Transurethral retropubic and transvesical intracapsular prostatectomy are rarely followed by loss of erectile power. These operations do not disturb the blood or autonomic nerve supplies to the penis and therefore should not be expected to interfere with erection. Retrograde ejaculation, however, is common following these procedures because of incompetency of the bladder neck.

2. Perineal intracapsular prostatectomy usually leads to loss of erectile power, for in this approach the parasympathetic nerves of the prostatic plexus which innervate the penile arterioles are in jeopardy. Postoperatively it is noted that the penis may become smaller than normal, unusually limber, and cold to the touch. These changes are caused by lack of parasympathetic nerve (dilator) impulses to the arterial supply of the corpora.

3. Radical (extracapsular) retropubic, perineal prostatectomy, abdominoperineal resection of the rectum, or prostatocystectomy almost surely destroys the prostatovesical plexus (containing sacral parasympathetic, sympathetic and somatic nerves). Inability to gain an erection should be expected after these procedures.

### 3. Endocrine disorders

#### a) Testes

Few diseases of the testes developing after adolescence have a deleterious effect upon sexual power. Even in Klinefelters's syndrome and bilateral cryptorchidism androgenic activity is well maintained. Bilateral removal or destruction of the testes by injury or infection may lead to a small decrease in the amount of 17-ketosteroids in the urine, but even this may have no effect upon sexual power, which is controlled by reflexes in the lower part of the spinal cord and depends upon normal penile arterial blood supply. Diminution in the excretion of testicular androgens may, however, effect a loss of sexual desire which responds quite readily to the administration of testosterone preparations.

#### b) Adrenals

Advanced disease of the adrenal cortex (e.g., Cushing's syndrome, Addison's disease) may at times cause loss of sexual desire and power.

#### c) Pituitary

Some diseases of the pituitary gland (e.g., acromegaly) may be associated with impotence.

#### d) Pancreas

Possibly one third of diabetics lose the power of erection even though no degenerative changes in the nervous system can be elicited. Improvement often occurs when the disease is brought under medical control (RUBIN and BABBOTT).

### 4. Effects of drugs

Certain drugs, administered for the control or treatment of various diseases may have an adverse effect upon erection. Estrogens, used in control of cancer of the prostate, cause testicular atrophy, leading often to both loss of power of erection and loss of desire. Parasympathetic blocking agents (e.g., methantheline bromide) used in the treatment of peptic ulcer or spastic bladder may negate the action of parasympathetic impulses to the arterioles of the corpora. Ganglionic blocking agents (e.g., mecamylanine hydrochloride) and antihistamines may have a similar effect. Tranquilizing agents as well as sedatives may impair the power of erection.

## IV. Examination of the patient for organic etiological factors

### 1. History

#### a) Sexual function

The duration of the complaint should be ascertained.

#### α) Erection

What degree of erection develops? Is it usable?

Does the erection persist or does it gradually fade away without accompanying orgasm?

Is the duration of erection short because of prematurity of ejaculation?

Is there difficulty in stimulating an erection from psychic stimuli? Does it require manual stimulation by the patient or his sexual partner?

If masturbation is practiced, is the erection of good quality? Is it well maintained to the time of orgasm?

Are nocturnal erections experienced? Are they of good quality? Does ejaculation of semen take place? Is the sensation of orgasm present?

### β) Ejaculation

At the time of orgasm, is semen delivered normally? If not, is the urine next voided cloudy?

Is ejaculation premature? What time elapses from insertion to orgasm? Does this period of time afford the sexual partner satisfaction?

Is ejaculation delayed unduly? Do ejaculation and orgasm fail to occur after prolonged intercourse?

### γ) Orgasm

Is the sensation of orgasm normal? If not, what sensations or reactions are felt?

### δ) Sexual desire

Is it normal? How often does it develop?

## b) Vesical function

(Since the parasympathetic innervation of the bladder is closely related to that controlling sexual power, some clues may be gained by surveying this function.)

Is urination normal in all respects?

Is the normal urge to void seldom experienced? Is the stream of poor size and force? Is straining required to initiate and continue it?

## c) Diseases of, injury to, or operations on the nervous system

Are there symptoms suggesting infections, toxic or degenerative disease of the nervous system (e.g., Parkinsonism, diabetes, tabes, syringomyelia)?

Can symptoms of neurogenic disturbances be elicited which are attributable to injury of the nervous system?

Has sympathectomy been performed?

## d) Symptoms of obstruction of the bifurcation of the aorta (Leriche syndrome)

Is there fatiguability or aching in the legs or buttocks with walking or even standing?

Are the legs and feet cool?

## e) Endocrine function

### α) Testes

Are the testicles descended? Have they sustained injury (i.e., direct, surgical, torsion, infection)?

### β) Adrenals

Are there symptoms suggesting malfunction of the adrenal glands (i.e., obesity, weakness, pigmentation, etc.)?

### γ) Pituitary

Is there a history suggesting severe hypopituitarism (with secondary effect upon the testes) or acromegaly?

### δ) Pancreas

Are there symptoms or signs of diabetes mellitus?

### f) Influence of drugs

Is the patient taking parasympathetic or ganglionic blocking agents, antihistamines, estrogens or sedatives?

## 2. Physical examination

### a) General

The general physical examination should include evidence of gross endocrinopathy (i.e., gynecomastia, pigmentation, body build, body weight, etc.).

### b) Genitalia

Evidence of congenital anomalies should be sought for, including severe chordee with hypospadias, cryptorchidism, and testicular atrophy.

### c) Vasculature

The arterial vessels of the lower extremity should be evaluated for signs of the Leriche syndrome which include diminished or absent pulsations of the iliac and femoral arteries; a bruit or systolic murmur over the aorta, iliac or femoral arteries; global atrophy of the legs and pallor of the legs and feet even when standing. The blood pressure may be higher in the arms than in the legs.

### d) Nervous system

The neurological examination should pay special attention to peripheral reflexes.

Muscle power, including that in gait and in the tone of the anal sphincter.

Sensation, with particular reference to perianal or "saddle" anesthesia.

The size and force of the urinary stream. (A normal stream rules out any significant damage to the neurological components governing potency.)

Repaired meningomyelocele or evidence of minor degrees of spina bifida (e.g., dimpling of the skin or a few hairs growing over the sacrum).

## 3. Radiography

### a) Osteograms

If spina bifida is suspected, radiograms of the bones of the spine and pelvis are indicated.

### b) Urograms

Should intravenous urograms be necessary, the postvoiding film may reveal residual urine (secondary to neurologic disturbance).

### c) Aortograms

Aortograms are needed to make the definitive diagnosis of the Leriche syndrome (thrombotic obliteration of the bifurcation of the aorta).

## 4. Estimation of residual urine for indirect evidence of neurogenic lesions

### a) Phenolsulfonphthalein (phenol red) test

The patient, without forcing fluids and after voiding urine, should be given 1 cc. (6 mg.) of the dye intravenously. If the one-half hour specimen is of small volume (i.e., 25—50 ml.) and the amount of dye recovered is 50 to 60%, there can be no appreciable amount of residual urine (see page 27).

### b) Passage of a catheter

This should be done immediately after the patient voids urine.

## V. Behavioral etiology of impotence

In nearly every case in which the presenting complaint is impotence, the root of the problem is behavioral rather than organic in nature. In seeking out the behavioral aspects of this ubiquitous but little discussed problem, it is helpful to know what constitutes average or normal sexual potency and to consider also some related abnormalities of male sexuality.

### 1. Normal sexual potency

There are many misconceptions about sexual ability in the male. There is no correlation between potency and virility. A man may be athletic and muscular, the picture of a virile male, yet be impotent. Another, living a sedentary life with an asthenic body habitus, may lead an active sexual life. The degree of sexual drive varies in men. Some have need for coitus daily; others once a month; others at longer intervals or not at all. Some authors believe there is a congenital absence of sexual desire in some men but this is more likely the result of infantile conditioning experiences rather than an inherent absence.

Considerable confusion arises as to the normal sexual pattern in men. According to KINSEY, married men in their twenties average coitus 3 to $3^1/_2$ times a week. Between 30 and 40 years the average is $2^1/_2$ times a week; between 40 and 50 years slightly less than twice weekly. Contrary to popular belief men do not have a change of life and the average 60-year-old man has coitus nearly once a week.

BERGLER states that normal intercourse should last 2 to 10 minutes with 60 to 100 insertive movements. Yet KINSEY found that 75% of men have orgasm in less than 2 minutes; many in 10—20 seconds after coital entrance, some even before entrance. This quick performance of the average male is usually most unsatisfactory for the wife. Unless she is already greatly excited the sexual act is over before she can begin to participate. To what extent this premature ejaculation causes lack of response in the female, and how much the wife's frigidity and lack of response occasions the prematurity of the husband, is worthy of more study. That there is an "intimate" reciprocal relationship goes without saying.

### 2. Conscious or nearly conscious factors

Some of the factors underlying impotence may be conscious or almost conscious so that the individual can almost grasp the reasons for his trouble. Just talking it over with his physician may help him to recognize these.

### a) The honeymoon and other stressful situations

Impotence in some degree is so common as to be expected on the honeymoon or during the early days of marriage. The young adult is prone to uncertainty and nervousness which interfere with his sexual functioning. If the wife's attitude is reassuring he may spontaneously correct this difficulty. However, its recurrence a few times at this early stage may produce a conditioned response with conscious or unconscious anticipation of failure and establish a pattern that continues through life.

When a married couple have been separated for a period by military service or other enforced separation, they build up strong sexual fantasies awaiting the moment of reunion. The emotional tension thus generated, combined with the strain and fatigue of travel, and meeting away from home in a strange community, can produce a duplication of honeymoon impotence.

Similarly in other stressful situations the average man may experience sexual failure. In the presence of family illness, financial crisis, or physical debility, he may find no interest or energy for love making. In "barrister's impotence", the ambitious, successful attorney or professional man bends all his efforts to his career, his books and studies taking his time even at home. Thus married to his work he has little or no drive for sexual expression. Despite the name "barrister's impotence" it is common to doctors, executives, professors and men of other professional categories.

### b) Fears and anxieties

Fear of detection in the act of intercourse is a common conscious cause of impotence and premature ejaculation. A squeaking bed, a bedroom next to parents or in-laws, the unavailability of contraceptives, these are but a few of the worries which may lead to failure. A woman may worry about the family wash, preparing lunch for the children, or the company coming to dinner, but she still can participate in coitus. A man beset by these problems is unlikely to have the frame of mind necessary for achieving or sustaining an erection.

To most men, failure in love-making is a disturbing situation, to some humiliating, to others shattering or even catastrophic. The fact that failure has occurred once, no matter what the reason, leads to the possibility or even anticipation it may happen again. The fear of failure impairs subsequent attempts and frequently brings more failures. This feedback may set up a self-perpetuating pattern of diminishing effort and increasing failure.

Fears of perversion or desires for "perverse" activity (conscious or unconscious) may underlie some cases of impotence. Many men and women have erroneous ideas as to what is right or wrong in "normal" sex behavior. It cannot be stressed too strongly that in happily married couples, there are no barriers— the use of the hands and mouth anywhere on the body is normal, that sucking, biting, pinching in moderation is usual. In preliminary lovemaking we make use of the sensual feelings we enjoyed as children in every part of the body as stimulants toward tumescence and eventual discharge in normal coitus. Most people experiment with mouth-genital contacts, feeling more or less guilty until they learn that it is a normal activity in lovemaking.

However, in some instances we may find that the male cannot become aroused except through mouth-genital contact or may be unable to complete the act without such stimulation. If this becomes the invariable pattern it suggests an underlying pathological state such as latent or overt homosexuality.

### c) Unsatisfactory spouses

Wolbarst has stressed the part the wife plays in the causation of impotence. Variety is the spice of sexual life. When it is permitted to develop into a routine affair the romance is gone. Male potency is highly susceptible to a wife's physical appearance and general emotional attitude. Obesity in a hitherto slim, attractive wife may cause the husband to lost interest. Sagging breasts, dry skin, thickening of the legs, loss of teeth, atrophic or patulous changes in the genitalia may inhibit sexual excitement in the male. The wife who is slovenly in appearance or personal hygiene or a slattern in caring for children and home can disgust her husband and squelch his ardor. If the wife nags and complains or is chronically ill, indisposed or confined to bed, her husband will hesitate to make any sexual approach.

The nature of a wife's sexual response throughout the years of marriage is very important. A woman, consistently unresponsive and submitting only as a wifely duty, is antagonistic to the sexual act and produces a reciprocal hostility in the husband. A man who consciously or unconsciously feels rejected by his wife has his pride recurrently hurt and may unconsciously seek refuge in impotence to assuage this grievous blow.

A paradox arises in the fact that many women, even those previously cold, have an increase of libido following the menopause. At a time when a man's sexual drive is diminishing for physiological reasons, his wife's drive may become greater. She may become incensed at his apparent disinterest in her, when she has strong sexual feelings, and domestic friction may arise.

### d) Inadequate sex education

It is amazing how much sex education, whether direct or by inference, stresses the likelihood of bad consequences following any indulgence. When parents, religious counselors, teachers, or even playmates stress the possibility of ill-effects, the impressionable boy may develop guilts and fears to plague him through his life. Guilt about masturbation, childhood sex play or adolescent homosexual acts can influence the entire psychosexual life and frequently give the guilt-ridden individual the anticipation of punishment by becoming impotent.

Early sex education stressing venereal disease may implant an excessive fear of disease or may color all sexual activity as being loathsome. Being taught that sex is unclean or nasty will interfere with later performance. Many men consciously think of the vagina as dirty or messy and liable to soil or injure the penis.

The youngster in his teens who is shy and ill-at-ease with girls is likely to be ashamed and afraid in intimacies as an adult.

As children we learn all sorts of sexual folklore and comments or quips heard on the street may have grave repercussions decades later. One patient as a youngster learned that men had a change of life at the age of 50. With this thought in the back of his mind it is not surprising that following his 50th birthday he suddenly became impotent with no conscious realization of the psychic origin of his difficulty.

## 3. Deep-rooted or unconscious factors

It must be realized that the emotional factors most significant in the etiology of impotence lie at a psychological level unconscious to the individual. The presentation of these factors, which is to follow, will be enhanced by review of the psychosexual development in the early years of life.

### a) Review of early psychosexual development

During the first year of life the child's existence revolves around the obtaining of food, and his oral activities color his personality. The extent of satisfaction or dissatisfaction with the feeding experience will affect his later human relationships. If the feeding experience is satisfactory, he will feel friendly and outgoing to the environment. If not satisfactory, the child will react with anger and become either demanding or clingingly dependent. In addition to food, the child learns about the world through his mouth—everything goes into it. The mother's attitude to this will begin to influence the rightness or wrongness of his mouth activities. In the early months of life, passive sucking is the primary oral activity; later, this gives way to active biting. The degree to which these are pleasurable will affect kissing and other mouth activities in later years.

The infant finds pleasure in body contact, in rocking and other rhythmic movement. This skin and muscle erotism will have profound effects in adult life. If body contact is unpleasurable to a person as an infant, as an adult he may find intimate physical contact disturbing and unpleasant with no conscious awareness of the reason.

During the second year of life considerable attention is focused on the child's acquisition of bowel control. The parental permissiveness or demand for conformity will influence the child's later development. Being trained too early or under too much pressure will cause the child anxiety. Attitudes of cleanliness or dirtiness are in large measure established at this time. If a predominant feeling of dirtiness colors the toilet training period, it will inevitably influence the sexual sphere owing to the anatomical proximity of the genital and excretory areas.

During the same period attention is also focused on acquiring bladder control. The male child becomes increasingly aware of his penis. Masturbation is a universal phenomenon at this age, and the parental reaction to it profoundly affects his later sexual life. Reproaching, scolding, or threatening the child produces feelings of guilt and anxiety. A verbal threat to cut off the penis or even the implication of such a threat as a punishment becomes a major factor in what is called castration anxiety. Even if no such threats arise, this form of anxiety will still be present because children becoming aware of the anatomic difference between boys and girls assume that the penis can be lost.

To accentuate castration fears, between 3 and 5 years of age the boy has an attachment for his mother—called the Oedipus complex—and a hostility to the father. He feels guilty and feels a need for punishment. If the home environment is relatively stable and healthy, the boy will break away from his maternal attachment and shift to a masculine identification with the father. If the father is rough, cruel, or violent in action, the boy will be afraid of him and unwilling to identify with him. He will have the feeling that men hurt women and so interprets the sexual act. When the mother is hypochondriacal or martyrlike and tells the boy how much she suffers or is maltreated, this feeling is reinforced. The mother who is overly affectionate or possessive will keep her son close to her and consciously or unconsciously try to prevent him from leaving her. His male identifications are impaired and in later years he will respond to her clinging by staying with her as a devoted son. In many cases such a man cannot marry or even go out with girls without guilt. If he does marry, his guilts and feelings of obligation to his mother impair a healthy relationship with his wife.

In some families the mother "wears the pants", dominates the household, and—consciously or unconsciously—is contemptuous or belittling of the husband. The little boy fears the mother and has no desire to identify with his weak, ineffectual father. He develops the idea that women are aggressive, destructive forces, creatures to be appeased at any price; and a fear of women develops. The mother who resents her son for any reason and rejects him produces feelings of unworthiness and an anticipation of hurt at the hands of a woman. Rejection, over-protection, or over-indulgence by either or both parents will affect the child and his male-female identifications. The struggle between love and hate, the degree of self-assertion or submission are all manifested in his subsequent emotional and sexual life.

## b) Excessive maternal attachment

The influence of the mother upon the child and developing youth is perhaps the most important causal factor in impotence. The overly loving, clinging or seductive mother envelops the boy in a web from which he may never extricate himself. Her apparent attachment or dependence upon him, aligning him on her side against the cruel, nonloving, or abusive husband, will impede the development of normal masculine identifications. The mother consciously or unconsciously thwarts his efforts to grow up and break away from her. Going with a girl friend or falling in love will therefore produce guilt. When he marries, the man unconsciously sees his mother in his wife and fails sexually.

A surprisingly large number of men differentiate between "good" and "bad" women. They tend to look upon sex as a "dirty" activity not to be performed with "nice, clean" women. "Fast" women are legitimate prey and many a man is potent in this area. However the idealized image of the "pure" mother is carried over to the "pure" wife not to be sullied by sex. Love relationships should be ethereal and not of the flesh. Such a man may be impotent with his wife but quite potent in extramarital affairs. His potency may be limited to particular women, such as redheads or blondes, short or stout, with large breasts or small breasts, depending to the degree they unconsciously may or may not remind him of his maternal love object.

Both the patient with ejaculatory impotence and the patient with premature ejaculation are afraid of the female, a fear which stems back to their relationship with the mother. The former unconsciously holds back and refuses to give of himself; the latter is afraid to refuse and gives too soon.

Ejaculatory impotence is reported by KAPLAN and ABRAMS. BERGLER has described this condition as "psychogenic oral aspermia". The patient with this problem can sustain an erection almost indefinitely and although the female partner may achieve orgasm, he himself cannot achieve climax. Sometimes nocturnal emissions are absent and masturbation brings no emission, while in other cases, these may be present. (Ejaculatory impotence may occur in individuals who have been potent for years when emotional problems have developed. One of our patients, previously potent, developed inability to ejaculate. He unconsciously diagnosed his condition when he stated, "I got tired of my wife taking me for everything I had." The patient thought he was describing his wife's inordinate financial demands upon him, but this also expressed the way he reacted to her sexually.)

KAPLAN and ABRAMS describe these individuals as passive, emotionally immature, unable to accept responsibility, and unable to be competitive or aggressive in a masculine way. They report a 21-year-old man whose presenting complaint was ejaculatory impotence. He could not masturbate to ejaculation but did have occasional nocturnal emissions. As a child he had been afraid of his father and overly protected by his mother. His mother would get into bed with him during childhood to kiss and hug him until he fell asleep. In marriage his love-making was usually confined to hugging and kissing his wife; when coitus occurred, he could not ejaculate. During his psychotherapy he began to masturbate to orgasm and eventually could function in the marital act. Unconsciously he considered the ejaculate as something valuable that he did not want to give up. With an understanding of his mother's seductive role, he gradually attained a healthy masculine orientation.

An excessive maternal attachment may produce an anxiety-laden relationship with any woman. The boy who shares his bedroom or bed with mother, sister, grandmother, aunt, or other close female relative will inevitably have sexual troubles in later years. Being thus thrown into intimate contact with a forbidden sexual object will produce chronic stimulation which is considered bad and is taboo. The youth will unconsciously inhibit his feelings of sexual arousal and curiosity to avoid conscious sexual impulses toward his mother, sister, or relative. Such inhibitions can pervade his relationships with all girls so that he feels no excitement with women and is completely incapable of achieving erection with them. In some cases he turns to men as an outlet which is free of this incest taboo.

### c) Sadomasochistic impulses

The fear of hurting or being hurt can be a powerful deterrent sexually. A child who has observed parental intercourse interprets the act as a fight, the father being violent to the mother. Sex is considered an aggressive assault and the man as an adult feels inhibited for fear of hurting the woman he loves. If the father is noisy, violent or rough in his daily activities, the child does not wish to identify with a destructive male and develops into a quiet, gentle, inhibited male. In a home where the mother is the dominant force, contemptuous or belittling of the husband, with conscious or unconscious hostility toward males, the youth gets the impression that women are aggressive, destructive forces. This fear of women will lead to failure in sex relations.

Some men may have desires to hurt women, to seek revenge for injuries previously suffered at their hands. Hostility in some degree is normally present in every human relationship. Some married people never argue or say a cross word yet may have an intense, deep-seated hatred for each other. The arousal of sadomasochistic impulses (desires to hurt and to be hurt) may lead to impotence in the male.

### d) Narcissism

The narcissistic male emotionally in love with himself cannot express love to a woman. He is the "Don Juan" who finds reassurance from his fears of impotence in endless affairs (but no lasting relationship). Very often he is able to have intercourse but cannot ejaculate—he simply cannot give anything of himself.

## VI. Related conditions or syndromes

### 1. Genital pain of psychological origin

Penile and testicular pain of variable intensity and location are not infrequent complaints. The pain may be stabbing, burning, aching, throbbing, or gnawing in nature. In most cases, no organic cause can be found (Sadger). However, psychiatric study will reveal a sexually repressed male with many anxieties about himself and his virility. Bergler reported a man who experienced drawing, piercing penile pain following unsuccessful coitus and feared that masturbation had damaged his penis. Hirsch stated that men with sexual "weaknesses" were prone to complain of penile pain, particularly on urination, hoping that the physician would find a physical reason for the sexual weakness in the course of his examination. Ferenczi described paresthesiae in the genital regions of impotent men.

A 40-year-old man who was under our care, three days after intercourse developed in the urethra severe pain not associated with urination. Following this pain, he had a nonspecific urethral discharge and an aching pain in his testes. Despite considerable urological treatment his complaints continued. On examination his genitals were normal, though the patient felt his testes were "swollen". The first glass of urine was clear; the second glass showed sperm. His symptoms had developed following extramarital intercourse which had occasioned him much guilt. Despite the use of a condom he had intense fear of venereal infection, a fear that was increased by the appearance of urethral discharge. All his life the patient had had mixed emotions about sexual activity, an intense drive which led to many extramarital episodes, and strong feelings that all sexual expression, even in marriage, was immoral. After coitus he always felt "drained out, exhausted" and would be aware of intense anger toward his sexual partner, with strong impulses to hurt her. Naturally these feelings recurred frequently in his marriage and were the source of much friction. In his childhood he had been aware of infidelity by both parents but had tended to blame his mother solely. He came to think that all women were seductive, seeking to take away a man's sexual virility and to leave him damaged. During intercourse, which he began at an early age, he felt intense guilt and anger toward the female. When he impregnated a girl friend, he felt obliged to marry her but had a strong feeling of being trapped.

Through psychiatric treatment he was able to verbalize his angers. Interestingly, he found that his hitherto idolized father was responsible for most of his mixed-up sexual ideas and that beneath his apparent attachment for his father was intense hatred. His fear of his father was so great that he did not realize the presence of the resentment. He had seen his father as a farmer castrating animals and had feared this fate for himself. In a symbolic way the testicular pain was self-punishment for his sexual misconduct. The patient made a good recovery and has been free of his urological symptoms for years.

## 2. Urethral discharge of psychological origin

Urethral discharge as a symptom of psychiatric disorder has been reported by Ross. These patients had a persistent or recurring urethral discharge showing no bacteria and few, if any, pus cells on examination. They had not responded to the administration of drugs. A study of their personalities, particularly their sexual lives, showed these men to be excessively conscientious, shy, and dependent, with extreme guilt about their sexual activity. Some were married men who had had one or more extramarital episodes, with profound guilt, often unconscious. In some the guilt increased with each successive lapse. The majority were unmarried men who had had limited sexual experience owing to their strong convictions that it was sinful and might result in some form of severe retribution. Fear of venereal disease and guilt about masturbation were common. The discharge appeared most commonly in the week following intercourse in the wake of guilt feelings associated with this lapse. One man developed a urethral discharge after only heavy "petting"; another following ejaculation without entrance. In a large group the urethral discharge did not appear until 1 to 2 months after intercourse, usually in relation to temptation to engage in intercourse again. Drinking increased the discharge in many cases, because the drinking increased sexual temptation and gave rise to further conflict and anxiety.

Of the 38 patients, 7 were considered to have a specific urethritis (gonorrhea) and 3 had a purulent discharge due to a nonspecific urethritis. The discharge

4*

became clear and mucoid under chemotherapy but persisted until psychiatric treatment was given. These individuals had personalities and guilt feelings similar to those of the patients with noninfectious urethral discharge. The occurrence of actual infection, in most cases gonorrhea, was a psychically depressing incident and aroused concern about sexual temptation and any subsequent contacts.

Ross suggested that nonpurulent urethral discharge or nonspecific urethritis occurs in men who are struggling to refrain from promiscuous sexual activity despite strong urges to do so. These men show a consistent background of strong sexual anxiety and guilt, with worries about masturbation and the general sinfulness of sex. He postulated that the persisting hypersecretion of the sex glands is due to persistent or recurrent sexual stimulation and equally strong inhibitions which preclude satisfying outlets.

In treating these individuals it is unwise for a doctor to recommend sexual activity as a cure since such uninhibited conduct would clash with their personal standards and might precipitate a serious personality disturbance. Gradual re-education, with reassurance that venereal infection is not present, is the method of choice.

Hirsch has pointed out that occasionally men have a mucoid secretion at the penile meatus while moving their bowels. This secretion is prostatic fluid forced out of the gland by the pressure of the fecal mass and the abdominal musculature. These individuals feel that this represents loss of sexual power or the presence of a venereal infection. Ungratified sexual excitement, however, is responsible for this prostatorrhea or spermatorrhea.

## 3. Sexual deviation

Not infrequently a patient will consult the urologist for help in problems of sexual deviation. Sometimes he will inform the doctor directly of his deviation and his wish to change to a more normal mode of life. At other times he will complain of some physical disturbance such as difficulty in urinating, or having a weak stream, or worry about his prostate or the size of his penis, hoping the physician will recognize the true nature of his concern. In nearly every case the patient will ask if he can become normal and lead an ordinary life including marriage and having children. He will seek any possibility of hormonal injection or implantation to correct his sexual "weakness".

With rare exception his body habitus is completely masculine, and there may be a complete absence of any feminine mannerisms. Occasionally a feminine habitus may be encountered, but it is doubtful that this in itself is solely responsible for the homosexual activity.

The varieties of sexual deviation are many, and the urologist should have some knowledge of these, particularly the two types for which patients most commonly seek help—homosexuality and transvestism.

### a) Homosexuality

In every individual's life development there is a short homosexual period, usually about the age of ten years, when boys and girls tend to associate with children of their own gender and have a strong antipathy toward the opposite sex. During group play at this time some overt homosexual acts may occur, but usually nothing develops beyond strong interest in and identification with other children of the same sex. Normally this homosexual phase is of short duration, and during adolescence heterosexual interests begin to develop.

The presence of mental or emotional disturbance in the family may adversely affect this normal transition to heterosexuality and cause a fixation at a homosexual level. Either or both parents may have desired a girl and could not accept the birth of a son, consciously or unconsciously moulding the child into what they wanted through hair style, clothing, and the types of play and behavior permitted or prohibited. The absence of a father in the home through death, divorce, or the nature of his work, will deprive a boy of male associations and may cause him to be overly attached to his mother. He patterns himself after his mother, identifies with her, and in later years seeks the male love objects she would desire as a woman. If the father is tyrannical, the boy shrinks from seeking a male role for himself and becomes a passive person. A dominating mother may make the boy feel threatened in the presence of women. Sexual stimulation by the mother, sister, or other female relative may invoke strong taboos against sexual arousal by any woman. Sexual seduction of the child may set the stage for an active homosexual life.

Depending upon the circumstances of their psychosexual development, homosexual males react in different ways in their sexual lives. Some are aggressive and court the sexual partner as though he were courting a female; others, with feminine identification, passively await being sought out and loved. The sexual act may involve mutual caressing of the penis with hand or mouth, or insertion of the penis in the anus or between the legs. In the past, the use of the words "active homosexual" and "passive homosexual" have been used in describing the sexual act. However, present day knowledge has largely discarded these terms, and emphasis is now placed on whether the individual's identifications are primarily masculine or feminine in the sex play.

Where homosexual activity has become the sexual outlet for the adult male, it must be recognized that in most cases a shift to heterosexuality is not possible. Neither the use of androgens nor intensive psychiatric treatment will effect such a change. Despite a conscious wish to change, most homosexuals are fundamentally content with their deviation since it solves serious emotional problems which might otherwise prove upsetting. They recognize the problem of actual or potential social ostracism but, in the absence of any motivation stronger than this external pressure, do not change with psychiatric treatment. Most are benefited by psychotherapy in terms of relieving their anxieties, but generally only limited goals are achieved. However, any homosexual individual seeking help should have the opportunity for psychiatric appraisal and be given treatment when this seems indicated.

### b) Transvestism

Transvestites are individuals who find their greatest sexual satisfaction in wearing the attire of the opposite sex. There is no physical or anatomical abnormality. For some, masturbation provides the means of sexual outlet; others are homosexual, and still others may be heterosexual. A 40-year-old professional man, married three times and the father of children by each marriage, found relief for his tension after his day's work in wearing female attire. While he found sexual intercourse with his wife most pleasurable, his need to "dress" as a woman was greater. He was willing to forego heterosexuality rather than abandon his transvestism, and this led to divorce in all his marriages.

Since the transvestism is psychologically important to the patient, he is unwilling to relinquish it. Neither urological nor psychiatric treatment is of much value in treating this condition. Some patients may request surgical castration to aid their sex reversal. This requires careful psychiatric evaluation.

## VII. Differential diagnosis of cause for impotence

By far the most common cause for impotence is behavioral, but before concluding this initially (though in some cases this cause becomes obvious almost immediately) the organic factors should be ruled out.

### 1. Vascular causes

With diminution in arterial blood supply to the penis, there is a progressive history of increasing difficulty with erections. Usually erection is normal, prompt in development, but it tends to fade gradually. The symptoms and signs of peripheral vascular changes should be obvious. Aortography is definitive.

### 2. Neurological causes

A proper history, physical examination, and radiological examination should uncover evidence of neurological abnormality.

### 3. Endocrinological causes

These should be obvious on medical survey. Diabetes mellitus commonly causes impotence even in the absence of neuropathy.

### 4. Pharmacological causes

The taking of certain drugs may be the underlying cause for sexual difficulty, particularly if the patient dates his disability from the time the drug was prescribed.

### 5. Behavioral causes

Impotence is caused by psychological or behavioral abnormalities in from 95 to 99% of cases. Though emotional instability is quickly noted, the organic etiological factors mentioned above should be ruled out. If normal nocturnal erections and emissions are experienced or if masturbation reveals normal function, the entire sexual mechanism (neurological and vascular) is normal. If a man develops normal erections but has premature ejaculation or has prolonged erections which do not culminate in ejaculation and orgasm, the abnormality is cerebral in origin. Certainly, if he is not aroused by his wife yet is by another woman, the cause must be psychological. Other clues have been discussed on pages 45 to 53.

## VIII. Treatment of impotence

The treatment of sexual problems in the male must depend upon their etiology.

### 1. Vascular causes (Leriche syndrome)

Once this diagnosis has been established, surgical intervention is indicated not only because of the sexual complaint but in order to relieve the vascular obstruction which is progressive and therefore increasingly disabling. It may culminate in gangrene.

### 2. Neurological causes

Unfortunately little can be done for men with impotence owing to nerve injuries. Delayed spontaneous improvement may occur some months after injury or surgical intervention (sympathectomy).

## 3. Endocrinological causes

In clinical practice, few cases of impotence are due to endocrinological abnormalities. Testosterone is often prescribed empirically; it seldom helps. If it does, its psychotherapeutic value must be considered.

## 4. Pharmacological causes

If the patient is taking parasympathetic or ganglionic blocking agents, estrogens, sedatives, or antihistaminics, they should be stopped if it is not contraindicated.

## 5. Behavioral causes

It has been shown that impotence has its origin in many diverse behavioral factors, some close to the surface, others deep-seated. In many cases, particularly those of the newly-wed, advice and reassurance by the physician may solve the problem. Male hormone may prove helpful, even though largely through suggestion. Prostatic massage, instrumentation, or operative measures may alleviate guilt feelings by symbolically serving as punishment for masturbation or previous sexual misconduct; it is doubtful that they have any direct curative influence. In most cases a trial period of androgen therapy is worthwhile since a few men seemingly recover on this regime. However, psychiatric treatment is usually the method of choice. Treatment must always give weight to psychic factors. Psychological treatment may consist only of advice, suggestion, and reassurance or may entail more intensive study of the personality. Elimination of fears and guilts are necessary to treat impotence effectively.

# IX. Prognosis of impotence

Some men with impotence develop no other symptoms, go through life with no conscious concern and may become eminently successful in all other spheres of their lives. Some react with feelings of inferiority and inadequacy which may color everything else they do. They may develop nervousness, depression, melancholia or even commit suicide. Some may have generalized nervous symptoms; others, symptoms in specific body organs—gastric distress, backache, or headache. A small number develop symptoms referrable to the genitourinary tract, such as penile or testicular pain, and nonspecific urethritis (or chronic prostatitis).

Except for arterial surgery in selected cases, organic treatment of impotence offers little to the impotent male.

If the sexual complaint is not severe or of long duration, simple explanations of psychosexual matters by the patient's personal physician may result in much improvement.

Psychiatric treatment for disorders of potency generally brings good results. Since impotence has its psychological roots at many different developmental levels it cannot be considered a specific disorder but rather as the external expression of many emotional problems of varying magnitudes. Infantile castration anxieties, hostile or non-giving attitudes toward women, intense narcissism or unconscious homosexual conflicts are common causal factors. Transient potency disturbances such as those following traumatic experiences respond most readily. Other disturbances may require years of psychoanalysis.

# References

*A. The effect of the psyche on vesical function*

ALKAN, L.: Anatomische Organkrankheiten aus seelischer Ursache. Stuttgart: Hippo-kratis-Verlag 1930. — AUERBACK, A., and D. R. SMITH: Psychosomatic problems in urology. Calif. Med. **76**, 23—26 (1952). — BLOMSTRAND, R., and F. LÖFGREN: Influence of emotional stress on the renal circulation. Psychosom. Med. **18**, 420—426 (1956). — BOWERS, J. E., P. E. SCHWARZ and M. J. LEON: Masochism and interstitial cystitis. Psychosom. Med. **20**, 296—302 (1958). — CASSIDY, W. L., N. B. FLANAGAN, M. SPELLMAN and M. E. COHEN: Clinical observations in manic-depressive disease. J. Amer. med. Ass. **164**, 1535—1546 (1947). — CHERTOK, L., P. ABOULKER and M. CAHEN: Perspective psychosomatique en urologie. Evolut. psychiat. **3**, 457—473 (1953). — CLANCY, F. J.: Urologic symptoms of psychogenic origin. Urol. cutan. Rev. **37**, 703—707 (1933). — CONE, R. E.: Psychosomatic problems in urology. J. Urol. (Baltimore) **56**, 146—150 (1946). — DÉJERINE, J., and E. GLAUCKLER: The psychoneuroses and their treatment by psychotherapy. Translated by S. E. JELLIFFE, 2. edit. Philadelphia and London: J. B. Lippincott Company 1913. — GREEN, M. R. and A. L. DEAN: Some psychiatric aspects of symptoms of genito-urinary disease. J. Urol. (Baltimore) **72**, 742—747 (1954). — JANET, JULES: Les troubles psycho-pathiques de la miction. Essai de psychophysiologie normale et pathologique. Paris: Li-brairie Lefrancois 1890. — MAYER, A.: Über gynäkologische Scheinkrankheiten (Pseudo-Retroflexio und Pseudo-Zystitis). Dtsch. med. Wschr. **55**, 1639—1640 (1929). — MENNINGER, K. A.: Some observation on the psychological factors in urination and genito-urinary afflic-tions. Psychoanal. Rev. **28**, 117—129 (1941). — MOMBAERTS, J.: Pathogenie et traitement des cystalgies la cervico-cystalgie oedemateuse. Proc. Soc. int. Urol. **1**, 403—450 (1949). — MONTASSUT, M., L. CHERTOK and P. ABOULKER: De quelques investigations psychiatriques en urologie. Sem. Hop. Paris **27**, 3002—3005 (1951). — Consultation psychosomatique en urologie. Extr. des Comptes rendus du Congrès des Médicins Aliénistes et Neurologistes, Luxembourg, July 21.—27., 1952. — MOSSO, A., and P. PELLACANI: Sulle funzioni della vescica. Repr. from: R. Acad. naz. Lincei **12**, 1—64 (1881). — Sur les fonctions de la véssie. Arch. ital. Biol. **1**, 97—128, 291—324 (1882). — SCHOTTSTAEDT, W. W., W. J. GRACE and H. G. WOLFF: Life situation, behavior patterns, and renal excretion of fluid and electrolytes. J. Amer. med. Ass. **157**, 1485—1488 (1955). — SMITH, D. R.: Psychologic aspects of urology in women. GP: **8**, 57—61 (1953). — General Urology. Lange Medical Publications, Los Altos, Calif., 2. edit., 1959. — STRAUB, L. R., H. S. RIPLEY and S. WOLF: Disturbances of bladder function associated with emotional states. J. Amer. med. Ass. **141**, 1139—1143 (1949). — An experimental approach to psychosomatic bladder disorders. N. Y. J. Med. **49**, 635—638 (1949). — TAUBER, E. S., L. G. LEWIS and O. R. LANGWORTHY: Vesical activity in schizophrenic states associated with catalepsy. Arch. Neurol. Psychiat. (Chicago) **39**, 14—23 (1938). — VAN DER HEIDE, C.: A case of pollakiuria nervosa. Psychoanal. Quart. **10**, 267—283 (1941). — VERNEY, E. B.: Some aspects of water and electrolyte excretion. Surg. Gynec. Obstet. **106**, 441—452 (1958). — WILLIAMS, G. F., and A. M. JOHNSON: Re-current urinary retention due to emotional factors. Psychosom. Med. **18**, 77—80 (1956).


*B. Functional enuresis*

BAKWIN, H.: Enuresis in children. J. Pediat. **34**, 249—262 (1949). — BEHRLE, F. C., M. T. ELKIN and P. C. LAYBOURNE: Evaluation of conditioning device in treatment of nocturnal enuresis. Pediatrics **17**, 849—854 (1956). — BOSTICK, J., and M. SHACKLETON: The maturation factor in enuresis. Med. J. Aust. **1**, 1042—1043 (1956). — BRODNEY, M. L., and S. A. ROBINS: Enuresis, the use of cystourethrography in diagnosis. J. Amer. med. Ass. **126**, 1000—1005 (1944). — BROOKFIELD, R. W.: Ephedrine in treatment of enuresis. Lancet **1937**, 623—625. — BROWNE, R. C., and A. FORD-SMITH: Enuresis in adolescents. Brit. Med. J. **1941**, 803—805. — CROSBY, N. D.: Essential enuresis: successful treatment based on physiological concepts. Med. J. Aust. **2**, 533—543 (1950). — DAVIDSON, J. R., and E. DOUGLAS: Nocturnal enuresis: A special approach to treatment. Brit. med. J. **1950**, 1345 to 1347. — DESPERT, J. L.: Urinary control and enuresis. Psychosom. Med. **6**, 294—307 (1944). — FRARY, L. G.: Enuresis: a genetic study. Amer. J. Dis. Child. **49**, 557—578 (1935). — GERARD, M.: Enuresis: Study in etiology. Amer. J. Orthopsychiat. **9**, 48—58 (1939). — GERARD, M. W.: Enuresis: a study in etiology. In F. ALEXANDER and T. M. FRENCH: Studies in Psychosomatic Medicine. New York: Ronald Press 1948. — HALLMAN, N.: On the ability of enuretic children to hold urine. Acta paediat. **39**, 87—93 (1950). — KARLIN, I. W.: Incidence of spina bifida occulta in children with and without enuresis. Amer. J. Dis. Child. **49**, 125—134 (1935). — KEIZUR, L. W., and C. V. HODGES: Control of enuresis by parasympathetic blocking agents. Northw. Med. Seattle **53**, 27—29 (1954). — MARSON, F. G. W.: Posterior pituitary snuff treatment of nocturnal enuresis. Brit. med. J. **1955**, 1194—1195. — MCGRAW, M. B.: Neural maturation as exemplified in achievement of bladder control. J. Pediat. **16**, 580—590 (1940). — MICHAELS, J. J., and L. SECUNDA: The relationship of neurotic traits to the electroencephalogram in children with behavior disorders. Amer. J. Psychiat. **101**, 407—409 (1944). — MOWRER, O. H., and W. M. MOWRER: Enuresis: A method for its study and treatment. Amer. J. Orthopsychiat. **8**, 436—459 (1938). — NASH, D. F. E.: Genito-urinary disorders in infancy and childhood with special reference to enuresis. Practitioner **159**, 188—196 (1947). — NICHOLS, L. A.: Enuresis, its background and cure. Lancet **2**, 1336—1337 (1956). — PINCK, B. D.: A physiological approach to enuresis. Amer. Practit. **7**, 1272—1277 (1956). — ROSENSON, W., and R. LISWOOD: Sodium chloride in the treatment of nocturnal enuresis in children. J. Pediat. **9**, 751—754 (1936). — SANFORD, S. P., and G. W. KLIMAN: Enuresis and spina bifida occulta. U.S. armed Forces med. J. **8**, 507—512 (1957). — SCHWARTZ, M. D., and A. H. STANTON: A social psychological study of incontinence. Psychiatry **13**, 399—416 (1950). — SEARS, R. R., E. E. MACCOBY and H. LEVIN: Patterns of child rearing. Evanston: Row, Peterson & Co. 1957. — SEIGER, H. W.: Treatment of essential nocturnal enuresis. J. Pediat. **40**, 738—749 (1952). — SHLIONSKY, H., L. R. SARRACINO and L. J. BISCHOF: Functional enuresis in the Army; report of clinical study of 100 cases. War Med. **7**, 297—303 (1945). — SPOCK, B.: Some common diagnostic problems in children. Med. Clin. N. Amer. **34**, 1078—1089 (1950). — STOCKWELL, L., and C. K. SMITH: Enuresis: A study of causes, types and therapeutic results. Amer. J. Dis. Child. **59**, 1013—1033 (1940). — SWEET, C.: Enuresis, a psychologic problem of childhood. J. Amer. med. Ass. **132**, 279—280 (1946). — THORNE, F. C.: The incidence of nocturnal enuresis after age of 5. Amer. J. Psychiat. **100**, 686—689 (1944). — TEICHER, J. D.: Enuresis: A critical review of the symptom. Calif. Med. **82**, 392—395 (1955).

## C. Impotence in the male

BERGLER, E.: Neurotic counterfeit-sex. New York: Grune & Stratton (1951). — BORS, E.: Neurogenic bladder. Urol. Surv. **7**, 177—250 (1957). — BORS, E., and A. E. COMARR: Effect of pudendal nerve operations on the neurogenic bladder. J. Urol. (Baltimore) **72**, 666—670 (1954). — DEYSACH, L. J.: The comparative morphology of the erectile tissue of the penis with especial emphasis on the probable mechanism of erection. Amer. J. Anat. **64**, 111—131 (1939). — EISENSTEIN, V. W.: Sexual Problems in Marriage. In V. W. EISENSTEIN editor: Neurotic Interaction in Marriage, chap. 7. New York: Basic Books 1956. — ENGLISH, O. S., and G. H. PEARSON: Emotional problems of living. New York: W. W. Norton 1955. — FERENCZI, S.: Further contributions to the theory and technique of psychoanalysis, chapt. 36. London: Hogarth 1950. — HENDERSON, V. E., and M. H. ROEPKE: On the mechanism of erection. Amer. J. Physiol. **106**, 441—448 (1933). — HIRSCH, E. W.: The Power to Love. New York: Knopf 1957. — HOTCHKISS, R. H., and J. FERNANDEZ-LEAL: The nervous system as related to fertility and sterility. J. Urol. (Baltimore) **78**, 173—178 (1957). — KAPLAN, A. H., and M. ABRAMS: Ejaculatory impotence. J. Urol. (Baltimore) **79**, 964—968 (1958). — KINSEY, A. C., W. B. POMEROY and C. E. MARTIN: Sexual behavior in the human male. Philadelphia and London: W. B. Saunders 1948. — KUNTZ, A.: The autonomic nervous system, 3. edit. Philadelphia: Lea and Febiger 1945. — LERICHE, R., and A. MOREL: The syndrome of thrombotic obliteration of the aortic bifurcation. Ann. Surg. **127**, 193—206 (1948). — MUNRO, D., H. W. HORNE jr. and D. P. PAULL: The effect of injury to the spinal cord and cauda equina on the sexual potency of men. New Engl. J. Med. **239**, 903—911 (1948). — O'CONNOR jr., V. J.: Impotence and the Leriche syndrome: an early diagnostic sign; consideration of the mechanism; relief by endarterectomy. J. Urol. (Baltimore) **80**, 195—198 (1958). — ROSE, S. S.: An investigation into sterility after lumbar ganglionectomy. Brit. med. J. **1953**, 247—250. — ROSS, W. D.: Urethral discharge as a symptom of psychiatric disorder. Psychosom. Med. **9**, 273—279 (1947). — RUBIN, A., and BABBOTT, D.: Impotence and diabetes mellitus. J. Amer. med. Ass. **168**, 498—500 (1958). — SADGER, J.: Über urethral-erotik. Jb. psychoanal. psychopath. Forsch. **2**, 409—450 (1910). — SEMANS, J. H., and O. R. LANGWORTHY: Observations on the neurophysiology of sexual function in the male cat. J. Urol. (Baltimore) **40**, 836—846 (1938). — TALBOT, H. S.: A report on sexual function in paraplegics. J. Urol. (Baltimore) **61**, 265—270 (1949). — The sexual function in paraplegia. J. Urol. (Baltimore) **73**, 91—100 (1955). — WALKER, K., and E. B. STRAUSS: Sexual disorders in the male. London: Cassell & Co. 1954. — WHITE, J. C., R. H. SMITHWICK and F. A. SIMEONE: The autonomic nervous system, 3. edit. New York: Macmillan Company 1952. — WHITELAW, G. P., and R. H. SMITHWICK: Some secondary effects of sympathectomy with particular reference to disturbance of sexual function. New Engl. J. Med. **245**, 121—130 (1951). — WOLBARST, A. L.: The gynecic factor in the causation of male impotence. N. Y. J. Med. **47**, 1252—1255 (1947). — ZEITLIN, A. B., T. L. COTTRELL and F. A. LLOYD: Sexology of the paraplegic male. Fertil. and Steril. **8**, 337—344 (1957).

# Neuromuscular Dysfunction and Paraplegia

By

J. COSBIE ROSS

With 28 figures

## A. Renal sympathecticotonia

Although a somewhat clumsy term, renal sympathecticotonica is preferable to the "nephralgia" of a bygone generation and to the inaccurate "renal asthma". The term indicates precisely what is believed to be the underlying pathology

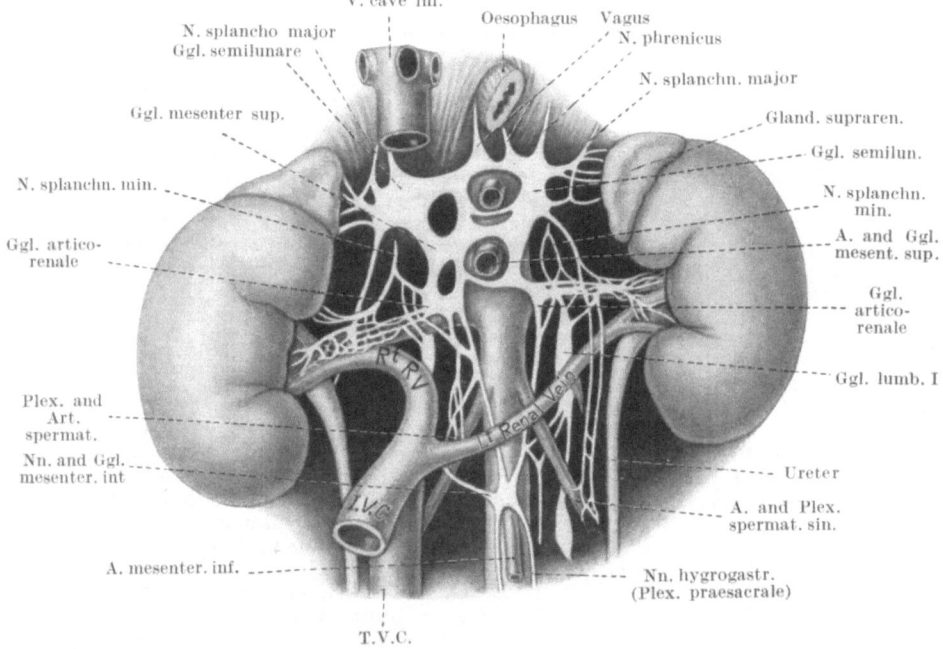

Fig. 1. Anatomy of the renal nerves. The inferior vena cava has been divided and the peripheral end has been turned down. (From Modern Trends in Urology)

of a nebulous condition (HARRIS 1930). Indeed, it seems evident that if renal denervation is successful in curing a patient with non-obstructive hydronephrosis, nephroptosis or otherwise unexplained pain of renal origin, that hyperactivity of the sympathetic nerve supply must have been the underlying cause.

## I. The renal nerves (Gray's anatomy 1935)

The renal plexus is derived from several sources, which include:
a) The aortico-renal ganglion.
b) The great splanchnic nerve via the semilunar ganglion.

c) Direct from the lesser and least splanchnic nerves.

d) Some branches from the vagus.

From the plexus as many as twenty nerves accompany the renal artery into the kidney substance (see Fig. 1). Should there be an aberrant artery this is also accompanied by renal nerves, an important point to remember when carrying out the operation of denervation. It is fortunate from the operative point of view that these nerves, derived from several sources, should converge on and are distributed around the renal artery where they are readily accessible. It is fortunate, too, that no nerves accompany the fragile and easily damaged renal vein.

OLDHAM (1948) points out that three important groups of nerves arise from the renal plexus and are distributed to the upper ureter, the left half of the colon, (through the inferior mesenteric), and the testis or ovary.

The renal nerves are largely vasomotor but some fibres are distributed to the unstriated muscle fibres encircling the pelvi-ureteric junction and the necks of the major and minor calyces

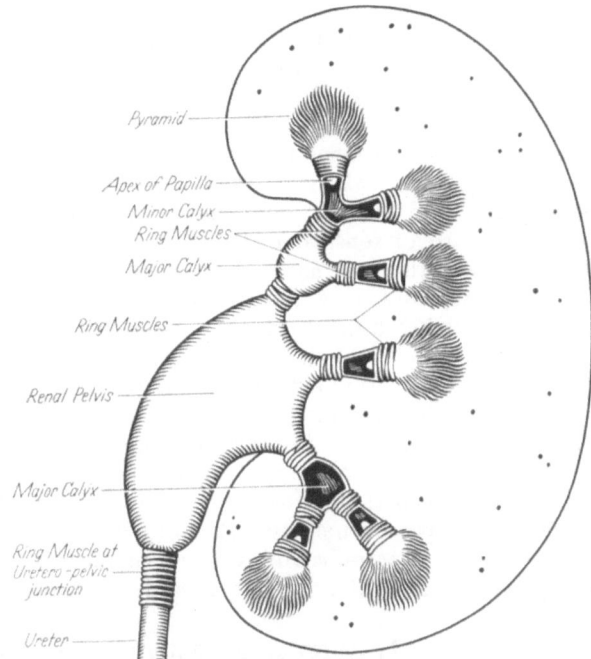

Fig. 2. Diagrammatic representation of the ring-muscle system modified from the original in KELLY & BURNAM, "Diseases of Kidneys, Ureters and Bladder". The anterior walls of all the minor calyces and the lower major calyx have been cut away to expose the tips of the papillae. (From the Liverpool Medico-Chirurgical Journal)

(see Fig. 2). A certain number of sensory fibres reach the papillae, calyces and pelvis but the parenchyma is relatively insensitive, although not completely so (OLDHAM 1940).

OLDHAM (1953) clearly indicates the function of the renal nerves in the following table:

| Nerves | Stimulus | Depression or section |
|---|---|---|
| Nerves to the blood vessels | Vaso-constriction<br><br>Decreased flow of blood through kidney<br><br>Anuria or oliguria | Vaso-dilation<br><br>Increased flow of blood through kidney<br><br>Increased urine of low specific gravity |
| Nerves to the pelvis and calyces | Contraction of sphincters<br><br>Increased intrapelvic pressure | Relaxation of sphincters |
| Sensory nerves | Pain | Anaesthesia of the kidney |

## II. The effects of denervation

As there are no secretory nerves the production of urine continues uninterruptedly even after all connection with the central nervous system has been divided. There are, however, certain modifications of the secretion which may be summed up as a moderate degree of diuresis. Hess (1930) and others have shown that the amount of urine secreted from the sympathectomised kidney is approximately one-fifth greater than on the normal side, the specific gravity being correspondingly lower. When indigo-carmine is injected intravenously the dye appears earlier on the operated side but the colour, as a rule, is not so intense. The jets of urine from the ureter are more frequent and possibly greater in volume. Above all, it is impossible to cause pain by distending the renal pelvis with fluid after an efficient sympathectomy has been carried out. There is some return of sensation after a period of time i.e. six months, but a high degree of anaesthesia remains. This, then is the logical basis for the renal denervation operation and over a period of years the effectiveness of the operation in suitable cases has been testified by Oldham (1936—1950—1953), Bauer (1944), Harris & Harris (1930), Wells (1935) and Woodside (1944). Complete relief may be expected provided the case is carefully chosen.

On theoretical grounds the operation has been advocated for reflex anuria, hypertension, for early tuberculous kidney and as a prophylactic measure to discourage the recurrence of urinary calculi. Practical experience, however, has clearly shown that all these conditions do not respond to renal denervation which should be confined to patients with persistent idiopathic renal pain and to early cases of non-obstructive hydronephrosis. It may possibly be justifiable to consider it also in renal ptosis and in essential haematuria.

### 1. Early non-obstructive hydronephrosis

In these not unfamiliar patients the degree of pain seems to be out of all proportion to the degree of hydronephrosis. It is probable that the hydronephrosis is due to a true neuromuscular dysfunction, causing spasm of the circular muscle fibres of the pelvi-ureteric junction and of the muscle fibres surrounding the necks of the calyces. The result of this spasm is raised intrapelvic and intracalyceal pressure leading to pain. Under normal circumstances the calyces, pelvis and ureter undergo a series of contractions and relaxations in a rhythmic manner approximately every ten to thirty seconds. Woodside (1944) has called the system the "renal heart". With the pelvi-ureteric sphincter closed the upper calyx empties itself into the pelvis and then remains contracted. This is followed in turn by the middle and lower calyces. With all the calyces closed the pelvi-ureteric junction relaxes and the pelvis empties itself into the ureter, approximately 1 cc. of urine being ejected from the pelvis per minute. This conception explains the early case of hydronephrosis in which the renal pelvis is dilated but the calyces still maintain their normal appearance as they are protected by the ring muscles. A solitary hydrocalyx is also explicable on these lines. On the other hand it must be pointed out that Lapides (1948) and Johnson (1952) believe that there is no central control and that movement of the urine is entirely dependant on mechanical pressure of the urine in each segment.

Non-obstructive hydronephrosis is a relatively common condition. Oldham found that 50% of his patients fell into this category.

Harris (1935) described three successive stages:

a) The stage of systole or irritability, in which the renal pelvis is small and contracted, with delayed emptying. The pain is intermittent and severe.

b) The stage of diastole or exhaustion, in which the pelvis is dilated but the calyces still retain their normal shape. The contractions of the pelvis are infrequent, irregular and incomplete. The pain consists of a dull aching type with exacerbations.

c) The stage of dilatation or paralysis. The hydronephrosis has developed fully and the condition is virtually one of retention with overflow.

Renal denervation for hydronephrosis is clearly indicated in stages a) and b), especially if no mechanical obstruction is present. A gross hydronephrosis requires a major plastic operation which can be usefully combined with sympathectomy. UNDERWOOD (1939) points out that every effort should be made to arrest the development of hydronephrosis at an early stage. He believes the life history of idiopathic hydronephrosis to be as follows:

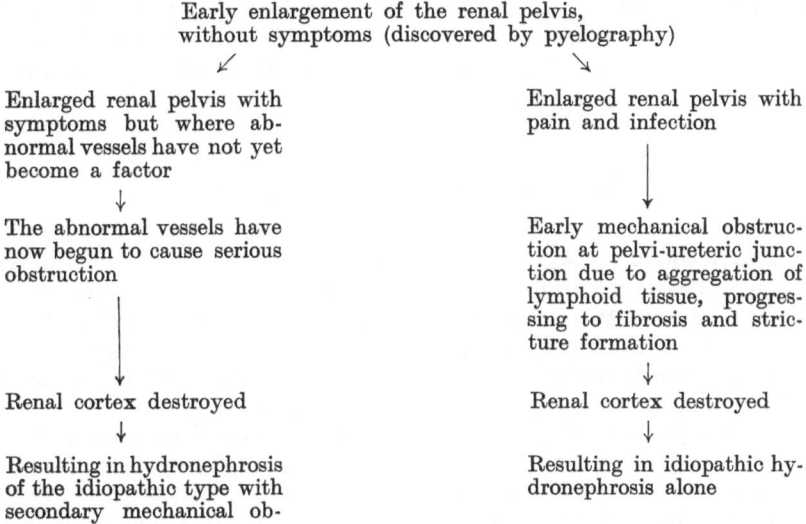

Early enlargement of the renal pelvis,
without symptoms (discovered by pyelography)

Enlarged renal pelvis with symptoms but where abnormal vessels have not yet become a factor

↓

The abnormal vessels have now begun to cause serious obstruction

↓

Renal cortex destroyed

↓

Resulting in hydronephrosis of the idiopathic type with secondary mechanical obstruction

Enlarged renal pelvis with pain and infection

↓

Early mechanical obstruction at pelvi-ureteric junction due to aggregation of lymphoid tissue, progressing to fibrosis and stricture formation

↓

Renal cortex destroyed

↓

Resulting in idiopathic hydronephrosis alone

BADENOCH (1953) quotes TUCKWELL as saying that good results have followed radicular denervation when it has been performed for bilateral hydronephrosis associated with hypertension. There are, however, two further conditions in which it is claimed that renal denervation is effective.

## 2. Renal pain or nephralgia

In this type there is a persistent and troublesome pain of undoubted renal origin but repeated and careful investigations reveal no abnormality whatsoever. It is suggested that renal denervation in these cases is similar to division of the sensory root of the fifth cranial nerve in trigeminal neuralgia.

## 3. Renal ptosis

HESS (1938), in a masterly review of the subject, points out that the average normal kidney has a wide margin of movement and that few patients with renal ptosis require operation. He believes that the symptoms are due not only to stretching of the renal nerves on the pedicle but also to circulatory disturbances due to dragging down of the suprarenal gland with the kidney. There may, therefore, be a few patients with intractable renal pain associated with a gross degree of ptosis in whom renal denervation is indicated. Papin (1929) says that the pain is also due to adhesions and that pain from the latter is constant and an indication for operation. Oldham states that out of a series of fifteen such cases there were only three failures. The writer considers it advisable to combine denervation with nephropexy in this condition.

## 4. Essential haematuria

Harris and Harris (1930) have suggested renal denervation in this condition on the grounds that the spastic condition at the necks of the calyces causes congestion and perhaps haemorrhage from adjacent blood vessels. V. J. O'Connor, quoted by Oldham, made a special study of twelve cases of essential haematuria and found extravasated blood beneath the renal papillae with slight erosions of the mucosa, causing oozing of blood into the pelvis. Both Harris and Papin have advocated denervation for essential haematuria and have reported successful cases. This view has not received wide acceptance but it would seem to be a reasonable procedure to perform a renal denervation when a kidney, from which bleeding had occured, appeared normal on exploration.

## III. Indications for operation

Before operation is even considered in this condition it is clear that the pain must be severe enough to warrant operation and must also have failed to respond to prolonged conservative measures. Not only must there be recurrent or persistent renal pain but there should also be tenderness in the renal angle. In the writer's experience these patients have already had several urological investigations with negative findings, or a non-obstructive, apparently idiopathic hydronephrosis has been revealed. The essential principles are that it must be clearly demonstrated that the pain is of renal origin and that distension of the renal pelvis, (after ureteric catheterisation), reproduces exactly the pain complained of by the patient. The pain may not be similar in degree but it must be identical as far as situation and character are concerned. Harris and Harris (1930) consider that supportive evidence is provided if the pain is relieved by an injection of eserine. The difficulty is that the urologist is usually entirely dependant on subjective evidence in this condition and this is the probable explanation for a percentage of unsatisfactory results encountered after the operation has been performed.

Underwood (1939) suggests connecting a ureteric catheter with a water manometer and recording the intrapelvic pressure on a tambour. The pressure should rise after the administration of a spinal anaesthetic. If the pelvis fails to contract down he does not advise sympathectomy.

After the operation it is possible to inject much larger quantities of fluid into the renal pelvis through a ureteric catheter than before and distension of the pelvis is rendered painless. Oldham (1948) points out that after a period of twelve months there may be some regeneration of the nerves but this is rarely sufficient to cause a return of renal pain.

Briefly, renal pain may be diminished or eliminated by the operation but, certainly in the author's experience, the effect on the hydronephrosis may be disappointing.

## IV. The operation of denervation

The operation may be carried out either by the periarterial or the radicular method of denervation.

## 1. Periarterial denervation

This operation, first described by PAPIN and AMBARD (1921), is the method advocated by OLDHAM. The procedure is facilitated by the fact that the renal nerves are distributed around the renal artery and few, if any, accompany the renal vein. The advantage of this operation, as opposed to the alternative radicular method, is that the nerve supply of the kidney only is disturbed. The disadvantage is that unless great care is taken the renal vein may be damaged, thus necessitating a nephrectomy. The kidney is exposed through the usual lumbar incision, removing the last rib. It is most important to free the pedicle and allow the kidney to be brought well up into the wound. Working from the aorta towards the kidney the artery is cleared of nerve filaments. The nerves are lifted off the artery by a blunt dissector, are divided at the inner end and gently freed from the artery, being again divided near the renal hilum. It is found to be safer (and to cause less venous bleeding) if the operator works towards and not away from the kidney. The artery is completely cleared of nerve fibres on all aspects for a distance of approximately one inch. It is not necessary to deal with the vein and indeed it is dangerous to do so as its wall is thin and readily torn. It is important to strip aberrant renal arteries, if any, and the upper ureter and pelvis are cleared of any obvious nerve strands. At the end of the operation the kidney is suspended simply by the renal artery and vein and the ureter.

## 2. Radicular denervation

In this operation the splanchnic nerves are divided and the first two lumbar ganglia are removed. Once more the last rib is removed through a lumbar incision and the kidney is drawn forward and inwards. The writer finds that it is best to identify the upper two lumbar ganglia in the first instance and then the great splanchnic nerve is found as it perforates the crus of the diaphragm, above and somewhat external to the lumbar chain. The great splanchnic nerve, which may be in several strands, leads to the aortico-renal ganglion which also receives the lesser splanchnic. The first and second lumbar ganglia are removed and a short length of the splanchnic nerves are resected. One great benefit of this operation, as compared with the periarterial denervation, is that it is safer in dealing with a solitary kidney.

# B. Neural disturbances of the ureter

Megalo-ureter due to neural disturbances must be clearly distinguished from that of obstructive origin. In a subject beset with confusion and obscurity it is best to confine neural lesions of the ureter to megalo-ureter and ureteric reflux. The latter subject is dealt with later in the section dealing with the complications arising from the paraplegic bladder.

## Megalo-ureter

Megalo-ureter is generally reputed to be due to a neuromuscular dysfunction or an achalasia of the ureterovesical orifice. Characteristically the ureter is grossly dilated but, as there is no actual rise of intra-ureteric or intra-pelvic pressure, the pelvis and calyces are not dilated and the kidney functions well, certainly until a late stage. As time goes on, however, constant reflux through the patulous ureteric orifices leads to hydronephrosis and increase of the hydro-ureter. Secondary infection, also, is a complication in the later stages.

Megalo-ureter due to achalasia can be distinguished from hydro-ureter due to mechanical obstruction by the fact that there is no back-pressure, no tortuosity of the ureter and by the later onset of hydronephrosis. Hydro-ureter due to mechanical obstruction often exhibits angularity and actual elongation.

Poole-Wilson (1952) points out that usually the condition is unilateral and that the urine remains for some time uninfected. On intravenous pyelogram the dilatation is more marked at the lower end although the whole ureter may be involved and distended. There is no residual urine after evacuation and, on cystoscopy, a catheter passes readily up the ureter except in cases where it is held up by mucosal folds. Radiographs taken after removal of the ureteric catheter show slow emptying of the opaque medium from the ureter.

# I. Aetiology

Up to date no satisfactory explanation of megalo-ureter has been proffered. The cause of the so-called achalasia remains obscure but the condition has been compared with cardiospasm and Hirschsprung's disease. On the other hand it has been more or less established that there are no ganglion cells in the ureteric wall and it is has been shown that ureteric contractions may take place when the tube has no neural connections whatsoever and is, in fact, completely detached from the body (Tinckler 1957). Tinckler goes on to say that "peristaltic movement in the isolated ureter is only reproduced when acetyl choline is added to the fluid perfusing the ureter during *in vitro* experiments. This finding supports the conception that purposeful coordinated activity of the ureter is dependent on neurogenic influence. It is in keeping with the suggestion that megalo-ureter, in the absence of demonstrable organic obstruction, is due to a local neurological fault".

Svenson et al. (1952) put forward the concept that a diminution of parasympathetic ganglion cells in the bladder wall was the fundamental lesion and caused an actual dysfunction of the bladder, which in turn caused megalo-ureter. Svenson believes that the condition is closely allied with Hirschsprung's disease and found that in half his patients with Hirschsprung's disease there was evidence of bladder dysfunction, consisting of an excessive capacity and of poor emptying contractions. In some of these patients megalo-ureter was also present. In six out of seven fatal cases he found evidence of an absolute diminution in the number and size of ganglia cells and nerve bundles in the bladder wall.

Murnaghan (1958) considers that the dilatation of megalo-ureter may be due to abnormal ureteric contractions, which in turn arise from a predominance of circular muscle at the lower end of the ureter in place of the normal longitudinal arrangement; he suggests that the normal opening mechanism of the ureteric orifice is impeded by the extension of circular muscle into the intramural ureter.

Innes Williams (1952) has pointed out the association of some cases of megalo-ureter with other congenital abnormalities. Spina bifida occulta should be considered as a possible factor when no other cause is apparent.

# II. Electromyo-ureterography

The electrical reactions of the muscular tissue in the ureter have been investigated during the last few years by Hanley (1953), Franksson & Petersen (1953), Milton & Robb (1954) and others. Hanley has devised an electrode, consisting of a ureteric catheter with two silver collars situated close together near the extremity of the catheter. Each collar is in contact with a fine insulated wire which runs in the catheter lumen and connected with the recording apparatus. MILTON & ROBB use a portable Ediswan electro-encephalogram for this purpose and have recorded waves of muscular contraction in the dilated part of the ureter in two cases of hydro-ureter. In the undilated, intramural part of the tube, however, no electrical evidence of contraction was obtained. MILTON & ROBB draw an analogy between their findings and SVENSON's (1950) demonstration that there were no ganglion cells in the undilated segment of colon distal to a megacolon. They conclude that the fundamental factor in the cause of megalo-ureter is that the undilated, distal, intramural part of the ureter fails to conduct normal waves.

G. W. MILTON (1957), in a critical survey, points out that if the electro-ureterogram is to occupy a useful place in clinical practice it must supply reliable information not available by such other methods as the ureterogram and recordings from a manometer in the ureter. Essentially, the method should provide a record of electropotential changes which take place in the smooth muscle of the ureteric wall. Unfortunately, the ureteric catheter with the two silver collars presents the difficulty that, owing to the electrolytic contents of the urine, there is likely to be shorting of the electrodes, one with the other. Also this shorting effect will not be constant owing to the varying amounts of urine present between the two collars. Further, difficulties of interpretation arise in a tracing obtained from structures which move against the electrode (ADRIAN & GELFAN 1933). It is obvious that there must be a considerable degree of movement between the electrode and the ureteric wall with each contraction. DRAPER & ZORGMOTTI (1954) have, in fact, recorded "movement potentials" from the ureter. MILTON goes on to say "Because of the irregularity of the electro-ureterogram and the absence of features which are regularly present in recordings from other smooth muscle, and because tracings similar to the electro-ureterogram may be obtained by movement of the electrical contacts, it is concluded that the electro-ureterogram gives a distorted outline of the electro-potential changes which occur in the ureteric wall.

If there is a condition in which the ureteric wall undergoes a type of fibrillation so that it contracts without any coordinated peristalsis, and if such a condition causes symptoms, and if at the same time the ureter does not become dilated because of the ineffective movement, then the electro-ureterogram might be the only diagnostic test available. This is because it will show the presence or absence of movement even when there are no pressure changes in the lumen. In this type of case the distortion of the wave form produced by movement artefacts would not constitute a serious objection. Otherwise, the information which is desired of the electro-ureterogram, namely a record of ureteric contractions and ureteric function, may be largely obtained, or at least inferred, by other methods which are not so difficult to interpret."

# III. Treatment

Treatment of megalo-ureter presents a difficult problem, mainly because of the obscurity relating to its cause. If the dilatation is not gross, and infection is absent or readily controlled, it is probably advisable to avoid operative measures and to keep the patient under regular observation, repeating the radiographs from time to time. Fortunately, megalo-ureter does not appear to progress rapidly and, indeed, sometimes remains static for years. Recurrent bouts of urinary infections may, however, compel more active measures. In advanced cases with gross infection nephro-ureterectomy will be necessary, but if the kidney is well preserved it may be possible to avoid nephrectomy by substituting a length of ileum for the diseased ureter. A number of other procedures have been advocated from time to time, including ureterolysis and excision of the lower quarter of the ureter and reimplantation into the bladder, either into the supero-lateral surface or into the site of the original orifice (Poole-Wilson 1952). If the view expressed above by Milton & Robb is correct then excision of the distal quarter of the ureter and reimplantation into the bladder would appear the correct procedure on theoretical grunds. Pursuing his view that the bladder is prominantly at fault, Svenson practices prolonged bladder drainage for megalo-ureter and is prepared to continue this treatment for six months. He claims clinical improvement of the patient and radiographic evidence of improvement of the dilated ureters. Bischoff (1957) prefers to retain the lower end of the ureter and has designed a plastic operation to shorten and narrow the tube by an oblique excision.

# C. Neural disturbance of the bladder
## I. Nerve supply of the bladder

The centre for micturition is situated in the sacral cord opposite the 12th thoracic and the 1st lumbar vertebrae. Both motor and sensory nerves reach the bladder by means of the nervi erigentes or pelvic nerves which arise from the cells in the lateral part of the anterior horn of the second, third and to a lesser extent, the fourth segment of the sacral cord. The nervi erigentes pass *through* the hypogastric plexus to reach the bladder in medial and lateral branches. Afferent fibres pass to the corresponding posterior root ganglia. Motor impulses cause detrusor contractions and sensory fibres convey sensations of pain (of over-distension), touch and the desire to void (Fig. 3). In addition the nervi erigentes are responsible for relaxation of the internal sphincter but the mode of action is still obscure. Relaxation may be due to a purely inhibitory (neural) action or may be achieved by mechanical means, due to the pull of those detrusor fibres which sweep over the posterior lip of the bladder neck into the prostatic urethra (Talbot 1948). On the other hand it may be that the true involuntary sphincter is not a ring but a double muscular loop which relaxes reciprocally when the detrusor contracts (Denny-Brown & Robertson 1933).

The second neural component which must be considered is the sympathetic but unfortunately the role of these nerves is ill-defined. The sympathetic nerves arise in the lateral grey column from T11 to L2, reaching the bladder by means of the hypogastric plexus and the presacral nerve. Two functions are attributed to the sympathetic nerves; firstly, it seems probable that they are responsible for contraction of the internal sphincter during ejaculation; secondly, the sympathetic nerves probably convey a sense of bladder fullness when the bladder is distended. Bors (1952) points out that intravesical tension can be appreciated by the patient as long as sympathetic fibres reach the cord above the level of the lesion. The sensation of distension becomes less the higher the lesion and disappears altogether at the level of T4 to T6. Petersén and Franksson (1955), in a study of the sensory innervation of the bladder, divided sensation into pain and touch, a sensation of fullness, the desire to micturate and the discrimination of right and left sides of the bladder. They found that painful sensations from the trigone were distributed to the first, second and third sacral segments, whereas other parts of the bladder were associated with the second lumbar to second sacral segments. Tactile sensation and the desire to micturate had a similar segmental distribution but fulness of the bladder was associated with higher segments, as high as the eleventh thoracic. The ability to discriminate between right and left sides of the bladder disappeared if anaesthesia ascended to the second lumbar segment. Finally, it is necessary to discuss the pudendal or perineal nerve, a somatic nerve arising from the pudic nerve which in turn arises from the 2nd, 3rd and 4th sacral segments. The pudendal nerve supplies the external sphincter muscle. It is said to be possible to contract the muscle voluntarily but not to relax it voluntarily.

McCREA and KIMMEL (1952 and 1954) have also described a possible additional pathway, reaching the bladder by a perivascular route.

## II. The act of micturition

Micturition is essentially a reflex act although it is under voluntary control under normal circumstances. The various stages may be tabulated as follows:

1. The intravesical pressure gradually rises, causing the "stretch reflex".

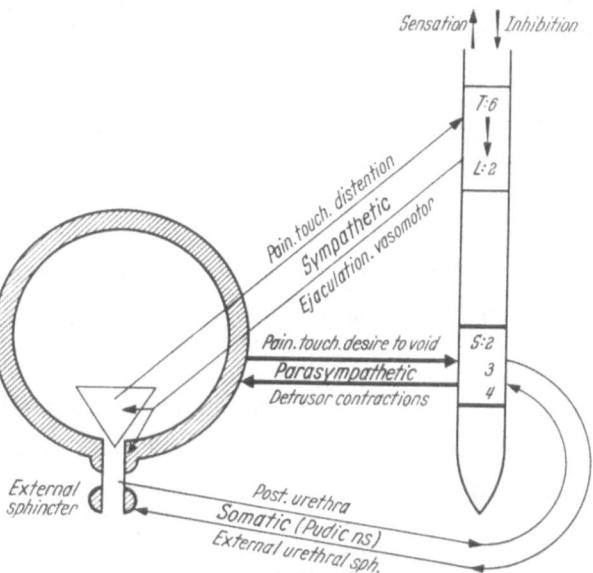

Fig. 3. Nerve supply of the bladder. (From the British Journal of Urology.)

2. An afferent impulse passes by the nervi erigentes to the 2nd, 3rd and 4th sacral segments of the cord.

3. In the absence of inhibition a motor impulse passes down by the nervi erigentes causing contraction of the detrusor and relaxation of the internal sphincter, the so-called "tug".

4. At this stage urine enters the prostatic urethra and its presence there initiates a second reflex which causes relaxation of the external sphincter.

Accessory factors include relaxation of the perineal muscles and a rise of intra-abdominal pressure.

The final outcome of these still somewhat obscure nervous processes is the act of micturition.

## III. Voluntary control of micturition

Micturition is primarily a reflex act but can be controlled by the cerebrum. LANGWORTHY et al. (1940) state that "there is evidence of cortical representation over the function of micturition" and that " the co-ordination of vesical function is dependant upon reflex arcs through the midbrain". It appears probable that inhibitory impulses from the cerebral cortex are in control between the acts of micturition and that the reflex act can only take place with the voluntary cessation of these inhibitory impulses. Impulses arising in the motor cortex and passing down the cord in the lateral columns cause contraction of the external sphincter. With regard to relaxation of this muscle it is generally believed that it is not possible to relax it voluntarily and that this can only be achieved by reflex action. While this view is held generally, MUNRO (1952) does not agree.

## IV. The neurogenic bladder

The neurogenic bladder arises as a result of injury or disease of the nervous system, severe enough to impede or interfere with the normal neural control of micturition.

### 1. Classification

There are two main groups, those due to traumatic paraplegia and those due to non-traumatic neural lesions of different types.

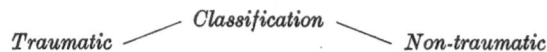

*Traumatic* —— *Classification* —— *Non-traumatic*

| Traumatic | Non-traumatic |
|---|---|
| 1. "Spinal shock" bladder | 1. Uninhibited neurogenic bladder |
| 2. Automatic or reflex bladder | 2. Atonic neurogenic bladder |
| 3. Autonomous bladder | 3. Idiopathic atony of the bladder |
| 4. Voluntary neurogenic bladder | |

#### a) Traumatic neurogenic bladder

##### α) "Spinal shock" bladder

The writer believes that this is the most accurate way of describing the condition of the bladder immediately after the spinal injury. There has been a tendency to describe this stage as "atonic neurogenic bladder" (PRATHER 1949) but this leads to confusion and it is preferable to reserve this term for non-traumatic lesions due to tabes dorsalis and lesions of the posterior roots affecting the 2nd, 3rd and 4th sacral segments of the cord.

The well-known term "spinal shock" has been in use for well over a century, being first used by MARSHALL HALL in 1843. MUNRO (1937) has defined it as "that condition which, when caused by spinal injury of any type, produces a suppression or alteration of the segmental reflex activity below the level of the cord injury". The bladder becomes greatly distended and a paralytic overflow-incontinence develops. The detrusor is paralysed and the internal sphincter is tightly contracted and fails to respond to any stimulus. On the other hand the external sphincter, like other muscles supplied by somatic nerves below the level of the lesion, may be relaxed. The only factor ensuring any evacuation of the bladder is the elasticity of its wall, the phase occurring in almost all patients and lasting from days to weeks, or even months. As the patient gradually recovers he ultimately develops an automatic or an autonomous bladder depending on the level of the injury (DONOVAN 1949). MUNRO (1952), however, points out that there are two intermediate stages, either of which may be so transient as to be overlooked. The two intermediate stages are as follows:

*1. Stage of ineffective and abortive emptying contractions.* The bladder capacity gradually diminishes and the intravesical tone rises but the internal sphincter remains contracted. Detrusor contractions appear but are feeble and sporadic, frequently discharging small amounts of urine.

*2. Stage of hypertonicity.* As time goes on the detrusor becomes more vigorous and the muscle remains in an almost constant state of contraction. As a result the curve of the basic tone is steep. Both sphincters relax physiologically at this stage.

It is obvious that it is only possible to follow these stages in recovery by means of cystometric and cysto-urethrographic examination. From stage (b) the bladder either progresses to the automatic type or relapses to atonicity.

### β) The automatic or reflex bladder

This type may be expected when the injury is situated at a higher level than the centre for micturition, which has escaped damage. The patient has no control over micturition; several ounces of urine are forcibly evacuated at intervals of two or three hours but sometimes as frequently as hourly. If there has been a complete injury of the cord an automatic or reflex bladder is the best end-result obtainable in the male because he can wear a rubber urinal. The female patient is more comfortable and more satisfactory with an expressible bladder. Provided there is no appreciable amount of residual urine this end-result may be regarded as satisfactory. Fig. 4 shows the cystometrogram seen in an automatic bladder. In Fig. 5 is shown the type of bladder associated with injuries at different levels.

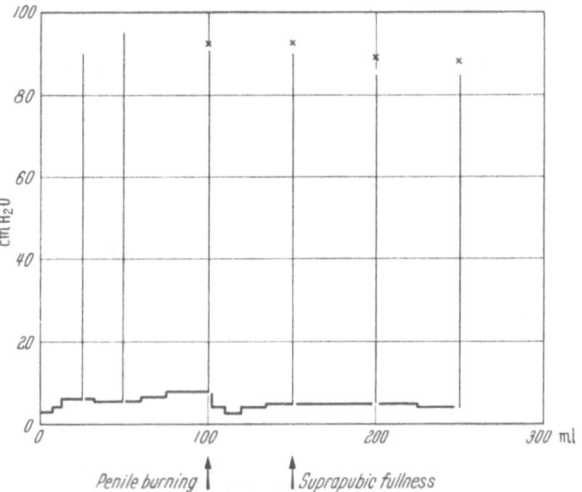

Fig. 4. Cystometrogram in the automatic or reflex bladder (injury at T3). X = leakage around the catheter. (From the British Medical Journal.) The vertical lines represent detrusor contractions

### γ) The autonomous bladder

When the second, third and fourth sacral spinal segments are completely destroyed or the nerves of the cauda equina are severed, an autonomous bladder may be expected. All that remains of the nerve supply of the bladder is the plexus situated between the mus-

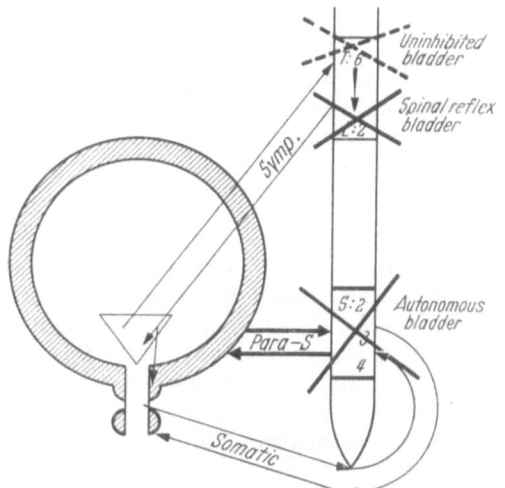

Fig. 5. Types of neurogenic bladder in relation to the level of the spinal cord lesion. (From the British Journal of Urology)

cular coats and any control exercised by this is feeble and ineffective. There are no proper detrusor contractions and there may be continuous dribbling of urine from the bladder. The cystometrogram (Fig. 6) shows a hypertonic basic intravesical pressure. As the internal sphincter is generally contracted a residual urine and secondary dilatation of the ureters are not uncommon. In compensation for all these difficulties, however, evacuation of the bladder may be facilitated by abdominal straining and manual suprapubic compression. Helpful also is the fact that the external sphincter muscle is paralysed.

### δ) Voluntary neurogenic bladder

This type has been described by Prather (1949) who pointed out that after a partial transection of the spinal cord there will probably be some degree of voluntary power and some degree of sensation, though neither may be apparent for some time after the injury. It is probable that in such patients voluntary control of micturition, although not perfect, may ultimately develop.

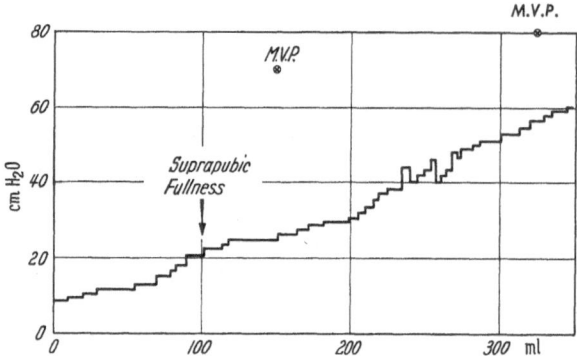

Fig. 6. Cystometrogram in the autonomous bladder (injury at L1). Residual urine = 14 oz. or 400 ml. *M.V.P.* = maximum voluntary pressure. (From the British Medical Journal)

### b) Non-traumatic

#### α) Uninhibited neurogenic bladder

The uninhibited neurogenic bladder may develop in the course of disseminated sclerosis, spinal tumour, subacute combined degeneration of the cord and sometimes in raised intracranial pressure. In all these conditions there is an incomplete or partial interruption of the pathways of the cord. The commonest example is, of course, enuresis.

On investigation there are usually early and uncontrollable detrusor contractions and sometimes spasm of the external sphincter. Symptoms include urgency, incontinence, frequency, enuresis and an inability to empty the bladder completely. An attack of acute or chronic retention of urine is sometimes seen in disseminated sclerosis.

### β) Atonic neurogenic bladder

The writer considers that this term should never be applied to traumatic paraplegia but should be reserved for the neurogenic bladder associated with tabes dorsalis, division of the posterior roots of the 2nd, 3rd and 4th sacral segments of the cord and for some forms of spina bifida. While the motor side of the reflex arc is intact there is an appreciable defect of sensation. Frequently these patients have a large residual urine or even an overflow incontinence. Cystometric estimations show a low-pressure curve, a high capacity, an absence of the desire to void and an absence of contractions.

Sometimes this type of neurogenic bladder is found after resection of the rectum for carcinoma and after Wertheim's radical hysterectomy, when it is probable that some of the branches of the nervi erigentes have been severed. The same clinical features are found, i.e. a chronic retention with a lack of appreciation when the bladder is full.

### γ) Idiopathic atony of the bladder

This obscure condition is encountered occasionally. It appears probable that there is some intrinsic neural defect in the bladder wall without any evidence of neural disease elsewhere. A typical example was seen recently by the writer and was eventually attributed to a transient birth palsy.

FRANKSSON and PETERSEN (1955) have pointed out the frequent association of atony of the bladder with chronic prostatovesiculitis and consider that hypotonia of the prostate, seminal vesicles and bladder may be caused by affection of nerve roots. It is possible that some cases of so-called idiopathic atony may be due to this cause.

Certain types of bladder dysfunction may be deduced from the nature and level of the lesion (COSBIE ROSS, GIBBON & DAMANSKI 1957). For example:

a) In lesions above the mid-dorsal region (including the cervical spine), the reflex arc is unscathed and, as a result, the detrusor acts with strong reflex contractions at a certain point of bladder filling, a condition similar to that seen in infancy. Voiding of urine around a blocked or displaced catheter strongly suggests a return of reflex activity.

b) The common injuries of the dorsi-lumbar spine often exhibit evidence of both upper and lower motor neurone lesions. If the bulbocavernosus and anal reflexes are present (and consequently the reflex arc is intact), an automatic or reflex bladder may be confidently predicted.

c) Cauda equina lesions result from fractures or fracture-dislocations of the first lumbar vertebra or lower. All reflexes below the level of the neurological lesions are permanently absent (including the bulbocavernosus and anal reflexes).

## 2. Investigation

These are long-stay patients and a single investigation is insufficient but must be repeated at intervals (COSBIE ROSS 1951). Urinary infections come and go and a hydronephrosis or a ureteric reflux may appear over a period of time. A full investigation includes:

a) Repeated microscopic examination of the urine and sensitivity studies.
b) Estimation of the residual urine.
c) Radiography of the urinary tract.
d) Cysto-urethroscopy.
e) Cystometry.
f) Cysto-urethrography.

### a) Examination of the urine

These patients frequently exhibit a mild degree of urinary infection and it is usual to find a few bacteria and a few pus cells in the urine, especially if there is an appreciable residual urine. This mild chronic infection can be eliminated for periods by means of treatment but is liable to an acute exacerbation.

### b) Residual urine

A consistently high residual urine is never satisfactory and inevitably leads to recurrent bouts of urinary infection and perhaps ultimately to renal failure. In this connection DAVID's (1921) experiments are of relevance. He found that injection of cultures of B. coli into the bladders of normal dogs produced no harmful effects, the organisms gradually disappearing without causing infection. If the dog had, however, an appreciable amount of residual urine, injection of cultures of B. coli into the bladder caused severe cystitis and renal infection. If the residual urine remains high, therefore, further therapeutic steps are necessary to deal with the obstructive factor, whatever it may be.

The residual urine must be considered in relation to the "bladder balance", or the ratio of residual urine to the bladder capacity. It should be the aim to prevent the amount of residual urine rising above six ounces.

### c) Radiography of the urinary tract

### d) Cysto-urethroscopy

At first the bladder mucosa appears atrophic and shows a fine trabeculation but, as time goes on, the trabeculae become coarser and more pronounced. With regard to the bladder neck, other methods of investigation may be more definite and helpful but it is sometimes possible to demonstrate a cuff of fibrous

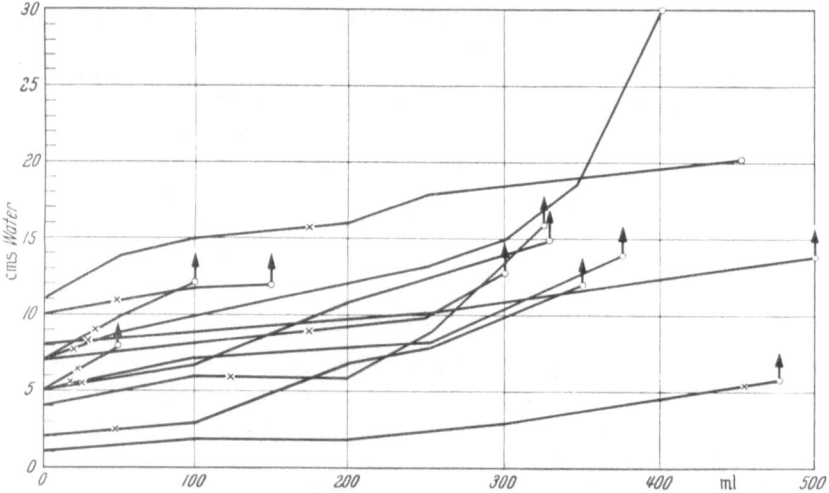

Fig. 7. Tracing of cystometrograms from twelve subjects with normal micturition (filling continued at 2—4 drops per second until emptying contractions ensued or discomfort became excessive). Arrow indicates emptying contraction. Asterisk shows first desire to void (Gibbon)

and muscular tissue, similar to a median bar and situated at the level of the internal urinary meatus. Chronic inflammatory changes, suggested by a bullous oedema of the trigone and by a fixity or lack of elasticity of the tissues in the immediate neighbourhood, are frequently present. These changes can best be appreciated when passing a cystoscope or a metal bougie and may be responsible for the development of the indurative cuff.

### e) Cystometry

Cystometry, or the study of the relationship between the intravesical pressure and the volume of fluid in the bladder, indicates bladder capacity, bladder sensation (especially the pain of distension), the maximum voluntary pressure and the presence of detrusor contractions. Watkins (1934) demonstrated the cystometric curves found in normal individuals. Fig. 7 illustrates a number of normal cystometrograms, the pressure rising to 15—20 cms. of water at a capacity of 300—400 ccs. when the bladder is filled at a constant rate of ninety drops a minute. The maximum voluntary pressure (M.V.P.) is dependant on the level of the lesion as it requires full activity of the abdominal muscles to be effective. If the lesion is sufficiently low to have spared the muscles of the abdominal wall the M.V.P. powerfully assists the reflex detrusor effort. Fig. 8 shows the type of cystometrogram found in the "spinal shock" bladder immediately after the injury. Although there is a more or less normal basic pressure curve (NESBIT & LAPIDES 1948), there is a complete absence of detrusor contractions. The cystometrogram found in the automatic or reflex bladder is shown in Fig. 4. It will be seen that detrusor contractions appear during the gradual filling of the bladder but micturition, demonstrated by leakage around the catheter, does not occur until a certain amount of fluid has been run into the bladder. The detrusor contractions are unaccompanied by any sensation. In the autonomous bladder there is usually a hypertonic basic curve with feeble detrusor contractions (Fig. 6).

It has been suggested that the cystometrogram is not of value but this is not the writer's opinion. For example, the presence of a large residual urine in spite of active detrusor contractions clearly indicates an obstruction at the bladder neck or at the level of the external sphincter. Again, it is only possible to diagnose the condition of hypertonic detrusor by means of the cystometrogram. In short, an accurate diagnosis in certain patients cannot be made without a cystometrogram which is, in addition, valuable in helping to assess progress in almost every case.

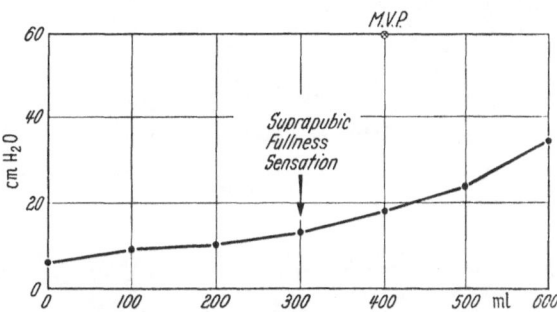

Fig. 8. Cystometrogram in "spinal shock" bladder, immediately after injury. (From the British Medical Journal)

Cystometry may be carried out at the bedside using the GIBBON catheter, this having the advantage that extra changes of catheter are obviated. GIBBON reports as follows: "Owing to the resistance to the inflow of fluid at a very fast drip, there is an artificial rise in the pressure shown on the manometer. We have, therefore, been filling the bladder intermittently, so that the resting vesical tone can be accurately measured. We have also noted, in a few cases that when the bladder does undergo a spinal reflex contraction, the pressures registered are relatively low as compared with our previous figures. This appears to be due to the ease with which the bladder contents are passed around the small tube. No doubt, this is to some extent a safeguard to the upper urinary tracts, especially in those cases with reflux along the ureters."

## f) Cysto-urethrography

The great value of this method of investigation has been shown by COSBIE ROSS and DAMANSKI (1953) and DAMANSKI and KERR (1957), its value resting on the fact that no other device reveals so accurately the condition of the bladder neck, the prostatic urethra and the relaxed or spastic state of the external and internal sphincters. This particular investigation is essential before arriving at a decision regarding further treatment in a patient with appreciable residual urine. Valuable information is also obtained by comparing the radiographs obtained before and after such procedures as resection of the bladder neck etc. DAMANSKI has described his technique as follows:

"A bladder syringe of 4 or 8 fl. oz. is used.

*Control Film.* A control film in antero-posterior projection is taken first. Later a soft rubber catheter is passed with strict aseptic precautions, the residual

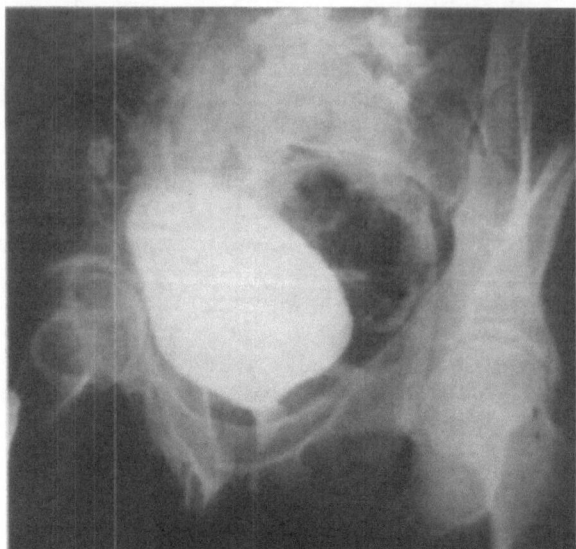

Fig. 9. Cysto-urethrogram showing a shelf or ledge at the bladder neck

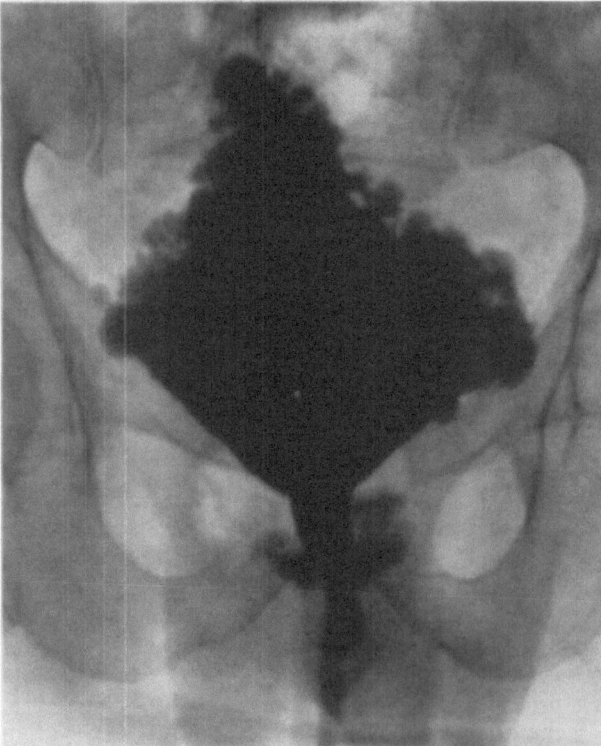

Fig. 10. Cysto-urethrogram demonstrating a rhomboid-shaped bladder with a fringe of small diverticula. Prostatic ducts and diverticula outlined by contrast medium. High degree of urinary infection and hydronephrosis. (From the British Journal of Surgery)

urine evacuated and the bladder filled with 8 fl. oz. of ten per cent sodium iodide. A contracted bladder may be incapable of holding the full quantity and only gentle pressure must be used on the injecting syringe.

*Resting films.* The first film is an antero-posterior exposure with the patient supine, the central ray being directed to the upper margin of the symphysis pubis at an angle of 5 degrees towards the feet. A right or left oblique exposure follows, the transverse axis of the patient's body being tilted at an angle of 50—60 degrees to the table, and the central ray being directed vertically through the upper margin of the symphysis pubis. The leg nearest to the table is flexed to an angle of approximately 45 degrees at the hip and knee-joints, the leg farther from the table being extended fully.

*Voiding films.* The two films at rest are followed by two films taken during micturition the patient being instructed to micturate by his usual routine.

*Retrograde filling films.* Frequently the voiding films are not satisfactory and retrograde filling of the urethra and bladder is necessary. A smooth-acting syringe is essential to obtain a steady flow of the fluid during the exposure.

*Film for backflow.* The examination is finished by taking an antero-posterior film of the renal tract to show any ureteric backflow. Finally all the contrast medium must be evacuated through the catheter."

The cysto-urethrogram may show a shelf or ledge at the bladder neck and, at the same time, it is found possible to distend the prostatic urethra with the opaque fluid (Fig. 9). This obstruction, which may be regarded as a form of median bar, should be dealt with by perurethral resection. On the other hand the cysto-urethrogram may show spasm of the external sphincter or of both sphincters, the whole length of the prostatic urethra being closed and impossible to dilate by the injection of opaque fluid from the external urinary meatus (Fig. 17a & b); this is a spastic obstruction and responds best to the operation of pudendal neurectomy.

Multiple vesical diverticula may be present and often indicate a long-standing obstruction at the bladder neck or at a lower level. There is usually an intractable infection and these patients often prove unsatisfactory in their response to treatment.

In patients with an established urinary infection the cysto-urethrogram may show dilated prostatic ducts and diverticula of the prostatic urethra (Fig. 10).

## 3. Treatment

### a) General aims of treatment

The treatment of paraplegia, especially of traumatic paraplegia, necessitates the collaboration and services of the neurosurgeon, plastic surgeon and the orthopaedist as well as the urologist. Neural damage occurs at the moment of injury when irreversible changes probably take place. Many of these spinal injuries involve an extensive conical area of the cord and not a narrow section or zone (ALLEN 1914). In paraplegia due to unstable fracture-dislocation at the thoraco-lumbar region HOLDSWORTH and HARDY (1953) advocate internal fixation by means of metal plates in order to prevent damage to roots which have escaped the original injury. These authors consider that torsional violence is especially prone to cause an unstable injury and they point out that not only are undamaged roots preserved but that stabilisation may encourage root recovery. It must, however, be pointed out that if the cord lesion is complete, stabilisation, apart from the question of roots, will not influence the course of events. Again, the possible value of preservation of roots must be weighed against the risk of carrying out an operation on a patient possibly suffering from shock and protein imbalance. The patient must be kept under careful and constant neurological observation so that if the lesion is incomplete and there is a tendency for the neural damage to spread upwards, a laminectomy may be considered. Laminectomy is, of course, essential in patients with penetrating wounds of the spine. There has been much written on laminectomy, but with a few exceptions, there is a certain agreement regarding the indication for the operation. WATSON-JONES (1955) emphasises the importance of nursing the patient in such a way that pressure sores, contractures and urinary infection are avoided. He advises laminectomy only under the following circumstances:

1. In the patient with a depressed fracture, especially at the thoraco-lumbar junction, with protrusion of bone into the spinal canal.

2. In incomplete lesions with progressively increasing neurological signs, suggesting the development of an epidural haematoma.

3. In cases where there is a block to the flow of the cerebrospinal fluid as proved by spinal puncture.

With regard to cervical fractures, WATSON-JONES advocates reduction by hyperextension for crush injuries of the vertebral bodies, followed by immobilisation in plaster of Paris for three months (see below). In cases of marked displacement of the upper segment of the spine, with locking, he reduces the dislocation by skeletal traction, using skull callipers, beginning with a weight of 15 to 20 pounds. Repeated radiographs are taken, the weight being reduced to 10 pounds as soon as the articular processes are disengaged. GUTTMANN (1949, 1954, 1955), who has carried out most valuable and pioneer work in this condition, is strongly opposed to plaster casts because he believes that they lead inevitably to pressure sores and are contrary to fundamental principles and rehabilitation. His method consists of placing the patient on sorbo packs with two or three pillows beneath the fracture, the so-called postural method, in order to encourage hyperextension and to restore the normal curvature. The patient is turned two-hourly, day and night, care being taken to ensure that the patient is moved "in one piece" by three or four orderlies. He believes that in complete transverse lesions remaining unchanged for 48 hours there is complete destruction of the cord, or at least most severe damage which is irreversible. GUTTMANN's indications for laminectomy are:

1. Incomplete lesions showing progression of the neurological signs, probably due to an increasing epidural haematoma.

2. Permanent block on Queckenstedt's test.

3. Constant, severe irritation of the spinal roots caused by displacement of bone fragments or by the prolapse of an intervertebral disc.

MAYFIELD (1933), on the other hand, applies plaster of Paris after reduction of dorsal and lumbar injuries by hyperextension. He advises laminectomy:

1. In partial lesions where indriven fragments of bone are retarding recovery or causing progressive paralysis.

2. In complete lesions where obstruction of the spinal canal is demonstrated.

In cervical injuries MAYFIELD treats both fractures and fracture-dislocations by skeletal traction, using Crutchfield tongs maintained for four to six weeks. MEIROWSKY (1954) is in favour of laminectomy in closed injuries where there is partial or complete blockage of the subarachnoid pathways.

MUNRO (1952) rejects the use of plaster of Paris casts in cord lesions because of the resultant high incidence of pressure sores. His method is similar to that of GUTTMANN, rolled blankets being placed between the boards and mattresses opposite the kyphos and being added to daily until some degree of hyperextension has been achieved. The patient is maintained in this position for 6 to 8 weeks or longer until solid weight-bearing repair has taken place. Two-hourly turning in bed is carried out night and day, using a drawsheet. Decompressive laminectomy is carried out for any block in the cerebrospinal pathways.

MUNRO treats cervical lesions with continuous traction and hyperextension with the help of Crutchfield tongs. COMARR (1955) and COMARR & KAUFMAN (1956) have reviewed a large number of patients with spinal injuries, finding that significant neurological improvement occured in 16% in patients subjected to laminectomy whereas 29% showed improvement in those in whom no operation was carried out. They attributed this disparity to the fact that patients requiring laminectomy had, as a rule, sustained more severe damage to the cord. COMARR & KAUFMAN considered that laminectomy should be carried out under the following conditions:

1. In the presence of a subarachnoid block or a bony encroachment on the cord. He adds, however, that it is not necessary or desirable to perform the

laminectomy immediately as the spinal block may be due to oedema which may subside if given time to do so (COMARR 1957).

2. In progressive neurological deterioration.

They believe that the absence of a cerebrospinal block indicates that neural structures are not seriously compressed and that maximum destruction has already taken place. In these circumstances nothing is to be gained by laminectomy. BOEHLER (1956) advises, in the dorsi-lumbar fractures, longitudinal traction on the arms and legs followed by hyperextension in a plaster of Paris jacket. Laminectomy is indicated in those cases in which the radiograph, taken after reduction, shows that a fragment of bone still lies in the lumen of the spinal canal.

To summarise the various views about the indications for laminectomy:

1. The operation is indicated in all penetrating wounds of the spinal cord (CAMPBELL & MEIROWSKY 1953). This relieves the cord, cauda and individual spinal roots from pressure produced by comminuted bone and disc fragments, blood clots and foreign bodies. It is advisable to perform the operation as early as possible but surgical shock, lower nephron syndrome and associated wounds of the abdomen and chest may necessitate a short postponement.

2. In the incomplete lesion in which there is an extension of the neural damage, presumably due to an epidural haematoma.

3. When there is evidence of a block of the cerebrospinal pathways.

4. When there is evidence of pressure on the cord or roots by displaced bony fragments.

Injuries of the cervical spine fall into two large groups, i.e. flexion and hyperextension injuries. Concerning the latter SCHNEIDER et al. (1954) point out that the common neurological pattern consists of a greater motor impairment in the upper than in the lower limbs, bladder dysfunction (usually retention of urine) and varying degrees of sensory impairment below the level of the lesion. Recovery also follows a certain pattern, with recovery of the lower limbs first, next bladder function and finally recovery in the upper limbs. Great interest has been taken in the group of patients with paraplegia due to hyperextension injuries with normal radiographic appearences (BARNES 1948, JEFFERSON 1948). TAYLOR (1951) and TAYLOR & BLACKWOOD (1948) have expressed the view that a simpler mechanism than rupture of the anterior common ligament is probably responsible for the cord damage in hyperextension injuries. TAYLOR considers that the forward bulging of the ligamentum flavum traps the cord and supports his view by post-mortem examination, in which gross destruction of the posterior columns of the cord was found with lesser damage to the anterior ones.

There appears much to support this view and several writers have warned against treating the neck in an extended position and have advocated a neutral position, neither flexed nor extended (WATSON-JONES 1955). DAMANSKI (1957) in reviewing 31 patients with quadriplegia, recorded that 12 of these were flexion injuries, (dislocations, compression-fractures and fracture-dislocations), while in the other nineteen there was a history of injury in hyperextension with no radiologically demonstrable injury to the bone.

DAMANSKI makes the following comparison between the two groups:

1. Flexion injuries to the cervical spine and cord are fewer in number, are predominantly complete neurological lesions, are more vulnerable in the early stages and often present most difficult bladder problems.

2. Extension injuries are more numerous, are usually incomplete lesions, are more resistant to complications during the early stages and rarely need operative measures to restore satisfactory bladder function.

Most authorities advise the use of a Schanz or light felt collar for some months after the initial phase.

The patient, then, is nursed on sorbo-rubber mattresses and his position in bed is changed two-hourly, to side, to back and then to the opposite side. All pressure points are attended to twice a day. Early mobilisation, so that the patient is sitting out of bed in a wheel-chair as soon as his general condition or the complications permit, should be the general aim (Damanski 1957). It is necessary to watch the plasma proteins, so that if there is a drop, the deficiency can be corrected by blood transfusions. The bowels are encouraged to function once (at precisely the same time of day), during twenty-four or forty-eight hours (Munro 1952). At first this is achieved by means of enemata but later these should become unnecessary and simple aperients, such as milk of magnesia or liquid paraffin, are all that is needed. The reflex is initiated by the fact that the patient is in position to defaecate. It may, however, be necessary to carry out digital removal of faeces on occasion. The urological measures must be correlated with the other services. For example, if it is found necessary to nurse the patient in the prone position following an operation by a plastic surgeon to cover a pressure sore over the sacrum, especial care is needed with the bladder as this particular position is unfavourable to micturition, whether automatic or otherwise.

Prather (1949) states the aims of treatment clearly and concisely. He says that "The patient should become ambulatory and free of urinary infection. A patient who has sustained a *partial* transection of the spinal cord should attain voluntary control of urination and be capable of emptying the bladder. A patient who has a *complete* transection of the spinal cord should attain involuntary periodic reflex voiding at satisfactory intervals and be capable of emptying the bladder". These are high ideals but anything less may lead to urinary infection and progressive deterioration of kidney function. Throughout the period of treatment (and in fact for the rest of the patient's life), a large intake of fluids, approximately six pints a day, is essential. Urinary antiseptics, especially antibiotics, are given only in short courses when specifically indicated by an exacerbation of urinary infection. Chemotherapy should not be given continuously.

### b) Stages of treatment

These may be indicated thus:

| | | |
|---|---|---|
| Initial stage | Neurological | Spinal shock |
| | Urological | Retention of urine |
| Intermediate stage | Neurological | Return of reflexes |
| | Urological | Establishment of bladder emptying |
| Third stage | Neurological | Physical rehabilitation |
| | Urological | Correction of high residual urine |
| Fourth stage | Follow-up | This is necessary indefinitely |

Treatment of the bladder begins in the "spinal shock" stage, which occasionally lasts days or weeks but more frequently lasts approximately two months. In the intermediate stage there ensues a course of bladder training when the degree of recovery of micturition is assessed. Should the recovery of micturition, automatic or otherwise, prove unsatisfactory, a further search is made to ascertain the cause and, as a result of this further investigation, additional measures i.e. alcohol block, resection of the bladder neck or pudendal neurectomy are necessary in order to achieve the ideal aim postulated by Prather.

## c) Initial urological treatment

In the past a large number of methods have been advocated at various time. The fact that many methods have been attempted indicates their defects. It appears to be a general principle in medicine that when a brilliantly successful form of treatment is introduced all other methods tend to be relegated. It is necessary to mention some of these methods:

### α) The passive method

BESLEY (1917) advocated leaving the bladder without either urethral or suprapubic drainage. The bladder empties itself by an overflow incontinence. This approach stands condemned not only because rupture of the bladder has been known to occur but mainly on the ground that irreparable damage may be sustained by the overstretched musculature. It is obviously impossible to carry out in women patients and, even in men, the constant leaking of urine leads to wet beds and pressure sores.

### β) Manual expression

While this procedure appears theoretically to have many advantages it is not, as a rule, successful. The reason for failure is that initially the bladder is large, atonic and flaccid, with a tightly contracted internal sphincter which permits only a small amount of urine to pass. There is a large quantity of residual urine. The method is, however, worth a trial and, should the internal sphincter be not contracted, may prove successful. Patients especially suitable for manual expression are those in whom the neural damage includes the spinal reflex arc subserving micturition (S2, 3 & 4) — the autonomous bladder. The external sphincter and the muscles of the pelvic floor are paralysed and, in addition, it is in this type of patient that the abdominal muscles retain their power.

### γ) Tidal drainage

This is the method advised by MUNRO (1952). He points out that the automatic filling and syphon-emptying of the bladder not only prevent infection but also the level of filling can be predetermined and altered during the course of treatment to suit the particular circumstances. There are, however, several objections to tidal drainage; firstly, it immobilises the patient in bed when the modern tendency is in favour of getting the patient up at the earliest possible moment; secondly, in the writer's opinion, the apparatus requires constant supervision and adjustment day and night to keep it functioning satisfactorily.

### δ) Suprapubic drainage

The lamentable results following spinal injury treated by catheterisation during the first world war led THOMSON-WALKER (1917) to suggest and practise suprapubic drainage. If, however, a de Pezzer catheter is used, only too often a small contracted bladder with a rigid fibrotic wall results, usually complicated by a urinary infection. The writer has had to deal with a number of such cases in which the bladder capacity was under two ounces, necessitating an operation for the closure of the fistula followed by a long and tedious period spent in increasing the bladder capacity. RICHES (1943) suggested a high oblique cystostomy using a fine catheter, inserted by means of a special introducer and, when suprapubic drainage is necessary, this is the method of choice. The narrow fistulous track closes within a matter of hours after removal of the catheter.

Suprapubic drainage would appear to be unnecessary save under exceptional circumstances in which the patient is treated initially under the most primitive conditions. When the patient can be admitted to hospital, or better still to a special centre, shortly after the injury, suprapubic drainage is unnecessary and undesirable.

### ε) Intermittent catheterisation

In the past intermittent catheterisation was rightly blamed for the large number of deaths due to urinary infection. Recently this method has been

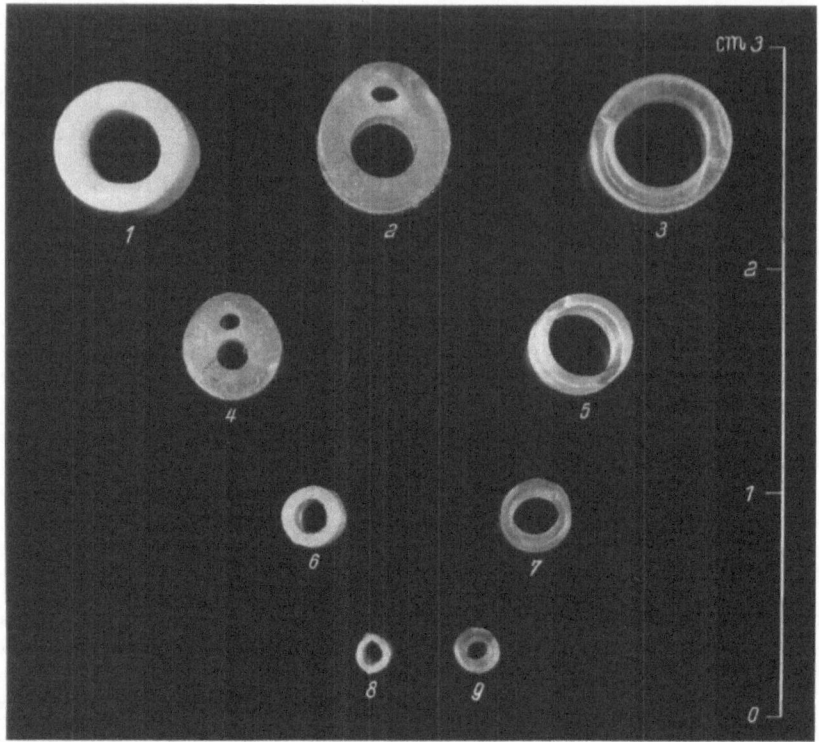

Fig. 11. Cross section of various catheters and tubes to show relative inside and outside diameters: 1. Jacques catheter (18 F). 2. Latex Foley catheter (18 F). 3. Portex tubing (18 F). 4. Latex Foley catheter (14 F). 5. Portex tubing (12 F). 6. Polythene tubing (7/8 F). 7. Portex tubing (9 F). 8. Polythene tubing (4/5 F). 9. Portex tubing (6 F)

advocated by GUTTMANN (1954), who uses the most careful "no touch" technique. In spite of the utmost care, however, infection develops inevitably after a period of approximately ten days. Both on logical and practical grounds it is obvious that this particular method is not likely to succeed except as a temporary measure.

### ζ) Continuous urethral drainage

For some years this method has been practised at the Liverpool Regional Paraplegic Centre. It is believed by the writer and others working there that continuous drainage has certain obvious advantages when compared with other methods. At the same time it is necessary to point out that the usual Foley type of catheter, even if made of latex rubber, is unsuitable and should not be used. The lumen is of small size in relation to the overall diameter (Fig. 11) and there is a tendency for the balloon to collect calcium salts which flake off into the bladder on deflation. The surface sometimes becomes sticky on boiling and the necessity for frequent irrigation and changes of catheter introduces the risk of infection.

For these reasons long "catheter-tubes" made of fine polythene (the GIBBON catheter, Figs 12 and 13) have been used at the Liverpool centre for some years

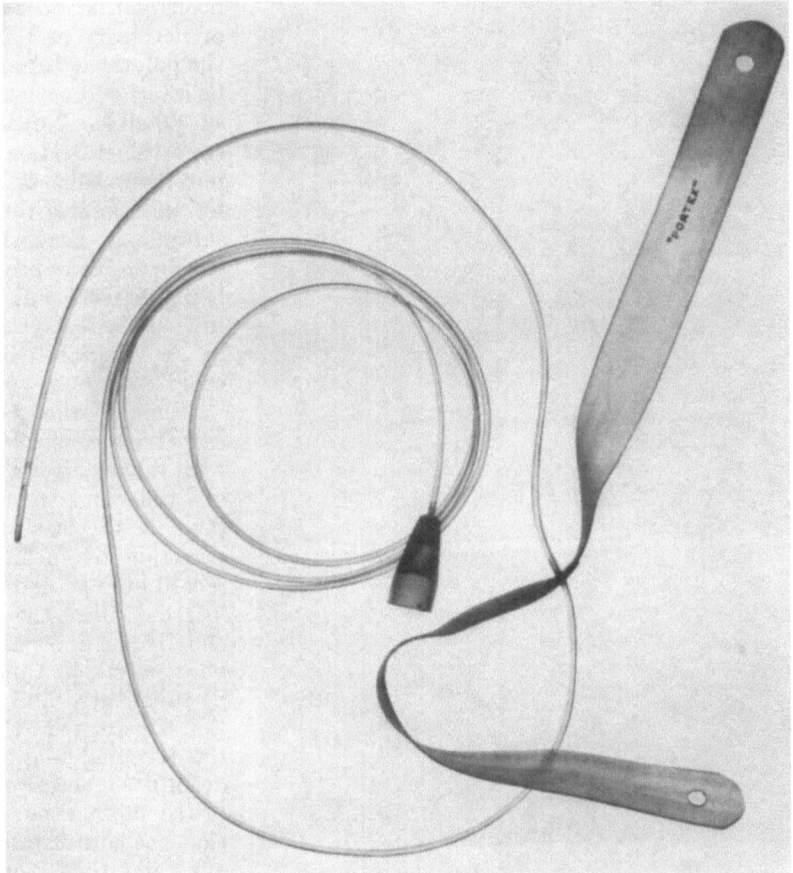

Fig. 12. GIBBON polythene catheter

(COSBIE ROSS, GIBBON & DAMANSKI 1957). The tubes possess the following advantages:

a) Urethritis is minimised or eliminated partly by the nature of the material, which is physically and chemically non-irritant, and also by the small calibre of the tube which has an overall diameter of 1.5 mm. or 2 mm.

b) Clinical urinary infection may be delayed for months and the urine remains sterile on culture for as long as a fortnight.

c) It is not necessary to change the catheter and drainage continues for many weeks with little interference. Cross-infection is eliminated and nursing-time saved.

d) Urethral pressure-sores and urethral fistulae are eliminated.

e) The tubing is extremely light so that there is little tendency for it to be displaced with the patient's frequent change of position. At the same time the tube is sufficiently rigid to resist compression and kinking.

f) The fact that there is a coil of tubing in the bladder cavity prevents difficulty arising in patients with quadriplegia who are so frequently troubled with priapism.

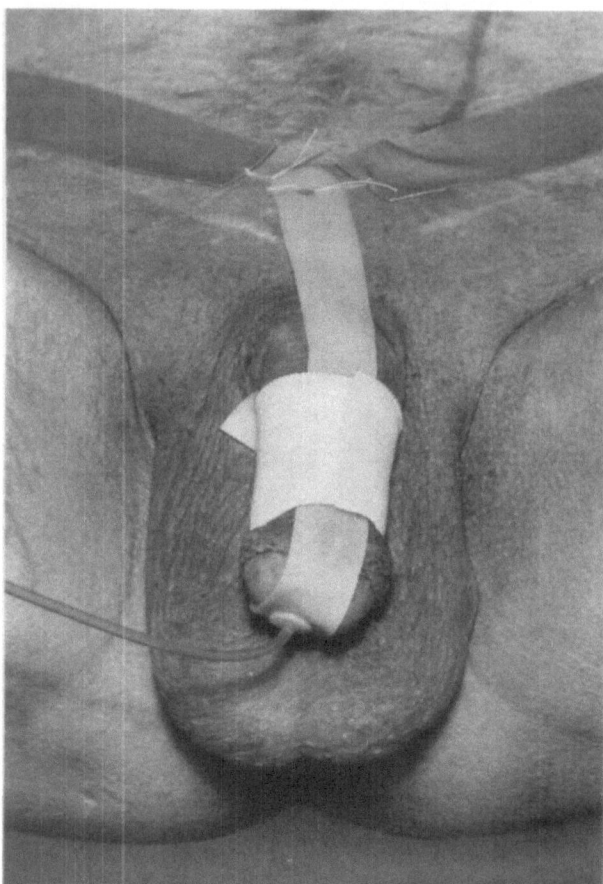

Fig. 13. Fine polythene catheter in use (GIBBON)

One of the great virtues of the method is that no irrigation is desirable or necessary and in fact the polythene tube should be interfered with as little as possible. Needless to say, the insertion of a polythene tube or catheter necessitates the most scrupulous attention to sterility, the procedure being carried out under full theatre technique in a special "bladder room".

Should the GIBBON catheter become blocked with mucus after a period of time it is usually possible to clear the obstruction by means of a record syringe and needle inserted into the distal end. If necessary, a larger bore polythene tube may be substituted and irrigation instituted through the terminal adaptor. If, despite the occasional use of chemotherapy, infection becomes established, a Foley-type catheter (No. 14 or 16) may be necessary in order to deal with accumulations of mucus by means of irrigation. It is often possible to return later to the fine plastic tube.

### d) Intermediate treatment

The initial stage of spinal shock is succeeded by the gradual return of uncontrolled reflex activity in those parts below the level of the neurological lesion. At this point bladder drainage is discontinued as soon as effective voiding develops, either by suprapubic expression or by detrusor contractions. Certain patterns of bladder function may be expected or deduced from the type and level of the lesion. For example (Ross, Gibbon & Damaski 1957):

1. In the cervical lesions, and as far down as the mid-dorsal region, the reflex arc is intact and therefore the detrusor muscle contracts strongly at a certain

point of bladder filling, a condition similar to the uninhibited voiding in infancy. A return of reflex activity is often suggested by the voiding of urine around a blocked catheter or polythen etube.

2. One of the most frequent injuries seen is in the dorsi-lumbar spine and, at this site, there is often a combination of upper and lower motor neurone lesions. The presence of the bulbocavernosus and anal reflexes indicates that the reflex arc is intact and that an automatic or reflex bladder may be expected.

3. Fractures or fracture-dislocations of the first, or lower lumbar vertebrae cause cauda equina lesions. All reflex activity below the lesion is permanently absent, including the bulbocavernosus and anal reflexes. Under these circumstances the patient must rely on abdominal straining and suprapubic pressure to empty the bladder. A compensating factor is that the lower the lesion the better are the abdominal muscles.

### e) Bladder training

Bladder training should begin when the reflex or automatic stage is reached (MUNRO 1952). The catheter is released at regular intervals by the clock with the object of training the detrusor and aiming at a bladder capable of retaining at least six ounces without reflex evacuation. After the catheter has been dispensed with, every effort should be made to achieve regular evacuations of the bladder (again by the clock) by control of fluid intake, which trains the sphincter. Micturition may be initiated by massaging the abdomen or by scratching the thigh, but the easiest method is for the patient to lift himself slightly in his chair, or, when confined to bed, by using the overhead bar and handle. No fluids should be given between 7 p.m. and 7 a.m. and drinks are given every hour during the remaining twelve hours, aiming at a three-hourly evacuation.

Bladder training is useless in the autonomous bladder and cannot be carried out in the stage of spinal shock or if the mass reflex is present. Other adverse factors include a suprapubic fistula, obstruction at the bladder neck, an over-stretched bladder and lack of co-operation on the part of the patient.

It is necessary for the bladder to be of the automatic type and of a reasonable capacity. Although suprapubic compression may be carried out by an attendant, it is obviously a great advantage if the patient has the use of his hands and can do this for himself. COMARR (1956) has devised an apparatus to assist the quadriplegic patient in this particular difficulty. It must be admitted, however, that some patients are not prepared to take the time and trouble necessary in bladder training, preferring to micturate into a two-chambered rubber urinal with a capacity of twenty-five ounces.

It is especially important to achieve an automatic bladder in females in view of the difficulty of wearing a urine-collecting apparatus. The only alternative is an expressible bladder.

### f) Final treatment

If satisfactory micturition is not achieved in spite of this careful and painstaking regime, a further search must be carried out to ascertain the cause. A high residual urine leads inevitably to persistent urinary infection, which may in time progress to renal failure and death.

Sometimes complete retention of urine persists but more often an automatic bladder is complicated by a high residual urine. An automatic bladder with an appreciable residual urine may be complicated by ureteric reflux, hydro-ureter and hydronephrosis with progressive renal deterioration. Severe degrees of infection, liable to lead to pyelonephritis and kidney damage, are also indications for further investigation and further measures. Incidentally, it is important that the specimen of urine for microscopy should be taken in the morning before the polyuria, induced by the forced diuresis, takes effect.

Similarly, the female patient who fails to achieve an expressible or well-trained reflex bladder obviously requires further measures.

Talbot (1957) has pointed out that it is usually the spastic bladder which proves troublesome and that the spastic bladder has certain characteristics. These include diminished capacity, raised intravesical pressure and repeated (and often ineffective) voiding efforts. He considers that following on, and directly due to the primary functional changes, there develop structural changes in the bladder such as hypertrophy and fibrosis of the wall and permanent diminution of capacity. The use of a catheter and urinary infection are contributory factors in causing spasticity of the bladder. Similarly, spasm of the muscles of the abdominal wall and lower limbs may cause increased intravesical pressure and sometimes stress incontinence. As Talbot says, it is extremely important to arrest the primary functional changes and to prevent irreversible structural developments taking place.

An appreciable number of patients with traumatic paraplegia require this reinvestigation and further measures, especially if those found to be progressing unsatisfactorily, or to have retrogressed, are included. The writer has found that approximately 25% of the paraplegic patients admitted to the Liverpool Regional Centre do not develop satisfactory bladder function as a result of the methods outlined above and consequently require some further procedure or procedures. In Talbot's (1954) series 22% failed to achieve adequate bladder emptying as a result of bladder drainage and bladder training. Comarr stated that only 20% were able to dispense with the catheter without further treatment. In such circumstances a complete reinvestigation and assessment are carried out, including cystometrogram, cysto-urethroscopy and cyso-urethrogram. In the writer's hands, the use of the cysto-urethrogram, carried out by the technique described by Damanski and Kerr (1957), has proved the most valuable single investigation. Expressed in the most simple terms the problem is to determine the ratio of the expulsive forces, that is detrusor contraction plus abdominal straining plus manual suprapubic compression against the resistance at the bladder neck. If the expulsive forces are efficient, and, in spite of this, the patient has a high residual urine, then there must be either a mechanical or spastic obstruction at the bladder neck or in the urethra. As a corollary to this, it is obvious that even if the expulsive forces are weak, satisfactory evacuation of the bladder may still be achieved by diminishing the degree of resistance at the bladder outlet (Cosbie Ross and Damanski 1953). This may be an over-simplification of the problem but the basic fact remains essentially correct. Many methods of dealing with such difficulties have been advocated during the last fifteen years but the writer has found the following four procedures of great value. These are:

1. Intrathecal alcohol block.
2. Resection of the bladder neck.
3. Pudendal neurectomy.
4. Division of the external sphincter.

Sometimes a single procedure is insufficient, possibly two, and in exceptional circumstances, three procedures are necessary before success is achieved. This is largely new ground and a certain element of trial and error is inevitable. However, at the present time the specific indications for the different procedures are becoming clearer and better defined.

It is also necessary, when it is impossible to halt progressive renal damage by any of the above procedures, to carry out a cutaneous ureterostomy or a transplant of the ureters into an ileal loop as a means of preserving the patient's life.

### α) Alcohol block

This procedure is advocated and practised by GUTTMANN (1954). As much as 5 to 10 cc. of alcohol are injected into the subarachnoid space, the larger doses only being permissable and safe in the event of there being evidence of a block of the cerebrospinal pathways. The method is used frequently because it is often necessary in patients with considerable spasticity of the skeletal muscles. This type of lesion is usually found in the higher or mid-thoracic injuries, but it is obvious that an alcohol block should only be given in complete lesions as the effect is indescriminate and destructive of neural tissues. As far as micturition is concerned the main object of giving an alcohol block is to obtain relaxation of the external sphincter muscle. There are certain disadvantages which include the following:

a) The effect of the alcohol is to damage neural tissue.

b) When the alcohol is given for skeletal spasticity it sometimes happens that the working of an efficient automatic bladder is disturbed by the abolition or diminution of detrusor contractions.

c) It has been contended that an alcohol block protects the upper urinary tract by reducing vesical hypertonicity. This is not supported by cystometric investigations of a large number of patients (GIBBON 1957).

Moreover the block is sometimes unsuccessful and it seems possible that it also abolishes erection and interferes with ejaculation.

In spite of these objections intrathecal alcohol block is a valuable therapeutic method in the correctly selected patient.

As an extension of this method may be mentioned MacCARTY'S (1954) "selective cordectomy", in which he removes the entire cord below the lesion in patients with a complete paraplegia, especially in those with high lesions. The purpose of this is to eliminate severe contractions of the lower limbs and to facilitate nursing care. EMMETT (1957) points out that, although this procedure inevitably converted an upper into a lower motor neurone lesion, subsequent micturition proved satisfactory, the bladder emptying every three to five hours with abdominal straining or manual expression or both. There was leakage of urine if the patient indulged in strenuous exercise with a full bladder. EMMETT attributes the fact that there is not a continuous leakage to passive resistance of the paralysed external sphincter and to the elasticity of the bladder neck*.

### β) Resection of the bladder neck

In 1945 EMMETT expressed the view that in spinal injuries the internal sphincter contracts simultaneously with the detrusor muscle, thus constituting an obstruction at the bladder neck to automatic micturition. For this reason he advocates bladder-neck resection in many of these patients. EMMETT (1957) states that the treatment of the lower motor neurone lesion is becoming exclusively resection of the bladder neck. He points out that nerve blocks and sections cannot hold out any hope of success in the lower motor neurone lesion because all nerves serving micturition are, by the very nature of the lesion, paralysed already, except in the rare mixed or incomplete injuries. The writer

---

* Recently, NATHAN (1959) and KELLY and GAUTIER-SMITH (1959) have reported satisfactory results in the treatment of spasticity, using 5% to 20% phenol in glycerol or myodil, given intrathecally, as an alternative to alcohol.

considers that it is possible to select patients suitable for resection by means of cysto-urethrography. If the technique described above is used it is sometimes possible to demonstrate a definite ledge or shelf at the bladder neck (Cosbie Ross 1951) (Fig. 9). It is this type of case which appears to respond best to resection. The writer resects about ten strips from five to eight o'clock using the Gershom-Thomson punch. At the Mayo Clinic it is the custom to resect the entire circumference of the bladder neck (Emmett 1957). It is not advisable to carry out an extensive resection as there is little thickness of tissue to be palpated between the resectoscope in the urethra and the finger in the rectum. It has been found unnecessary to resect around the clock from the point of view of the functional end-result and it is, moreover, possible to demonstrate radiologically that after the operation the shelf has disappeared and that the bladder neck is wide, shelving and unobstructed (Fig. 14).

On microscopic examination the strips resected consist of a mixture of muscular fibres and fibrous tissue, with the former preponderating. The fibrous tissue is probably of inflammatory origin and is responsible for the stiffness or induration so frequently observed at the bladder neck when passing a cystoscope. In the writer's series of 32 resections there were 20 successes and 12 failures.

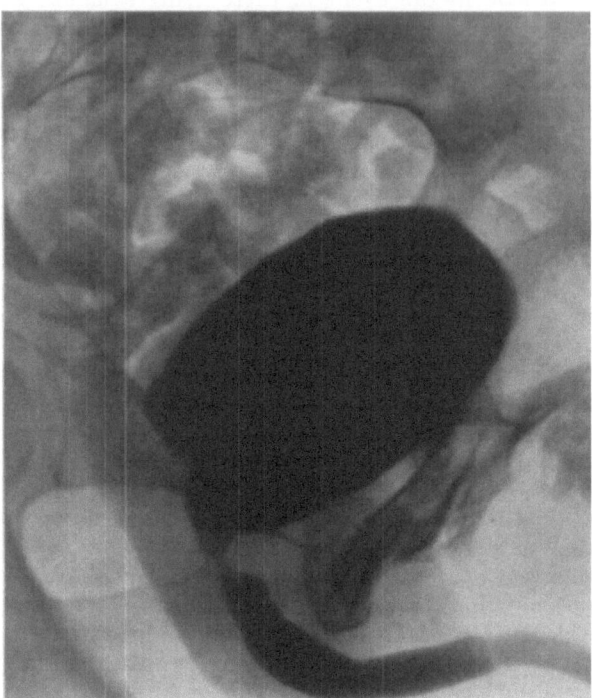

Fig. 14.   Cysto-urethrogram after resection of the posterior shelf (same case as Fig. 9)

It is, of course, possible to perform resection both in upper and lower motor neurone lesions (Cosbie Ross 1956).

### γ) Pudendal neurectomy

It may be, however, that investigation reveals the presence of a spastic obstruction of the external, or of both, sphincters. This is most clearly demonstrated by the cystourethrogram which reveals either an obstruction at the level of the external sphincter or complete closure of the whole length of the prostatic urethra. In such circumstances it is impossible to dilate the prostatic urethra by injection of opaque fluid from the external urinary meatus. This spastic obstruction is in the writers's opinion best treated by pudendal neurectomy (Cosbie Ross & Damanski 1953). At first the operation was confined to spastic obstruction at the external sphincter but its use was ultimately extended to those with spasm of both sphincters. It appears probable that motor impulses, carried by the pudendal nerve, supply the internal as well as the external sphincter, which explains the success in the latter group. Bors and others (1954) found striated muscle fibres at the bladder neck in nineteen out of twenty-one resections, the striated fibres being situated at 12 o'clock and not elsewhere in the circumference.

It is true that an intrathecal alcohol block may relax the sphincters but, at the same time, the injection adds a lower motor neurone lesion to the damage already present. The alcohol block also weakens detrusor contractions and, only too often, satisfactory automatic micturition has been temporarily or permanently suppressed by an alcohol injection given for spasticity of the skeletal muscles. Pudendal neurectomy is a more selective and more accurate procedure, the neural destruction being limited to a relatively unimportant nerve. The operation is indicated only in the upper motor neurone lesion and is more suitable for the automatic bladder. It is essential to ascertain that the reflex arc is intact and, in this connection, the following tests are of value:

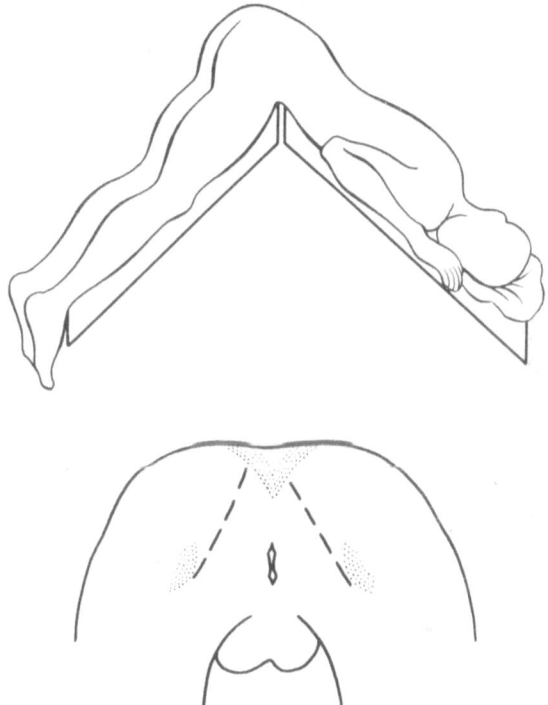

a) Bulbocavernosus test. A finger is placed on the perineum. If the glans penis is squeezed firmly, the examiner will feel the contraction of the bulbocavernosus (PURVES-STEWART 1945).

b) When a rectal examination is carried out, it is noted that the finger is tightly embraced, the "internal anal reflex" (MONRAD-KROHN 1948).

Fig. 15. Pudendal neurectomy. Position of the patient on the operating table and the incision in relation to bony landmarks. (From the British Journal of Urology)

c) A pin-prick in the perianal skin evinces a brisk contraction of the sphincter.

d) The presence of the tendo achilles reflex (COMARR 1957).

A possible objection to bilateral pudendal neurectomy is that erections are abolished, but as both erection and emission are reflex phenomena in this condition the loss is not great and the writer has encountered few patients, when the implications of the operation are explained to them, who made any objection.

## The operation (COSBIE ROSS & DAMANSKI 1953)

"The patient is placed on his face and the table angled at the pelvis so that the hips are flexed almost to a right angle (Fig. 15). An incision is made, starting at the border of the sacrum and running obliquely downwards and outwards over the outer part of the ischiorectal fossa. It is an advantage for the surgeon to stand on the contralateral side of the patient. Special care is necessary to prevent the incision encroaching on the tuber ischii as a scar in this position might lead to a subsequent pressure sore. The incision is deepened so that the operator is working on the inner aspect of the tuber ischii and the outer wall of the ischiorectal fossa. The neurovascular bundle is found in Alcock's canal at the upper limit of the ischiorectal fossa at a depth of approximately two to two and a half inches from the skin (Fig. 16). The pudendal nerve, arising from S2, 3 & 4 gives off the inferior haemorrhoidal branch in Alcock's canal, then dividing into the dorsal nerve of the penis and the perineal nerve, the artery lying between the two. The inferior haemorrhoidal nerve is usually found first and is a useful guide to the main nerve trunk. It is our present practice to trace the pudendal nerve to the edge of the sacrum and there divide it, resecting a short length. The greatest care is necessary to ensure that the entire nerve has been divided, because we believe that one of our failures was attributable to the fact that the nerve divided high up and an important branch had escaped division. Although the branch to the external anal sphincter is also divided this does not appear to matter in patients with spinal injuries. Bleeding points are dealt with by diathermy and the wound is sutured without drainage. A similar procedure is carried out on the opposite side. All wounds healed satisfactorily and by first intention in spite of the occasional proximity of unhealed pressure sores."

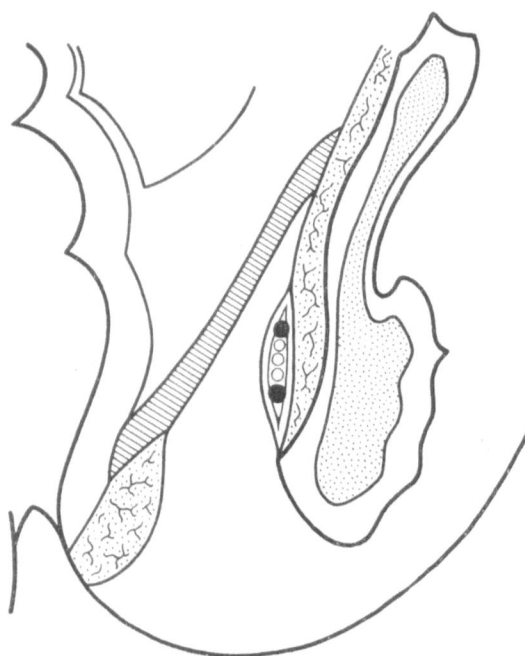

Fig. 16. Neurovascular bundle in Alcock's canal. (From the British Journal of Urology)

To emphasise the importance of making sure that the whole nerve has been divided it must be pointed out that BORS and COMARR (1954), in a series of fifty dissections, found a solitary trunk in sixteen, two branches in twentythree and three branches in eleven. If the cysto-urethrogram is repeated a few days after the operation, and compared with the earlier radiographs, it will be seen that the prostatic urethra is widely opened up, there is no obstruction at the external sphincter level, voiding occurs in a powerful stream and the residual urine is largely eliminated (Figs 17 & 18). Furthermore it is possible to dilate the prostatic urethra by injection of the opaque fluid from the external meatus.

Pudendal neurectomy is, then, a safe and reliable procedure in patients with a spastic obstruction. The operation puts considerably less strain on the patient than resection of the bladder neck.

### δ) Division of the external sphincter

Experience has shown that in spite of bladder training, alcohol block, resection of the bladder neck and pudendal neurectomy there remains a small group, a hard core, in which there is failure to achieve an efficient automatic

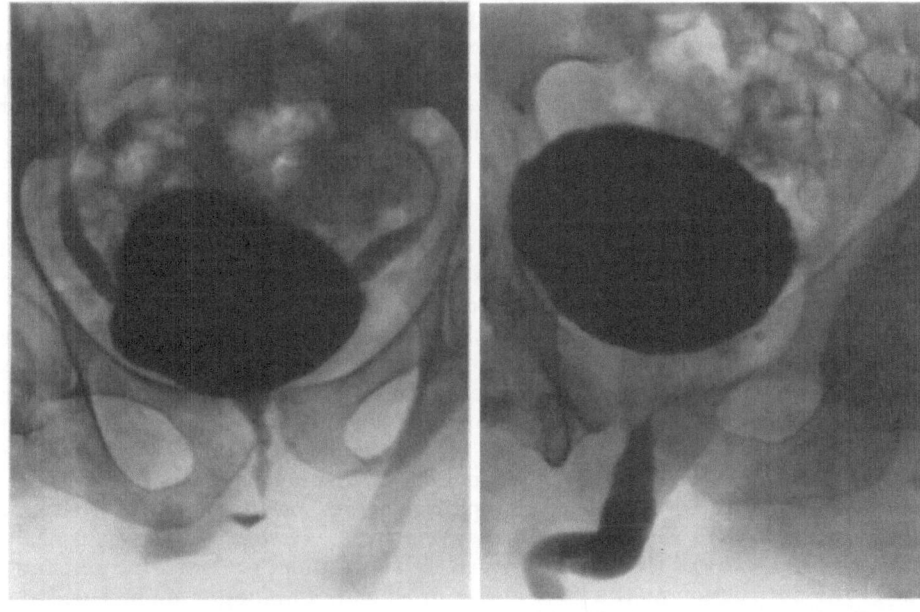

Fig. 17a and b. a Cysto-urethrogram (anteroposterior view) before pudendal neurectomy. Patient unable to pass opaque fluid on X-ray table despite filling with about 8 ozs. His usual residual urine was 10 to 14 ozs. Note the narrow trickle filling the posterior urethra when injecting fluid from the external meatus. b Oblique view, before pudendal neurectomy. Complete urinary retention: on attempts at voiding a few drops penetrated into the posterior urethra: there was also some ureteric reflux. (From the British Journal of Urology)

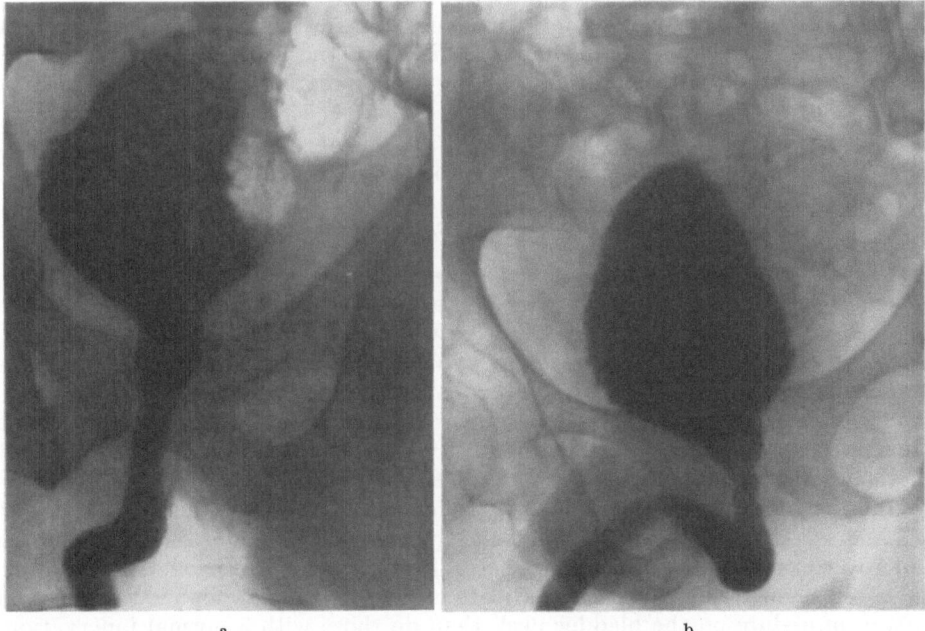

Fig. 18a and b. a Anteroposterior view, after pudendal neurectomy. Patient voiding opaque fluid in a powerful stream. Note the wide lumen of the posterior urethra. b Oblique view, after pudendal neurectomy. Patient voiding satisfactorily. The whole posterior urethra is widely open: the ureteric reflux has disappeared. (From the British Journal of Urology)

bladder because of an organic obstruction remaining at the external sphincter. This point is well illustrated in a recent paper by Bors (1956), in which he points out that 80% of patients with quadriplegia, still in hospital, remained on permanent catheter drainage. Quadriplegia presents an especially difficult problem because abdominal straining is weak or absent owing to loss of power in the abdominal muscles: also the patient may not be able to carry out supra-pubic compression. It is clear, therefore, that something must be done to avoid that counsel of despair, "catheter life". The view that the obstruction may be located at the external sphincter level was first suggested by Watkins (1936), who thought that the obstruction was due to deformity and lack of elasticity of the urogenital diaphragm. Cystographic studies by Damanski and Kerr (1957) in a large series of patients with paraplegia have confirmed that a persistent and troublesome obstruction in the region of the external sphincter does occur in a small percentage. The writer suggests that failure of pudendal neurectomy to relieve this condition is probably due to some degree of fibrosis in the sphincter muscle. The operation of division or resection of the external sphincter was described by the writer in 1956 and he believes that the procedure had not previously been used for this particular purpose (Cosbie Ross, Gibbon & Damanski 1957). The idea of dealing with the external sphincter surgically is not new as Donovan (1949) put forward the suggestion that extensive punching-out of the obstruction at the level of the urogenital diaphragm might be carried out. He did, however, add that he feared this would be followed by incontinence of urine.

It must be emphasised that division of the external sphincter should be reserved for the patient with chronic retention who has failed to respond to more orthodox methods, such as alcohol block, resection of the bladder neck and pudendal neurectomy. It is a method to be used to avoid the catheter life in these difficult patients. Frequent exacerbations of urinary infection, ureteric reflux, diverticulosis of the bladder and filling of the prostatic ducts on cysto-urethrography are all conditions making the operation even more necessary and urgent.

Contra-indications include advanced hydronephrosis and a gross urinary infection which cannot be, at least temporarily, controlled by chemotherapy.

### The operation

The cold punch has been used in the majority of patients, several strips being resected from the postero-lateral aspect of the external sphincter. In one patient the external sphincter was exposed and divided by an open perineal approach but without improvement. When the perurethral procedure was subsequently carried out on this patient a satisfactory result was obtained. On two occasions the external sphincter was divided by a Colling's knife through a urethroscope and it may well be that this will prove the safest and most efficient method. The resection may cause troublesome venous bleeding for which diathermy has not proved very effective. It has been the writer's practice to insert a large catheter (Ch. 24—26) immediately on completion of the resection in order to control the bleeding by pressure. Post-operative care is most important. It is well known that paraplegic patients usually develop a more severe reaction to any procedure on the bladder neck than do those with a normal innervation. This severe reaction is probably due to neurological changes affecting the contractability of the blood vessels and the bleeding time. A chronic urinary infection is also an adverse factor.

These adverse factors apply even more forcibly to the external sphincter area so that post-operative care is most important, continuous observation being necessary for several hours in order to prevent, or to deal quickly with, clot-retention. It is not always easy to decide if the bladder is distended owing to spasticity of the abdominal muscles. In such a case an increase or reappearance of autonomic hyperreflexia, (headache, feeling of throbbing, patchy redness of the skin above the level of the paralysis, congestion of the face, profuse sweating and cutis anserina) is a helpful sign of clot-retention.

Antibiotic prophylaxis is used before, and for a few days after, the operation. The large catheter is changed to Gibbon's polythene tube as soon as the gross haematuria has cleared. Biopsy of the resected strips have shown either infiltration of chronic inflammatory cells or inflammation and fibrosis.

*Addendum.* Since writing the above, further experience with this operation suggests that two posterolateral cuts with a Colling's knife are not usually followed by troublesome bleeding, provided the two areas to be divided are first dealt with by the coagulating diathermy current. This appears to be the safest method of dealing with the external sphincter.

## Results

Out of a series of ten patients the results were eminently satisfactory in eight. There were two deaths, one of which was due to a particularly heavy, and largely uncontrollable, preoperative urinary infection. The other had an advanced hydronephrosis with a paper-thin renal parenchyma. It is clear, now, that neither of these patients should have been subjected to this particular procedure and it would have been better to implant their ureters into a segregated ileal loop.

The eight successful patients all showed some degree of stress incontinence which, far from being harmful, proved beneficial. A urine-collecting appliance was worn and a penile clamp occasionally. The operation had converted a chronic retention to an easily expressible bladder. These eight individuals have been spared the "catheter life" and, possibly, subsequent damage to the upper urinary tract. Figs. 19 & 20 show the cysto-urethrogram before and after the procedure. It should be emphasized that the operation does not cause complete incontinence of urine. The studies of CAINE (1957) have shown that there is an elasticity of the tissues which helps to preserve continence even in the absence of any effective control by the external sphincter muscle. Similarly, LANG-WORTHY and others (1940), as a result of experimental studies, pointed out that a "collapsed" urethra offers a resistance to the escape of urine and prevents total incontinence even after section of sacral roots, sympathetic trunks and pudendal neurectomy.

LAPIDES and others (1957) believe that the smooth muscle of the bladder is directly under voluntary control, and that striated muscle is unnecessary during the act of micturition. It is also suggested that urinary continence is independent of the external sphincter.

LAPIDES (1958), in an experimental study carried out to investigate the anatomy and physiology of the internal sphincter, suggests that it is essentially a tubular structure consisting of smooth muscle and elastic tissue. He considers that the internal sphincter is synonymous with the female urethra and the male posterior urethra. His experiments further suggest that the internal sphincter prevents incontinence by virtue of the resistance it presents to urinary outflow, the resistance varying directly with the inherent tension of the urethral wall and length of the urethra, and inversely with the radius of the urethral lumen.

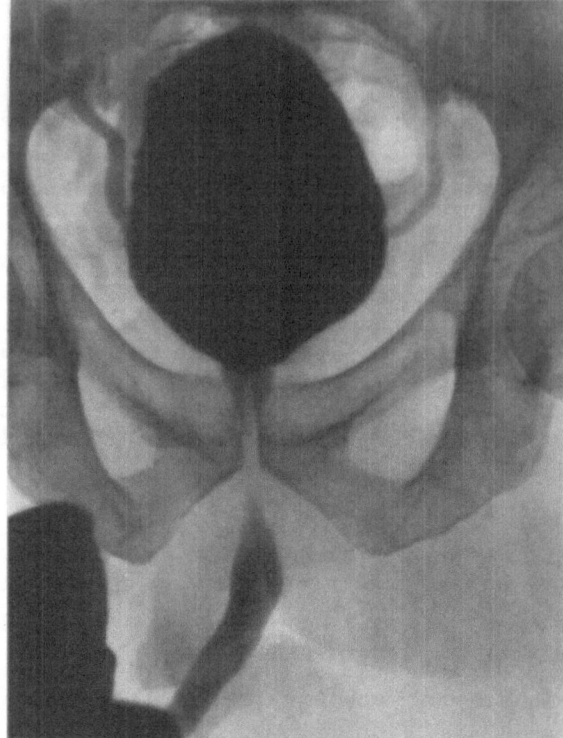

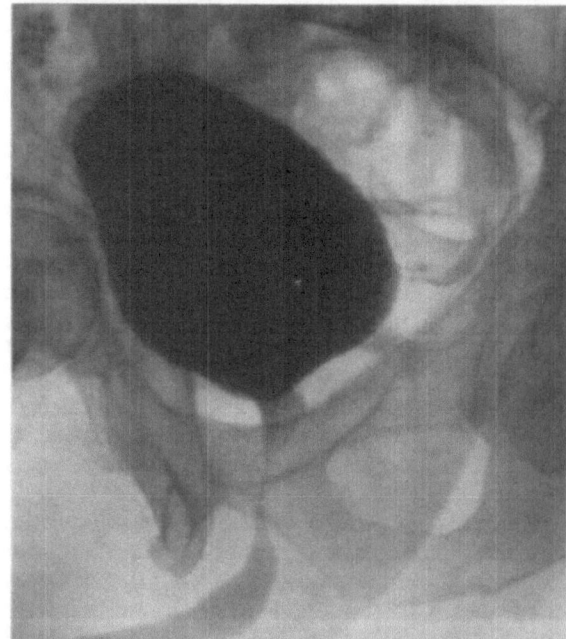

Fig. 19. Cysto-urethrogram before division of the external sphincter

## g) Treatment of non-traumatic lesions

The general principles of treatment of traumatic paraplegia apply (up to a point) to non-traumatic conditions affecting the central nervous system.

a) *Tabes dorsalis*. As it is the sensory part of the reflex arc which is defective in this condition the patient fails to appreciate the fact that his bladder is overfull. The most effective treatment is bladder drill, especial emphasis being laid on routine evacuation by the clock. On occasion, resection of the bladder neck may be necessary.

b) *Transverse myelitis*. There is no essential difference between this condition and a traumatic lesion, treatment being on similar lines.

c) *Disseminated sclerosis*. Bladder complications may be extremely troublesome, leading to a large residual urine or even to complete retention. The usual investigations are carried out and, according to the indications, a bladder-neck resection or a pudendal neurectomy is performed.

## h) Other methods of treatment

The methods outlined above are those advocated and practised by the writer but numerous other procedures have been advised over a period of years. These include:

### α) Various nerve blocks

Although some authors advise a preliminary procaine injection before undertaking operative procedures, MUNRO (1952) tends to rely on the injection alone and is opposed to destructive neural operations. In the troublesome condition of hyperactive detrusor, MUNRO advocates stretching the bladder wall and temporary denervation of the detrusor by injection of 5—10 ccs. of procaine into the sacral foramina, care being taken *not* to inject the third sacral segment simultaneously on both sides. The injection may have to be repeated on several occasions, the necessity for doing so being influenced by the cystometrogram. MUNRO points out that it should be possible to increase the bladder capacity, to flatten the curve of the basic tone, to diminish or eliminate the residual urine and to achieve more effective and better spaced detrusor contractions.

### β) Spinal root section

It has been suggested that sometimes a reflex bladder fails to develop because of a lack of satisfactory working of the reflex arc itself. It is envisaged that disorganised and conflicting stimuli, arising in the cord below the level of the lesion, affect the sacral centre. Workers holding this view (BRENDLER et al. 1953) advise a preliminary test of spinal anaesthesia at T10—12, or a sacral procaine block, in order to create a similar though temporary condition. If there is:

a) An increase of bladder capacity to 300 ccs.

b) Ability to void with moderate assistance.

c) A residual urine of less than 100 ccs.

d) No development of incontinence.

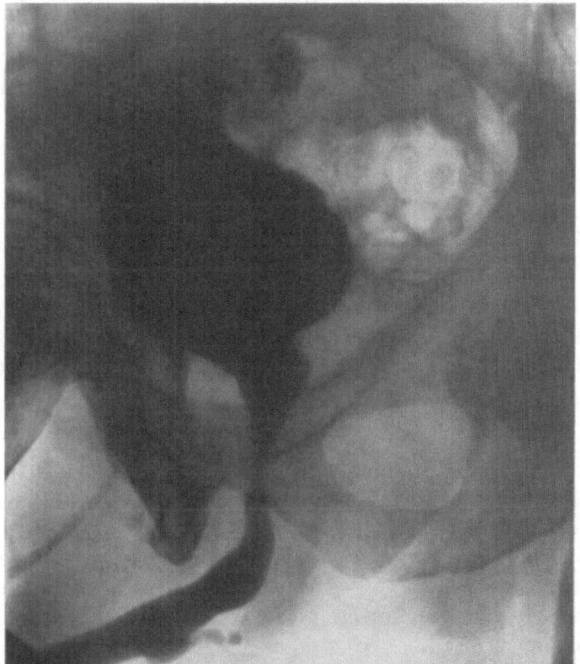

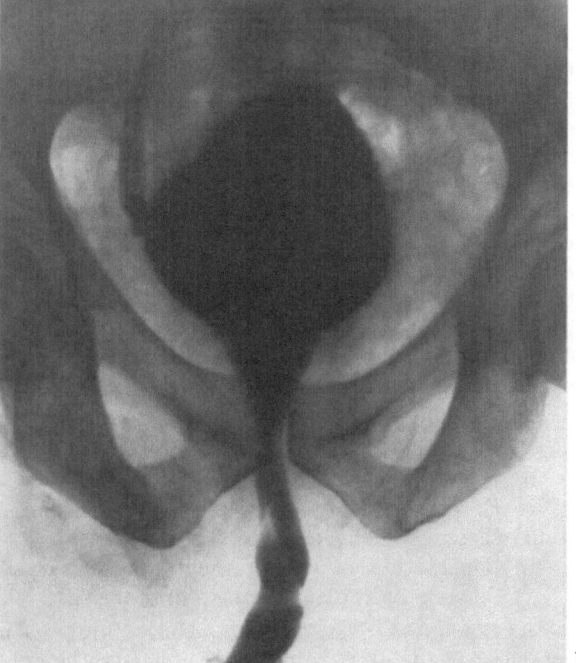

Fig. 20. Cysto-urethrogram after division of the external sphincter

then BRENDLER considers that rhizotomy is indicated. He divides both anterior and posterior roots from S1—S5 either alone or as part of a more extensive rhizotomy from T12 to S5. BRENDLER claims that the results of this procedure are satisfactory, but, out of twelve patients, no less than eight remained on catheter drainage. Meirowsky (1952) aims at dividing the correct number and distribution of sacral nerve roots to restore a "normal" balance to the bladder and the sphincters. The method can be used both in complete and incomplete lesions, care being taken not to divide roots likely to produce muscular weakness of the skeletal muscles; for example, division of the second sacral root causes some degree of weakness and division of the first sacral considerable muscular weakness.

### γ) Denervation of the bladder

If this procedure, i.e. division of the nervi erigentes or pelvic nerves could be carried out accurately and effectively it might be possible to overcome all spasticity of the internal sphincter and detrusor. It is not, however, a standardised surgical procedure at present (Leadbetter and others 1955).

### δ) Division of the anterior commissure

In 1954 Bors and his co-workers reported finding striated muscle fibres at the bladder neck in nineteen out of twenty-one resections, the interesting fact being that the striated muscle fibres were found only at 12 o'clock (at the anterior commissure) and not at any other part of the circumference. It would seem, therefore, that in cases of persistent spasticity of the internal sphincter, a myotomy of the striated muscle at 12 o'clock should also be carried out when a resection is performed.

### ε) Various neurectomies

In carrying out experiments on spasticity Abramson (1953) found, by means of the electromyograph, that the pelvic floor relaxes before the detrusor contracts. In spasticity associated with an upper motor neurone lesion he observed that the spastic condition extended also to the muscles of the pelvic floor as well as to the external sphincter. Similarly, in the lower motor neurone lesion, in which the muscles of the pelvic floor are denervated, there is little resistance to micturition which can be efficiently performed by assisting the act by means of suprapubic pressure. As a result of these studies it appears clear that spasticity of the muscles of the pelvic floor is a factor which has not been sufficiently considered and assessed up to the present time. Support is given to this view by the ciné films of normal micturition, shown by Caine & Edwards (1957), in which the base of the bladder is clearly seen to descend as the detrusor muscle contracts. Similarly, Hinman et al. (1954) state that by means of cineradiography and serial radiography they have demonstrated this sequence of events in nulliparous females:

    a) Isometric detrusor contractions and opening of the internal sphincter.
    b) Relaxation of the perineal muscles.
    c) Emptying contractions of the detrusor.
    d) Closure of the external sphincter.
    e) Contraction of the perineal muscles and elevation of the bladder base.
    f) Closure of the internal sphincter with relaxation of the detrusor.

Abramson & Hirschberg (1952) further suggest that the motor effects resulting from interference with muscular contraction, whether by neurectomy or tenotomy or by ankylosis or amputation, are not the only factors which account for the relief of spasticity. It is possible that the sensory effect is at least of equal importance. It is suggested that sensory stimuli occur in the muscle itself, either by stretch, or by what would be appreciated by a normal individual as cramp, and this constant flow of afferent impulses tends to perpetuate and enhance the spasticity. These afferent impulses may be eliminated, or at least diminished, by such operations as tenotomy and obturator neurectomy. BORS and COMARR (1953) have observed bladder function to return in one patient after division of the obturator nerve; they agree that contraction of the pelvic floor, which

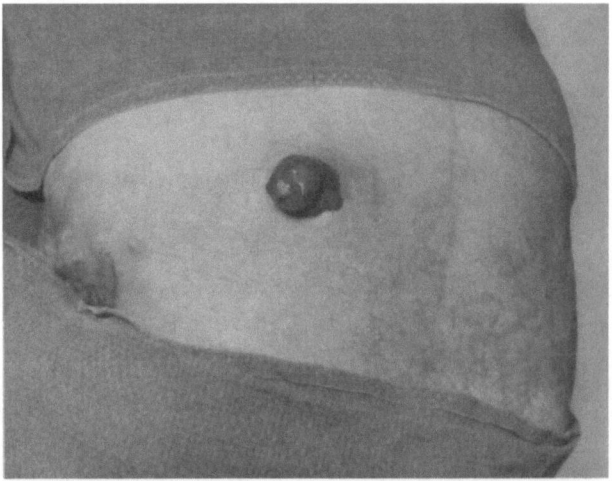

may help to prevent automatic micturition, possibly arises from any spastic muscle in the body.

DAMANSKI (1957) has noted that on several occasions, in an upper motor neurone lesion, that the bulbocavernosus and anal reflexes may be present a short time after the injury in spite of the fact that the legs are flaccid. In such cases both sphincters are closed, thus explaining why the bladder is not expressible. It may well be that the beneficial results after division of the external sphincter muscle are not altogether due to a direct attack on an obstructive factor but are also due to a diminution of afferent impulses from a spastic muscle, largely immobilized by means of a myotomy.

BORS has carried this concept a step further. He attempts to abolish sensory impulses by the injection of local anaesthetic solutions into the bladder and by pudendal

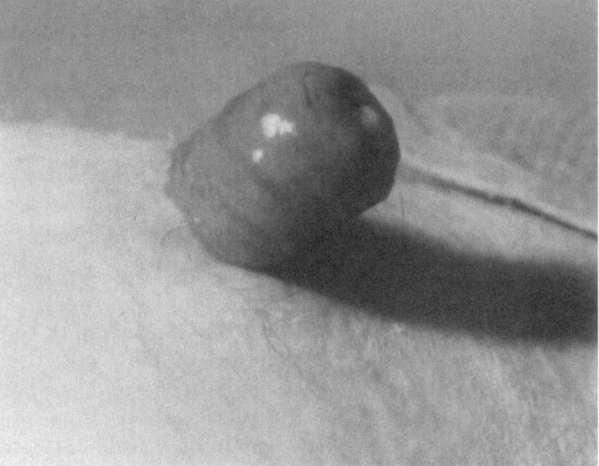

Fig. 21. Implantation of the ureters into a segregated ileal loop

and sacral nerve blocks. He considers that, if this procedure is repeated on several occasions, the spasticity may disappear, automatic micturition becoming possible.

CIFUENTES and YOUNGER (1952 and 1958) consider that presacral and hypogastric neurectomy is of value in the neurogenic bladder, especially if there is an open or funnel-shaped bladder neck.

### ζ) Urinary diversion

With the increasing knowledge of this condition, and the greater efficiency of its treatment, diversion of the urine is becoming less necessary and is only now performed in the exceptional case. In the patient with an intractable obstruction at the external sphincter level it is not safe or wise to attempt division of the sphincter if the renal function is poor. Under such circumstances the implanting of the ureters into a segregated loop of ileum may be a life-saving measure, possibly preventing further renal damage (Fig. 21). Alternately, a cutaneous nipple ureterostomy may be fashioned, bringing the ureters through jug-handle grafts which have been prepared three weeks previously (see Fig 22).

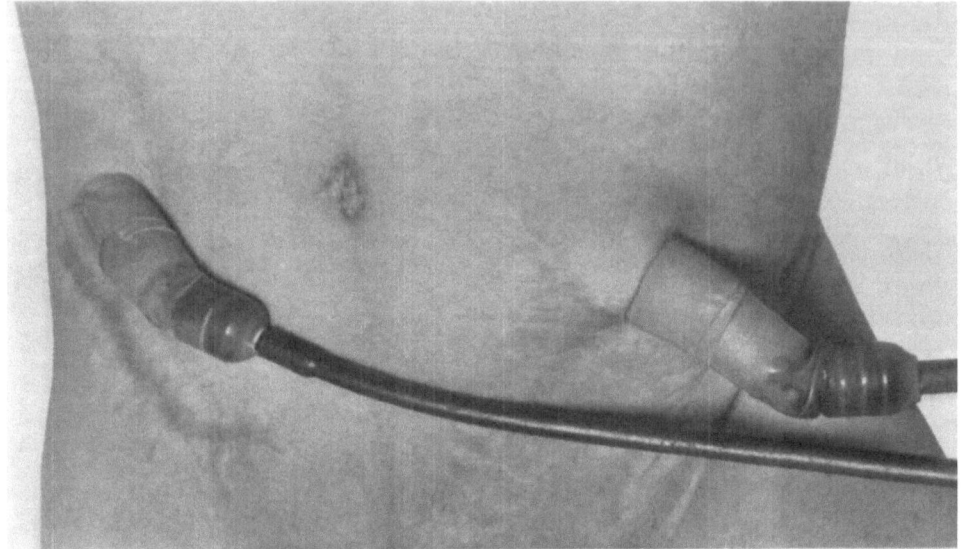

Fig. 22. Bilateral nipple or 'spout', ureterostomy

### η) Other methods

It is possible that some form of sling operation would be of benefit to the patient with a constant dribbling incontinence. These patients, as a rule, wear a rubber urinal during the day but it is a great convenience to them if they can enjoy a short period, sufficient to shave and dress, after getting out of bed.

MAY of Munich (1950) has recently described an operation in which he sutures the inner half of the rectus abdominus muscle to the bladder wall. He claims satisfactory results which he thinks may be due to "neurotisation" of the paralysed bladder musculature from the normal rectus.

## 4. General prognosis

GUTTMANN (1954), in discussing 1000 patients treated at the Stoke Mandeville centre over a period of ten years, pointed out that the death rate for cases of traumatic paraplegia arising from World-War II was still under 10%, the survivors having already lived from nine to fourteen years following their injury. This figure compares very favourably with the 80% mortality rate after the first World War. The death rate for nontraumatic cases was considerably lower, i.e. 3.6%. The prognosis is satisfactory in view of the fact that many of these patients receive other severe injuries in addition to the traumatic paraplegia. It has been suggested by SPURLING (1948) that some of these patients now have a chance of living their normal life-span. The most serious threat to the survival of the paraplegic is progressive damage or deterioration of the upper urinary tract, on this factor depending the long-term prognosis. Relatively long-term surveys of this type have been carried out in the United States by TALBOT and BUNTS (1949), TALBOT & LYONS (1950), and HUTCH and BUNTS (1951). The result of these surveys has suggested that whereas infection and dilatation of the upper urinary tract and stone formation reach their peak within the first two years, loss of renal function, as judged by intravenous pyelography, becomes more common after the third year. Nephrostomy and ureterostomy have frequently been necessary in their series of patients to arrest renal deterioration; plastic operations have been performed upon the lower end of the ureter (HUTCH 1952) in an attempt to restore valvular action.

DAMANSKI & GIBBON (1956), in reviewing patients treated at the Liverpool Regional Paraplegic Centre, found that one third had developed hydronephrosis. They go on to say, "We have also shown that stone formation, an important factor in the mortality rate, is largely preventable and that dilatation of the upper urinary tracts is reversible at least in the early stages. We believe, therefore, that if paraplegics are to benefit to the full from the advantages offered by the spinal injuries centres, two conditions must be fulfilled. First, delay in admission must be reduced to the minimum. Ideally the patient should be transferred as soon as he is fit to travel. Whatever increase might be necessary in the number of beds available would be temporary, as the turn-over would soon be increased two-fold or three-fold. Secondly, it is clear that the paraplegic must be followed up at least as carefully as the case of vesical papillomatosis, in whom also the clinical features lag far behind the pathological changes. The follow-up investigations should be done at the regional centre where a few beds should always be available for the purpose. Deterioration in bladder function, hypertonia, trabeculation and ureteric reflux indicate the need for special care. There is a natural reluctance on the part of some of the patients, especially those in full employment, to return sometimes over a long distance for a routine checkup when everything appears to be going well. It is our duty to impress on them all before their discharge that their chance of survival may well depend on their willingness to co-operate whole-heartedly in their follow-up examinations. Finally there are certain cases in which renal function deteriorates progressively. Sometimes this is due to failure to establish an efficient bladder mechanism. Occasionally one or both kidneys may fail despite apparently good bladder function or in spite of prolonged bladder drainage. It may be that some of these patients could be saved by ureterostomy or even nephrostomy and that such operations should be performed more frequently than has been the practice in the past."

It is clear, then, that the important factors in deciding the prognosis include early admission to a special centre and the establishment of an effective bladder-emptying mechanism with a minimal residual urine. In spite of these criteria being attained regular follow-up investigations are necessary for the rest of the patient's life to detect and to deal with early signs of renal deterioration. It is obvious, also, that the prognosis immediately becomes infinitely worse if it is necessary for the patient to continue with an indwelling catheter permanently. No effort should be spared to avoid this most undesirable outcome. Incidentally the level of the lesion does not appear to exercise a great effect on the incidence of urinary complications. The only exception to this is the fact that reflux is more common in the high than in the low lesion. This has been pointed out by BORS & COMARR (1952) who attributed the high incidence of reflux in high

lesions to loss of sympathetic innervation of the trigone and hypertonia. DA-
MANSKI & GIBBON (1956) refer to the difference in the incidence of reflux in the
high and the low lesions. They consider that hypertonia, although a common
finding in cases of reflux, and a possible cause, does not account for this difference of incidence.

The whole question of prognosis is closely bound up with the complications
which are dealt with in the next section.

In conclusion, although a great deal of laborious investigation and careful
clinical research remains to be done in this distressing condition, already much
has been achieved in rehabilitating these unfortunate patients, making it possible
for them to take their place in the community and for them to live comfortable
and relatively happy lives.

## 5. Complications

The complications are numerous but undoubtedly the two most menacing
ones are infection and hydronephrosis, with or without hydroureter. Such
conditions as pressure sores and osteomyelitis are not dealt with here.

### a) Infection

Urinary infection has proved to be the most intractable and persistent
complication. It seems almost impossible to keep the urine permanently sterile
and there always appear to be a few pus cells and stray bacteria present on
microscopy. The route of the infection is interesting because in many cases
reflux cannot be demonstrated; hence the pathway in these cases must be
either by the blood stream or by the lymphatics. The early period of catheterisation appears to initiate the complication which may be perpetuated by a residual
urine. The first factor may be rendered considerably less dangerous by the
use of the Gibbon polythene tube-catheter which not only constitutes a closed
system but also remains in situ for weeks if necessary, without requiring changing
or bladder irrigation (see section on initial treatment).

The second factor must be dealt with by the elimination of residual urine
and of all obstructive factors. As a routine measure, and one which must be
continued indefinitely, the patient should drink at least six pints of fluid during
the twenty-four hours. During an acute attack of infection, treatment consists
of chemotherapy according to the sensitivity of the organisms concerned. It
is not, however, a sound practice to continue urinary antiseptics during the
quiescent periods, reliance being placed then on forced diuresis.

Finally, all authorities agree that the general condition of the patient is of
great importance in this respect, especially with regard to the elimination of
pressure sores, concerning which the experimental studies of DAVID (1921) are
of interest. Similar organisms were found in pressure sores and in the urine
following the introduction of B. coli into the bladders of dogs.

### b) Urinary calculi formation

FLOCKS (1946) has pointed out the three important and known aetiological
factors i.e. infection, stasis (due to recumbency) and hypercalciuria. PRATHER
(1953) stated that the "combination of renal calculi and renal infection is the
great enemy of recovery in those who have suffered spinal cord injury". This
opinion, however, requires some modification today. Renal infection remains
a menace but renal calculus has become of considerably less importance. The
incidence of renal calculus has declined from 12% (1945—1950) to 1% (1950 to

1955) according to COMARR (1955). As a result of limiting infection by forced diuresis, early mobilisation of the patient and the elimination of residual urine, the formation of urinary calculi has diminished considerably. An additional safeguard is to keep the urine acid and it has been shown that, if the urine can be kept at a pH of approximately 6, stone formation is unlikely as calculi found in paraplegics are usually of the alkaline type. For this purpose acid sodium phosphate or ammonium chloride may be given, but TALBOT (1953) finds cranberry juice is as effective and better tolerated. It appears possible that stone formation might be virtually eliminated if all paraplegics were admitted promptly to a spinal unit (DAMANSKI & GIBBON 1956). An interesting fact has been pointed out by COMARR (1955) that renal calculi are more frequently encountered in patients with a lower motor neurone lesion and are also more frequent in complete neurological transections. At the same time it must be emphasised that stones in the kidney may develop with extreme rapidity, necessitating a routine review at regular intervals, especially as there may be no clinical indications of their presence apart from recurrent bouts of pyrexia. The stones are often pultaceous in consistence and may not show easily on the radiograph. There is no doubt if renal calculi are present the prognosis is made correspondingly more grave. Prophylactic measures have been indicated elsewhere. It is important to preserve renal tissue and a conservative approach to this problem is necessary in the paraplegic patient. A nephrectomy should only be performed as a last resort and as a life-saving measure; it is wise to avoid operation until the patient is ambulatory. It is necessary to remove stones under the following circumstances:

a) A renal calculus obstructing the pelvis and causing hydronephrosis.

b) A ureteric calculus, impacted and causing obstruction.

c) All vesical calculi (by lithotrity).

It is not necessary to remove a small stone impacted in a calyx. Following the removal of multiple stones it is advisable to irrigate the kidney pelvis with Suby's solution through a TRESIDDER nephrostomy tube (1957).

### c) Hydronephrosis and hydro-ureter

Hydronephrosis still constitutes a formidable problem and DAMANSKI and GIBBON (1956) found it to be present in a third of the group of patients whom they kept under review for a number of years. Hydronephrosis, which is usually accompanied by, and often preceded by hydro-ureter, may develop as early as two months or as late as eight and a half years after the injury. Generally, however, the condition first appears, if it is going to appear, within the first three years after the original spinal injury. Various authors have recorded a high incidence of hypertonia and trabeculation. Hydronephrosis is important, not only on account of the possibility of a progressive renal failure, but also because it has been found that the slightest degree of dilatation of the ureters and kidneys seems to be sufficient to prevent more than a temporary sterilisation of the urine in spite of antibiotics (COSBIE ROSS, GIBBON & DAMANSKI 1957).

Of the series reported by DAMANSKI and GIBBON (1956) approximately one third were unilateral and two-thirds bilateral. The seriousness of the condition is emphasised by the fact that nine of the bilateral cases eventually died of uraemia and two others remained in a state of nitrogen-retention. On the other hand 50% of these patients with hydronephrosis improved under treatment, but, when kept under review for a period of years, a high incidence of relapse

was found. Warning signs of an impending hydronephrosis are deterioration
of bladder function, hypertonia, trabeculation and ureteric reflux. A study
of the patients emphasises the extraordinary lability of the upper urinary tracts
in the paraplegic. A hydronephrosis may develop without obvious cause and,
in other cases, remarkable recoveries may take place. HUTCH (1957) asks "why
may a person who sustains a transection of his spinal cord develop hydroureter
and hydronephrosis and die in uraemia ?". He believes that the numerous,
powerful and erratic nervous impulses arising in the distal stump of the spinal
cord are fundamentally responsible because they cause the bladder to become

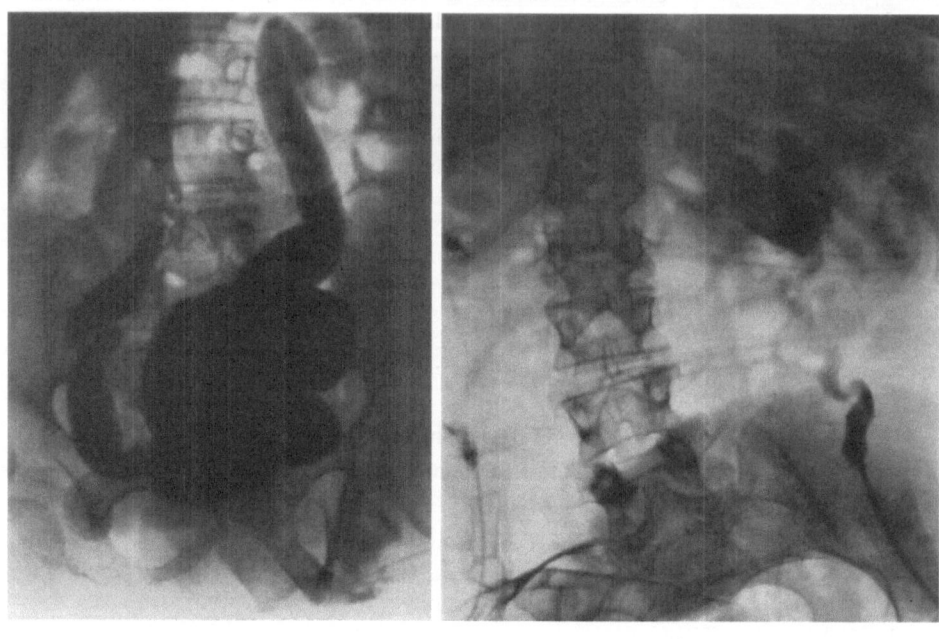

a                                                   b

Fig. 23 a and b. a Cystogram before bilateral ureterostomy. Bilateral ureteric reflux with gross dilatation.
b Retrograde pyelogram fourteen months after ureterostomy showing reduction in ureteric dilatation. (From
the British Journal of Urology)

contracted and trabeculated, resulting in sacculation of the bladder wall at the
site of the intramural ureter. As a result of these two factors, i.e. small capacity
spastic bladder and sacculation, hydro-ureter and hydronephrosis develop.
Hence HUTCH advises sacral rhizotomy of the 2nd, 3rd & 4th nerves (both
anterior and posterior roots) and has shown an increase in bladder capacity
and a diminution of the hydronephrosis; in some complete lesions the distal
stump of the cord was removed.

If the hydronephrosis is progressive, and fails to respond to measures ensuring
efficient bladder-emptying, it is clearly necessary to carry out diversion of the
urine into a segregated ileal loop (Fig. 21), or by means of a nipple ureterostomy
(Fig. 22). The radiograph in Fig. 23 a shows a preoperative cystogram exhibiting
ureteric reflux, with gross dilatation. Fig. 23 b is a retrograde pyelogram fourteen
months after nipple nephrostomy, showing reduction in ureteric distension.
YATES-BELL (1949) advocates a course of pituitrin in cases of hydronephrosis
without organic obstruction in paraplegia. The course consists of $1/_2$ cc. of
pituitrin intramuscularly each day for two weeks, $1/_2$ cc. on alternate days for two

weeks and a maintenance dose of $^1/_2$ cc. once a week for six weeks. He considers that improvement in the appearance of the pyelogram can be achieved in certain patients.

### d) Ureteric reflux

In the series of patients mentioned above (DAMANSKI & GIBBON 1956) reflux was observed in approximately one-fifth of the cases. While there is little doubt that backflow is harmful to the upper urinary tract, the actual relationship is far from clear. Of all the complications associated with the paraplegic bladder there is none concerning which further research is more necessary. The essential problem lies in the fact that although a high intravesical pressure may exaggerate the effects of reflux, backflow may develop during free drainage of the bladder.

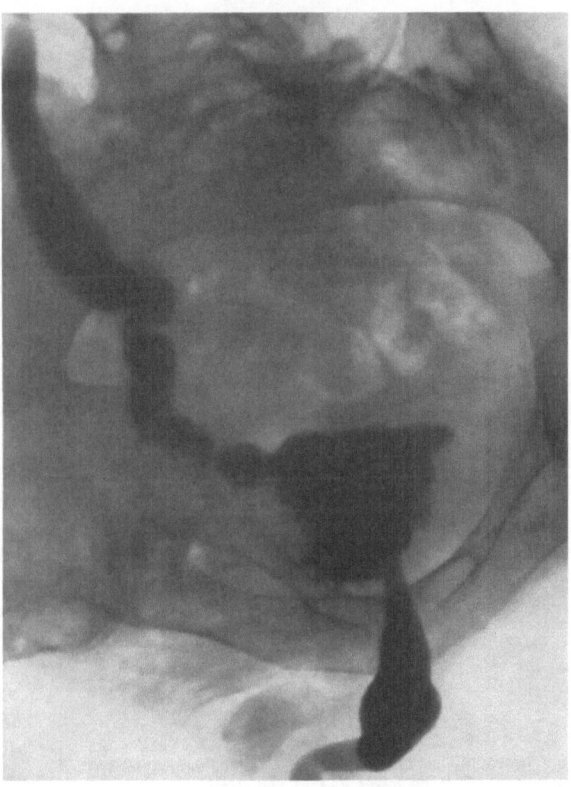

Fig. 24. Radiograph showing a saccule at the lower end of the ureter

HUTCH (1952) has suggested that the saccule, sometimes seen at the lower end of the ureter (Fig. 24), tends to destroy the valvular action. HUTCH has also described a constriction in the same situation (Fig. 25) but the writer has not found that either the saccule or the constriction causes any obstruction to the passage of a ureteric catheter. The obstruction appears to be functional and not organic. HUTCH (1957) writes "I believe basically, that both reflux and obstruction at the ureterovesical junction are the result of the same defect and this defect is the extravesicalization of the intravesical ureter. I also believe that the escape of the intravesical ureter into the extravesical space may be brought about by many different diseases of the bladder wall. In those diseases in which the bladder wall is very trabeculated such as the upper motor neurone paraplegic or a patient with obstruction to his urinary stream at or below the bladder neck, a discrete saccule will form around the intravesical ureter thus allowing it to fall into an extravesical position. In those conditions in which the bladder is flaccid rather than spastic I believe that a general thinning of the bladder wall occurs in such a way that the oblique course of the ureter through the bladder wall cannot be supported. In either event there occurs an extravesicalization of the intravesical ureter. This defect may allow reflux to occur because there is no longer any firm bladder wall for the intravesical ureter to be compressed against as the bladder fills. In the same manner the same defect may produce obstruction in the lower ureter because the intravesical segment has no circular fibres in its wall and is incapable of conveying peristalsis therefore, if this segment of ureter becomes part of the extravesical ureter it serves as a functional obstruction to the flow of urine from the ureter into the bladder.

I believe that the best way to deal with this condition is by some procedure which will effectively correct the disease of the bladder wall. If disease of the bladder wall is due to obstruction at or below the bladder neck the relief of this obstruction often results in a reduction in vesical trabeculation and a spontaneous repair of the damage at the ureterovesical junction. In paraplegics where the vesical trabeculation is the result of impulses reaching the bladder wall from the distal stump of the spinal cord, cutting these sacral nerves which convey this impulse will free the bladder and allow it to return once again towards normal. Some of the most dramatic results in the treatment of hydro-ureter and hydro-nephrosis in paraplegics have been brought about in this manner by cutting the sacral nerves. In the event that the disease in the bladder wall is not amenable to any correction by any procedures we know to-day, such as bladder flaccidity or in those cases in which the spastic bladder has been treated and a reflux and hydro-ureter persists then we must try a plastic

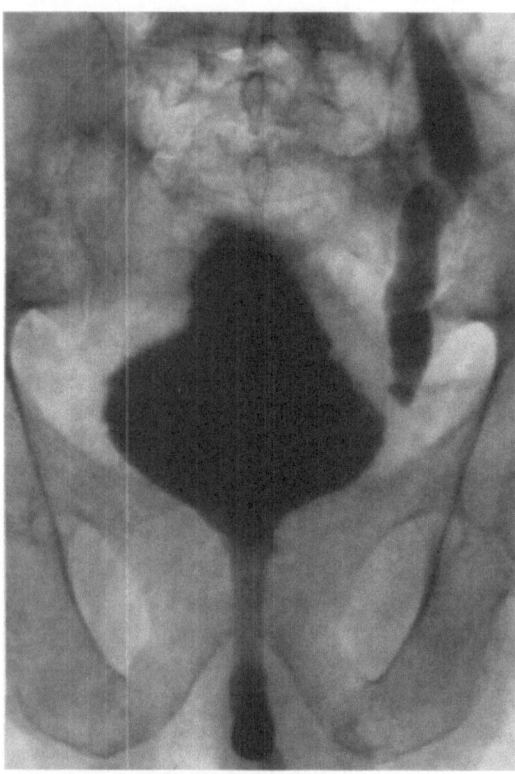

Fig. 25. Radiograph showing the "pseudo-constriction" at the lower end of the ureter

operation designed to bring the intravesical ureter back into its normal position such as the operation I outlined for reflux in 1952."

In support of his views HUTCH (1955) reported a detailed study of the ureterovesical junction in two stillborn infants with complete atresia of the urethra, trabeculation of the bladder, hydro-ureter and hydronephrosis. It was shown that there was a herniation of the bladder mucosa through a defect in the bladder wall where the bladder was penetrated by the ureter. It was further demonstrated that the intravesical ureter had been displaced into this herniation.

TALBOT (1953) suggests that the pan-ureteritis may be a factor in the causation of reflux. Reflux is a condition which may develop without any obvious reason and may as mysteriously disappear. Again, it is possible for reflux to exist for a considerable time (in fact indefinitely) without causing any damage to the upper urinary tract. This, however, is rather the exception than the rule. In view of these facts it is clear that reflux, in itself, does not necessitate drastic measures but only if it is causing damage to the upper urinary tract.

If there is merely retrograde filling of the lower third of the ureter, operative measures are not necessary, and such patients do not necessarily show any sign of renal deterioration over a period of years. In view of the association of reflux with hypertonia and trabeculation it is important to ensure that the bladder is easily expressible or that there is an efficient automatic bladder without an appreciable residual urine. Figs. 17 and 18 show the disappearance of reflux following pudendal neurectomy carried out for this purpose.

HUTCH (1952) has described a plastic operation on the lower end of the ureter to correct reflux. TALBOT (1953) advocates cutaneous ureterostomy but only when there is evidence that the reflux is causing some renal damage.

### e) Renal failure without hydronephrosis

This condition is by no means infrequent and in the twenty-five deaths due to traumatic paraplegia recorded by REINGOLD (1953) in no less than six was death due to pyelonephritis. DAMANSKI and GIBBON (1956) record five cases of pyelonephritis in their long-term survey. All five developed within three years of injury and there was often hydronephrosis on the contralateral side. Reflux was observed in two of DAMANSKI & GIBBON's series. Although many patients with pyelonephritis eventually succumb to uraemia recovery of renal function may occur and did so in two of the five patients mentioned above, which illustrates the vital importance of following up and constantly reassessing these patients; at the same time, it emphasises the difficulties of giving an accurate prognosis.

### f) Amyloid disease

This is an infrequent complication but occasionally develops in patients with deep-seated and intractable pressure sores or chronic suppuration elsewhere, especially in bone. Amyloidosis is often associated with suppurative pyelonephritis but there is some doubt as to which is the primary condition. Deposits of amyloid tissue are found both in the glomerular tufts and in the interstitial tissue of the kidney. Deposits are also found in the liver, spleen, pancreas and adrenal glands. The Congo-red test is positive and there is a heavy albuminuria with consequent hypoproteinaemia. The albumen-globulin ratio may be reversed.

### g) Urethral complications

Periurethral abscess and urethral fistula are occasional complications but are less frequent now than formerly. GRIFFITHS (1956) reported twenty-three cases of urethral fistula admitted over a period of years to Stoke Mandeville, dividing them into fistulae arising from intra-urethral causes and those due to extra-urethral pressure from the edge of a urinal or a hard mattress. The former condition is, of course, almost always due to an indwelling catheter, especially if a large and stiff catheter is used, the catheter causing a pressure-sore frequently situated at the peno-scrotal junction. The writer believes that the use of the fine GIBBON polythene catheter will eventually eliminate urethral complications. At the Liverpool Regional paraplegic centre few urethral troubles have been encountered since the use of the GIBBON catheter. As with urethral fistulae in non-paraplegic subjects, those in the bulbous urethra tend to heal spontaneously; on the other hand fistulae at the peno-scrotal junction usually require operation but heal well as a result.

It is often found advisable to perform circumcision as early as possible in the interests of hygiene and in order to facilitate the management of the indwelling catheter (DAMANSKI 1957).

## h) Epididymitis

If epididymitis occurs as a complication it is thought that the infection reaches the epididymis by means of the lumen of the vas from the posterior urethra, although a blood-borne or lymphatic infection is also possible. It is surprising that the condition is not seen more frequently in view of the wide gaping bladder necks often present. Attention is drawn to the condition by pyrexia, swelling of the epididymis, oedema and reddening of the scrotum. Epididymitis usually subsides with supportive treatment combined with chemotherapy and it is unusual for drainage to be necessary. Should the inflammatory reaction be severe, however, and vascular thrombosis occur, the testis may subsequently slough and require removal.

## i) Sexual complications

Neural control of the sexual act follows very closely the nerve supply of the bladder. Parasympathetic fibres arising from the 3rd and 4th sacral segments pass to the genital organs by means of the nervi erigentes and can produce erection by means of dilatation of the vessels of the corpora cavernosa (METTLER 1942). Sympathetic fibres reach the bladder wall by means of the hypogastric plexus, stimulation of these nerves causing contraction of the seminal vesicles and common ejaculatory ducts, leading to ejaculation, which is facilitated by contraction of the perineal muscles innervated by the somatic pudendal nerve. Thus, as a result of spinal injury, erection and emission become reflex phenomena. TALBOT (1949) found that if the injury was at T11, or higher, 75% of patients had erections, but when the injury was at a lower level the number with erections fell to 50%. Similarly, destruction of the 2nd, 3rd and 4th sacral segments may abolish erections altogether. During the period of recovery from spinal injury, erection of the penis and priapism are frequent complications, especially in complete cervical lesions.

As a result of an investigation carried out by HORNE and others (1948) it was considered that a spinal cord injury did not preclude fertility. STEMMER-MANN and others (1950) carried out testicular biopsies in sixteen young paraplegic patients, finding the histology to be normal in six; in the remaining ten there was some atrophy of the germinal epithelium.

## k) Changes in blood chemistry

These are complicated and much work has been carried out to reduce the changes, and their correction, to mathematical formulae. GUTTMANN & ROBINSON (1954) have summarised the changes as far as serum protein is concerned pointing out that, following injury to the spinal cord, there is a rapid fall in serum protein values, which consists in a lowered serum-albumin concentration and an increase of the alpha globulin content. Their work suggests that these changes take place a short time after the injury, the albumin-globulin ratio rarely returning to a normal value even after a considerable lapse of time.

In discussing the metabolic response to injuries in general, and with special reference to bony injuries, CUTHBERTSON (1954) pointed out the increased urinary output of nitrogen, sulphur and phosphorus, the loss of nitrogen amounting to as much as 137 g. during the ten days following fracture of both bones of the leg. He also demonstrated, by precipitation methods of investigating the blood plasma, that there was a rise in globulin and a slight fall in the albumin fraction. CUTHBERTSON described the period of depressed vitality and diminished metabolism which may ensue immediately after a serious injure as the "ebb" period.

This "ebb" is followed by the "flow" period which reaches its peak between the fourth and eight day after the injury, when there is an extensive catabolism of protein. As a direct result there is a loss of body nitrogen which cannot be corrected by a high protein intake or a high caloric diet at the height of catabolic response (CUTHBERTSON 1936); presumably an excess of food intake at this particular stage is wasted in any endeavour to restore nitrogen balance. He further suggests that labile protein is catabolised to provide energy or amino-acids to facilitate healing and that glycogen and fat deposits will also be utilised. The protein deficiency, complicated by a secondary anaemia, may cause wide-spread troubles and predispose to pressure sores and infection generally. For-tunately, blood transfusion, using several pints of blood, affords an easy and efficacious method of dealing with the protein defect (BROWNE 1945, KREMEN 1948). KLEINMAN (1953) points out that the caloric and protein requirements of patients with traumatic paraplegia are exceptionally high and that the diet should provide for 3500 to 5000 calories per day; approximately 200 grams of protein must be included in the daily requirement. He adds that, on account of various biochemical factors, glucose may not be readily available and energy is therefore obtained from the fatty acid pool. As a result of the loss of protein, these patients lose a great deal of weight after spinal injury, the average loss being 49 pounds. It is possible to give additional protein either intravenously or through a RYLE'S tube into the stomach, but from what has been said above there appears to be considerable doubt as to whether any such measure is effective during the early stages of disturbed metabolism after the injury. The administration of methionine is said to limit the nitrogen loss (STEVENSON 1946).

The effect of serious injury on carbohydrate metabolism is complicated and presents the anomaly that, although there is an excessive loss of carbohydrate, energy is not produced correspondingly (GREEN & STONOR 1954). The hyper-adrenalinaemia, which accompanies the injury, mobilises the carbohydrate and converts the cellular store to glucose which is deposited in the extracellular space (STONOR & others 1952). In addition, gluconeogenesis is promoted by the secretion of adenocortical hormones and thus glucose utilisation is inhibited. Both these mechanisms appear to conserve carbohydrate and to slow down carbohydrate metabolism (GREEN & STONOR (1954). FREEMAN (1949) emphasises the importance of early mobilisation in order to avoid loss of calcium and osteo-porosis.

### l) Oedema of the lower limbs

It is well known that deep venous thrombosis and swelling of the lower limbs are seen not infrequently in the paraplegic patient. In a study of 99 patients BORS and others (1954) showed, by means of phlebography, unilateral or bi-lateral deep venous occlusion in over 58%, the veins of the thigh being affected more frequently than those of the lower leg and pelvis. Venous throm-bosis was found more often in patients with flaccid than with spastic paraplegia. In spite of this high incidence of thrombosis, BORS and his co-workers found that swelling and oedema of the lower limb only occured in 14% of patients and that pulmonary embolism was extremely rare.

### m) Autonomic hyperreflexia

This troublesome and difficult complication, first described by HEAD & RIDDOCH in 1917, tends to occur in patients with high lesions and is often asso-ciated with a spastic bladder. Distension of the bladder in certain patients with cervical or upper thoracic lesions may cause headache, hypertension, bradycardia, sweating and cutis anserina (GUTTMAN & WHITTERIDGE 1957). The reaction subsides as the bladder empties and can sometimes also be caused by the administration of an enema. HUTCH (1955) discusses this condition and advises the use of spinal or caudal anaesthesia for operations involving filling and emptying the bladder. Some of his patients responded to a subarachnoid alcohol block and in one, in which an anterior and posterior rhizotomy from D10 to S5 was carried out for peripheral spasm, the autonomic hyperreflexia was abolished. TALBOT (1957) advocates the use of ganglion-blocking agents, such as hexamethonium or ansolycin in the first instance. If these fail a thorough trial of repeated nerve blocks is carried out before contemplating root section.

### n) Gynaecomastia

Gynaecomastia was at one time a troublesome complication and BORS (1948) reported a 10% incidence in a large series of spinal cord injuries. COOPER and others (1950) pointed out such factors as a lowered metabolism, hypoproteinaemia with reversal of the normal albumin-globulin ratio, testicular atrophy and a decreased output of 17 ketosteroids.

The fact that gynaecomastia is not seen frequently now is probably due to better feeding and to the correction of the hypoproteinaemia and anaemia by repeated blood transfusion.

## 6. Incontinence in paraplegia

It is necessary in this regard to draw a distinction between incomplete and complete lesions of the cord.

### a) Incomplete lesions

It is possible for such patients to enjoy almost normal bladder sensation and control.

A difficulty arises, however, in patients with incomplete paraplegia of hyperextension origin as they may have little power left in their hands and superimposed arthritic stiffening makes their actions even more clumsy. Experience has shown that these men find difficulty in unbuttoning their clothes and in handling the penis so that it is necessary to wear an appliance during the day and also to have a glass, metal or plastic urinal available when in bed.

In a second category are found those with poor or absent motor power in the legs. Even with normal or somewhat diminished bladder sensation and control it is found to be difficult for this type of patient to leave the wheel-chair to urinate so that a rubber urinal is used during the day.

The third group includes those who can move about freely but have some precipitancy of micturition. In such cases it is only necessary to wear an appliance on long journeys or on social occasions.

### b) Complete lesions

In complete lesions the bladder may be of the reflex or non-reflex type.

Patients with reflex bladders may be trained to evacuate by the clock, the urinary stream usually being forceful and the volume variable. There may be some warning but there is, of course, no control. If it is possible to visit the W. C. at regular intervals, (implying getting out of the chair and the use of walking callipers) appliances may be dispensed with.

In the non-reflex type any change of position, any spasm of abdominal or leg muscles or coughing and laughing initiate bladder emptying. The amount thus evacuated varies in amount and may be only a few drops. It is usually desirable for these patients to wear an appliance both by day and night. It is possibly in this type of patient that the various operations for stress incontinence may have their place. As mentioned previously, however, owing to the resistance or elasticity of the structures at the bladder neck, a constant dribbling incontinance is not common.

### c) Appliances

DAMANSKI (1958) reports on this subject as follows:

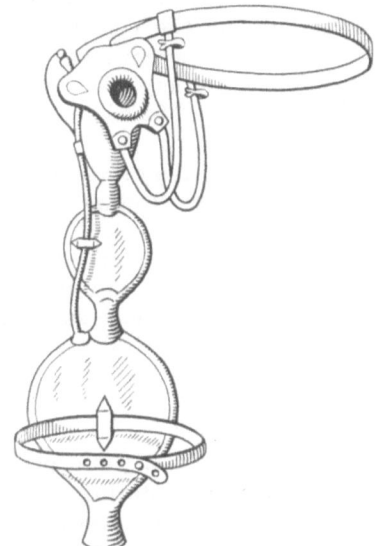

Fig. 26. Rubber urinal (ALLEN and HANBURY)

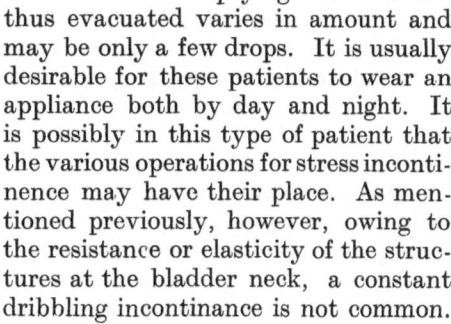

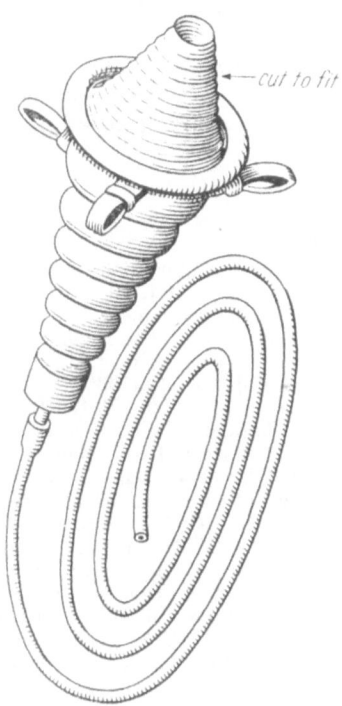

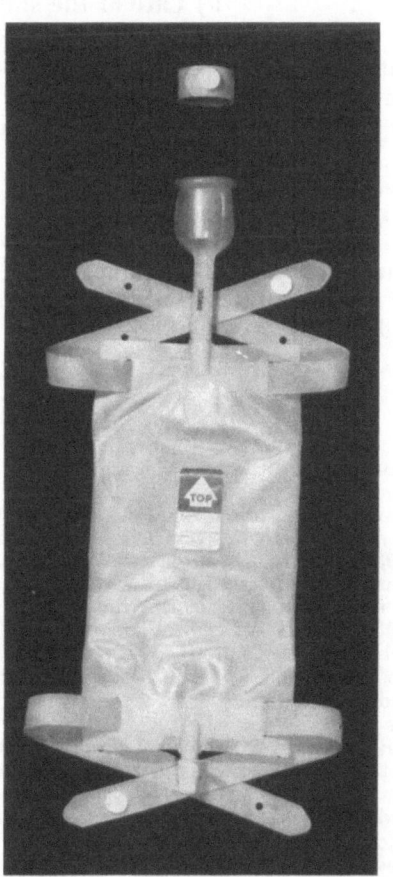

Fig. 27. "Simplic" male incontinence appliance (FRANKLIN)

Fig. 28. Bardic incontinence apparatus (C. R. Bard Inc.)

"The patients at the Liverpool Regional Paraplegic Centre use rubber urinals shown in Fig. 26 during the day. This is a two-chambered appliance with a non-return valve between the chambers and a permanently inflated collar, the patient emptying the apparatus by means of the tap at the lower end. Cleaning should be carried out daily and it is necessary to have two urinals, one for use on alternate days. Cleansing is effected by first rubbing the urinal between the hands in order to break up the sediment inside; it is next necessary to remove the phosphatic sediment by $1/2\%$ acetic acid and finally the organic impurities are removed by a standard solution of hydrogen peroxide. The Simplic urinal (Fig. 27) is also used, mainly in bed.

At night, if the patient is being nursed from one side to the other, it is best to have a bottle by the penis. If the patient is in the prone position a bedpan or large receiver is placed in a gap between the mattresses."

In many clinics in the United States the "Bardic" type of appliance (Fig. 28) is preferred (BISHER 1951). As a simple alternative the writer has found that, provided the patient is confined to bed, a length of Paul's tubing secured to the penis by sleek strapping and led to a Winchester beside the bed has proved effective and has kept the patient dry.

### d) Care of the skin when using an appliance

The genitalia must be kept scrupulously clean, especially in those patients with adductor spasticity. This is best done with a mild, non-irritating soap and water, followed by talcum powder. Silicone creams have proved disappointing as the skin becomes greasy, the grease affecting the rubber.

In patients with a tendency to priapism especial care is necessary to ensure that the pressure of the urinal does not cause an ulcer, or indeed a fistula (GRIFFITHS 1957), at the peno-scrotal junction.

When being dressed or undressed many patients find the penile clip useful, but it is important for the patient not to forget to remove it, as pressure-necrosis, or a urinary fistula may result if the clip is left in situ too long or adjusted too tightly.

## References

### A. Renal sympatheticotonia

BADENOCH, A. W.: Manual of urology, p. 471. London: Heinemann 1953. — BAUER, G.: Late results of denervation of kidney for renal pain. Acta chir. scand. **90**, 460 (1944). — *Gray's Anatomy* edit. T. B. Johnson, p. 1134. London: Longman's Green & Co. 1935. — HARRIS, S. H.: Proc. roy. Soc. Med. **28**, 1479 (1935). — HARRIS, S. H., and R. G. S. HARRIS: Renal sympathetico-tonus, renal pain and renal sympathectomy. Brit. J. Urol. **2**, 367 (1930). — HESS, ELMER: Renal sympathectomy. Penn. med. J. **33**, 741 (1930). — Management of nephrotic patients. Urol. cutan. Rev. **42**, 703 (1938). — JOHNSON, T. H.: Peristalsis of upper urinary tract as demonstrated by new X-ray technique. N. Y. J. med. **52**, 189 (1952). — LAPIDES, J.: Physiology of the intact human ureter. J. Urol. (Baltimore) **59**, 501 (1948). — OLDHAM, J. B. Renal pain and its treatment by denervation of the kidney. Lpool med.-chir. J. **44**, 81 (1936). — The diagnosis of renal pain. Med. Press. **203**, 528 (1940). — Kidney and ureter denervation of the kidney. Brit. Surg. Prac. **5** (1948). — Denervation of the kidney. Ann. roy. Coll. Surg. Engl. **7**, 222—245 (1950). — Modern trends of urology, edit. by E. W. RICHES. London: Butterworth & Co. 1953. — PAPIN, E.: Arch. Mal. Oct. u. Dec. 1929. Quoted in the Med. Echo **8**, 31 (1930). — PAPIN, E., et L. AMBARD: Ètude sur l'énervation des reins. Arch. Mal. Reins **1**, 1 (1921). — UNDERWOOD, W. E.: Idiopathic hydronephrosis. Proc. roy. Soc. Med. **32**, 1681 (1939). — WELLS, C. A.: Renal sympathectomy. Proc. roy. Soc. Med. **28**, 1505 (1935). — WOODSIDE, C. T. A.: The renal heart. Ulster med. J. **13**, 123 (1944).

### B. Neural disturbances of the ureter

ADRIAN, E. D., and S. GELFAN: Rythmic activity in skeletal muscle fibres. J. Physiol. **78**, 271—287 (1933). — BISCHOFF, P.: Mega-ureter. Brit. J. Urol. **29**, 416—423 (1957). — DRAPER, W., and A. W. ZORGMOTTI: N. Y. St. J. Med. **54**, 77 (1954). — FRANKSSON, C., and I. PETERSEN: Electromyographic recording from the normal human urinary bladder, internal urethral sphincter and urethra. Acta physiol. scand. Suppl. **106**, 150—156 (1953). — HANLEY, H. G.: The electro-ureterogram. Brit. J. Urol. **25**, 358—365 (1953). — MILTON, G. W.: Personal communication 1957. — MILTON, G. W., and W. A. T. ROBB: Electrical studies in hydro-ureter: Report of two cases. Brit. J. Urol. **26**, 274—278 (1954). — MURNAGHAN, G. F.: Personal communication 1958. — POOLE-WILSON, D. S.: Proc. roy. Soc. Med. **45**, 835—844 (1952). — SWENSON, O.: A new surgical treatment of Hirschsprung's disease. Surgery **28**, 371—383 (1950). — SWENSON, O. E., H. E. MacMAHEN, W. E. JAQUES and J. S. CAMPBELL: A new concept of the aetiology of megalo-ureter. New Engl. J. Med. **246**, 41—46 (1952). — TINCKLER, L.: Personal communication 1957. — WILLIAMS, D. I.: Discussion on the chronically dilated ureter. Proc. roy. Soc. Med. **45**, No 12, 840—843 (1952).

## C. Neural disturbance of the bladder

### Nerve supply of the bladder

BORS, E.: Segmental and periferal innervation of the urinary bladder. J. nerv. ment. Dis. **116**, 572 (1952). — DENNY-BROWN, D., and E. G. ROBERTSON: On physiology of micturition. Brain **56**, 149 (1933). — McCREA, L. E., and D. L. KIMMEL: A new concept of vesical innervation and its relationship to bladder management following abdominoperineal proctosigmoidectomy. Amer. J. Surg. **84**, 518—523 (1953). — J. urol. (Baltimore) **71**, 549 (1954). — PETERSÉN, I., and C. FRANKSSON: Sensory innervation of the urinary bladder. Urol. int. (Basel) **1**, No 2, 108—119 (1955). — TALBOT, H. S.: Cystometry and the treatment of vesical dysfunction in paraplegia. J. Urol. (Baltimore) **59**, 1130 (1948).

### The act of micturition

DONOVAN, H.: Bladder in paraplegia. Postgrad. med. J. **25**, 383 (1949). — FRANKSSON, C., and I. PETERSÉN: Chronic prostatovesiculitis and affections of the spinal nerve roots. Urol. int. (Basel) **1**, No 3, 171—187. — LANGWORTHY, O. R., L. C. KOLB and L. G. LEWIS: Physiology of micturition. Baltimore: Williams & Wilkins Company 1940. — MUNRO, D.: Treatment of the urinary bladder in cases with injury of the spinal cord. Amer. J. Surg. **38**, 120 (1937). — Treatment of injuries to the nervous system, p. 94. Philadelphia: W. B. Saunders Company 1952. — PRATHER, G. C.: Urological aspects of spinal cord injuries. Springfield, Ill.: C. C. Thomas 1949. — ROSS, J. COSBIE, N. O. K. GIBBON and M. DAMANSKI: Recent developments in the treatment of the paraplegic bladder. Lancet **1957**, 520.

### Investigation

DAMANSKI, M., and A. S. KERR: The value of cysto-urethrography in paraplegia. Brit. J. Surg. **44**, 398—407 (1957). — DAVID, V. C.: The management of the urinary tract of paraplegic patients. J. Amer. med. Ass. **76**, 494 (1921). — NESBIT, R. M., and J. LAPIDES: Tonus of the bladder during spinal "shock". Arch. Surg. **56**, 138 (1948). — ROSS, J. COSBIE: Management of the bladder in spinal injuries. Brit. med. J. **1951**, 616. — ROSS, J. COSBIE, and M. DAMANSKI: Pudendal neurectomy in the treatment of the bladder in spinal injury. Brit. J. Urol. **25**, 45 (1953). — WATKINS, K. H.: Clinical value of bladder pressure estimations. Brit. J. Urol. **6**, 104 (1934).

### Treatment

ABRAMSON, A. S.: Proc. Sec. Ann. Clin. Paraplegia Conf., Vet. Admin. Hosp., Long Beach, Calif., 1953, pp. 28—29. — ABRAMSON, A. S., and G. G. HIRSCHBERG: Studies on spasticity. Bull. Hosp. Jt. Dis. (N.Y.) **13**, 164. — ALLEN, A. R.: Remarks on the histopathological changes in the spinal cord due to impact. J. nerv. ment. Dis. **41**, 141—147 (1914). — BARNES, R.: Paraplegia in cervical spine injuries. J. Bone Jt Surg. B **30**, 234 (1948). — BESLEY, F. A.: A plea for the non-catheterization of the urinary bladder. J. Amer. med. Ass. **69**, 638 (1917). — BOEHLER, L. The treatment of fractures, 1. New York and London: Grune & Stratton 1956. — BORS, E.: The challenge of quadriplegia. Bull. Los. Angeles neurol. Soc. **21**, 121 (1956). — BORS, E., and A. E. COMARR: Proc. Sec. Ann. Clin. Paraplegia Conf., Long Beach, Calif. 1953, p. 32. — BORS, E., and A. E. COMARR: Effect of pudendal nerve operations on neurogenic bladder. J. Urol. (Baltimore) **72**, 66 (1954). — BORS, E., A. E. COMARR and I. M. REINGOLD: Striated muscle at the bladder neck. J. Urol. (Baltimore) **72**, 191 (1954). — BRENDLER, H. et. al.: Spinal root section in treatment of advanced paraplegic bladder. J. Urol. (Baltimore) **70**, 223 (1953). — CAINE, M.: Personal communication 1957. — CAINE, M., and D. EDWARDS: Periferal control of micturition, a oine-radiographic study. Brit. J. Urol. **30**, No 1, 34 (1958). — CAMPBELL, E., and A. MEIROWSKY: Chapter on penetrating wounds of the spinal canal in: Surgery of trauma. Philadelphia, London and Montreal: J. B. Lippincott Company 1953. — CIFUENTES, L., y C. YOUNGER: Disfuncion vesical neurogenia tratada for receccion de los nervos presacro e hipogastricos. Arch. esp. Urol. **8**, Nun 1 (1952). — CIFUENTES, L.: Personal communication 1958. —

Comarr, A. E.: The immediate and early case of traumatic paraplegia. Meeting of South Calif. Chapt. Amer. Coll. Surg., Palm Springs, Calif. (Jan.) 1955. — A self-managed bladder training device for tetraplegics. J. Urol. (Baltimore) 76, 200 (1956). — The problems of cord bladder rehabilitation. J. Urol. (Baltimore) 77, 232—237 (1957). — The practical cure of spinal cord injuries. J. Indian med. Prof. 1957. — Comarr, A. E., and A. A. Kaufman: A survey of the neurological results of 858 spinal cord injuries; a comparison of patients treated with and without laminectomy. J. Neurosurg. 13, 95 (1956). — Damanski, M.: Personal communication. 1957. — Treatment of spasticity. Discussion at Scientific Meeting, Stoke Mandeville 1957. — Donovan, H.: Care of urinary tract in paraplegic patients; review of 82 cases. Lancet 1947, 515. — Emmett, J. L.: Transurethral resection in treatment of true and pseudo cord bladder. J. Urol. (Baltimore) 53, 545 (1945). — Treatment of the chronic phase of the cord bladder. Symposium on cord bladder. Amer. Ass. of Genito Urinary Surg., Hot Springs (May) 1957. — Gibbon, N. O. K.: Personal communication 1957. — Guttmann, L.: Discussion on the treatment and prognosis of traumatic paraplegia. Proc. roy. Soc. Med. 40, 219 (1947). — Surgical aspects of the treatment of traumatic paraplegia. J. Bone Jt Surg. B 31, 399 (1949). — Statistical survey on one thousand paraplegics. Proc. roy. Soc. Med. 47, 1099 (1954). — Initial treatment of traumatic paraplegia. Proc. roy. Soc. med. 47, 1103 (1954). — Scientific Meeting, Stoke Mandeville 1955. — Hinman, jr. F., G. M. Miller, E. Nickel and E. R. Miller: Vesical physiology demonstrated by cineradiography and serial roentgenography. Radiology 62, 713—719 (1954). — Holdsworth, F. W., and A. Hardy: Early treatment of paraplegia from fractures of the thoraco-lumbar spine. J. Bone Jt Surg. B 35, 540 (1953). — Jefferson, G.: Paraplegia in cervical spine injuries. J. Bone Jt. Surg. B 30, 232 (1948). — Kelly, R. E., and P. C. Gautier-Smith: Intrathecal phenol in the treatment of reflex spasms and spasticity. Lancet 1959 I, 1102—1105. — Langworthy, O. R., J. E. Drew and S. A. Vest: Urethral resistance in relation to vesical activity. J. Urol. (Baltimore) 43, 123 (1940). — Lapides, J.: Personal communication 1958. — Lapides, J., R. B. Sweet and L. W. Lewis: Role of striated muscle in urination. J. Urol. (Baltimore) 77, 247 (1957). — Leadbetter, W. F., and F. G. Shaffer: Ileal loop diversion: Its application to the treatment of neurogenic bladder dysfunction. Trans. Amer. Ass. gen.-urin. Surg. 47, 130—139 (1955). — MacCarty, C. S.: The treatment of spastic paraplegia by selective spinal cordectomy. Amer. J. Neurosurg. 11, 539—545 (1954). — May, F.: Sonderdruck aus der Z. Urol. Sonderheft (Arbeitsgemeinschaft medizinischer Verlage). — Mayfield, F. H.: Injuries of the spinal cord, p. 30. Cl. C. Thomas 1953. — Meirowsky, A. M.: The management of the paraplegic patient. J. Tenni. med. Ass. 47, 431 (1954). — Meirowsky, A. M., C. D. Scheibert and D. K. Rose: Indications for neurosurgical establishment of bladder automaticity in paraplegia. J. Urol. (Baltimore) 67, 192—196 (1952). — Monrad-Krohn, G. H.: The clinical examination of the nervous system, p. 219. London: H. K. Lewis & Co. 1948. — Munro, D.: Treatment of injuries to the nervous system, p. 84. Philadelphia and London: W. B. Saunders Company 1952. — Nathan, P. W.: Intrathecal phenol to relieve spasticity in paraplegia. Lancet 1959 I, 1109—1102. — Prather, G. C.: Urological aspects of spinal cord injuries. Oxford: Blackwell Scientific Publ. 1949. — Purves-Stewart, J. The diagnosis of nervous diseases, p. 545. London: Arnold & Co. 1945. — Riches, E. W.: The methods and results of treatment in cases of paralysis of the bladder following spinal injury. Brit. J. Surg. 31, 135 (1943). — Ross, J. Cosbie: Treatment of the bladder in paraplegia. Brit. J. Urol. 28, 14—23 (1956). — Annual meeting of the Brit. Ass. Urol. Surg. 1956. — Ross, J. Cosbie, N. O. K. Gibbon and M. Damanski: Recent developments in the treatment of the paraplegic bladder. Lancet 1957, 520. — Resection of the external urethral sphincter in the paraplegic-preliminary report. Trans. Amer. Ass. gen.-urin. Surg. 49 (1957). — Schneider, R. C., G. Cherry and H. Pantek: Syndrome of acute central cervical spinal cord injury with special reference to the mechanisms involved in hyperextension injuries of the cervical spine. J. Neurosurg. 11, 546 (1954). — Talbot, H. S.: Third Ann. Clin. Paraplegia Conf. 1954, p. 65. — The management of the spastic bladder in paraplegia. Scientific meeting, Stoke Mandeville 1957. — Taylor, A. R.: The mechanism of injury to the spinal cord in the neck without damage to the vertebral column. J. Bone Jt Surg. B 33, 543 (1951). — Taylor, A. R. and W. Blackwood: Paraplegia in hyperextension cervical injuries with normal radiographic appearances. J. Bone Jt Surg. B 30, 245 (1948). — Thomson-Walker, J.: The bladder in gunshot and other injuries of the spinal cord. Lancet 1917, 173. — Watkins, K. H.: The bladder function in spinal injury. Brit. J. Urol. 23, 735—759 (1936). — Watson-Jones, R.: Fractures and joint injuries. Edinburgh & London: E. & S. Livingstone 1955.

*Prognosis*

Bors, E., & A. E. Comarr: Vesico-ureteral reflux in paraplegic patients. J. Urol. (Baltimore) 6, 691—698 (1952). — Damanski, M., and N. O. K. Gibbon: The upper urinary tract in the paraplegic. Brit. J. Urol. 28, 24—36 (1956). — Hutch, J. A.: Vesico-ureteral reflux in the paraplegic: cause and correction. J. Urol. (Baltimore) **68**, 457 (1952). — HUTCH, J. A., and R. C. BUNTS: Present urological status of the war-time paraplegic. J. Urol. (Baltimore) **66**, 218 (1951). — SPURLING, R. G.: Conference on care of paraplegics, Washington, D. C. 1948 (cited by Bors in Veterans Administration Technical Bulletin on Spinal Cord injuries, Dec.). — TALBOT, H. S.: A report on sexual function in paraplegics. J. Urol. (Baltimore) **61**, 265 (1949). — TALBOT, H. S., and R. C. BUNTS: Late renal changes in paraplegia. Hydronephrosis due to vesico-ureteral reflux. J. Urol. (Baltimore) **61**, 870—882 (1949). — TALBOT, H. S., and M. K. LYONS: Later renal changes in paraplegia: destructive lesions. J. Urol. (Baltimore) **63**, 667 (1950). — TALBOT, H. S., D. P. PAULL and G. R. READ: Late renal complications of paraplegia: treatment of vesico-ureteral reflux by skin uretero-stomy through a pedicle flap. J. Urol. (Baltimore) **70**, 216 (1953).

*Complications*

BISHER, W.: An improved urinal for paraplegics. J. Urol. (Baltimore) **77**, No 2, 322 (1951). — BORS, E.: Spinal cord injuries. Veterans Adm. techn. Bull. **10**, 503 (1948). — BORS, E., C. A. CONRAD and T. B. MASSELL: Venous occlusion of lower extremities in paraplegic patients. Surg. Gynec. Obstet. **99**, 451—454 (1954). — BROWNE, J. S. L.: Conference on Metabolic aspects of bone and wound healing, Proceedings of the 9th meeting, New York, Feb. 2—3, 1945, p. 15. New York: Josiah Macy Jr. Foundation 1945. Quoted by Cuthbertson. — COMARR, A. E.: A long term survey of the incidence of renal calculosis in paraplegia. J. Urol. (Baltimore) **74**, 447 (1955). — COOPER, I. S., G. S. MACCARTY and E. H. RYNERSON: Gynaeco-mastia in paraplegic males. Amer. J. Neurosurg. **7**, 364—367 (1950). — CUTHBERTSON, D. P.: Further observations on the disturbance of metabolism caused by injury, with particular reference to the dietary requirements of fracture cases. Brit. J. Urol. **23**, 505—520 (1936). — Inter-relationship of metabolic changes consequent to injury. Brit. med. Bull. **10**, 33—37 (1954). — DAVID, V. C.: Management of the urinary tract of paraplegic patients. J. Amer. med. Ass. **76**, 494 (1921). — FLOCKS, R. H.: Early calcium lithiasis. J. Amer. med. Ass. **130**, 913 (1946). — FREEMAN, L. W.: The metabolism of calcium in patients with spinal cord injuries. Ann. Surg. **129**, 177 (1949). — GREEN, H. N., and H. B. STONOR: Effect of injury on carbohydrate metabolism and energy transformation. Brit. med. Bull. **10**, 38—41 (1954). — GRIFFITHS, H. I.: Personal communication 1956. — GUTTMANN, L., and D. WHITTERIDGE: Effects of bladder distension on autonomic mechanisms after spinal cord injuries. Brain **70**, 361—404 (1947). — HEAD, H., and G. RIDDOCH: The automatic bladder, excessive sweating and some other conditions in gross injuries of the spinal cord. Brain **40**, 188—963 (1917). — HORNE, H. W., D. P. PAULL and D. MUNRO: Fertility studies in the human male with traumatic injuries of the spinal cord and cauda equina. New Engl. J. Med. **239**, 959 (1948). — HUTCH, J. A.: Vesico-ureteral reflux in the paraplegic: cause and correction. J. Urol. (Baltimore) **68**, 457 (1952). — A study of hyperactive autonomic reflex initiated by bladder distension in patients with lesions in the cervical and high thoracic cord. J. Urol. (Baltimore) **73**, 1019—1025 (1955). — A pathological study of uretero-vesical junctions of two stillborn infants with complete urethral atresia. J. Urol. (Baltimore) **74**, 795 (1955). — Personal communication 1957. — Treatment of hydronephrosis by sacral rhizotomy in paraplegics. J. Urol. (Baltimore) **77**, 123 (1957). — KLEINMAN, A. M.: Injuries of the spinal cord, p. 244, edit. by G. C. PRATHER and F. H. MAYFIELD. Ch. C. Thomas 1953. — KREMEN, A. J.: The problem of parenteral nitrogen administration in surgical patients. Surgery **23**, 92 (1948). Quoted by Cuthbertson. — METTLER, F. A.: Neuroanatomy. St. Louis: C. V. Mosby Comp. 1942. — PRATHER, G. C., and F. H. MAYFIELD: Injuries of the spinal cord, p. 147. Ch. C. Thomas 1953. — REINGOLD, I. M.: Proc. Sec. Ann. Clin. Para-plegia Conf., p. 1., Long Beach, Calif. 1953. — ROBINSON, R.: Serum protein changes follo-wing spinal cord injuries. Proc. roy. Soc. Med. **47**, 1109—1113 (1954). — ROSS, J. COSBIE, N. O. K. GIBBON and M. DAMANSKI: Resection of the external urethral and phencter in the paraplegic-a preliminary report. Trans. Amer. Ass. gen.-urin. Surg. **49**, 193—198 (1951). — Recent developments in the treatment of the paraplegic bladder. Lancet **1957**, 520. — STEMMERMANN, G. N., L. WEISS, O. AUERBACK and M. FRIEDMAN: Study of the germinal epithelium in male paraplegics. Amer. J. clin. Path. **20**, 24 (1950). — STEVENSON, G., P. P. SWANSON, W. WILLMAN and M. BRUSH: Nitrogen metabolism as influenced by caloric intake, character of diet and nutritional state of animal. Fed. Proc. **5**, 240 (1946). — STONOR, H. B., C. J. THRELFALL and H. N. GREEN: Studies on mechanism of shock. Carbohydrate meta-bolism in nucleotide and ischaemic shock. Brit. J. exp. Path. **33**, 131 (1952). — TALBOT, H. S.: A report on sexual function in paraplegics. J. Urol. (Baltimore) **61**, 265 (1949). — Proc. Sec. Ann. Clin. Paraplegia Conf., p. 20, Long Beach, Calif. 1953. — Proc. Sec. Ann. Clin. Paraplegia Conf., p. 15, Long Beach, Calif. 1953. — TRESIDDER, G. C.: Nephrostomy. Brit. J. Urol. **29**, 130—134 (1957). — YATES-BELL, J. G.: Pituitrin therapy in hydro-nephrosis. Proc. roy. Soc. Med. **42**, 541—546 (1949).

# Urogenital allergy

Carl E. Burkland

## A. Introduction

### I. General considerations

Diseases now known to be manifestations of allergy or altered reactivity have
undoubtedly existed throughout human history, but their nature and relationship to each other have been understood only in the past fifty years. There
are records dating from antiquity of a casual relationship between exposure to
innocuous substances and the production of minor or severe clinical disorders.
Before the present century it was not suspected that such a diversity of disease
conditions could be caused by allergic hypersensitivity; nor was there any
suspicion that a vast number of environmental substances, which are in themselves
relatively harmless, can produce distresssing and even fatal disease through their
capacity to induce the allergic state. It has been estimated that approximately
ten per cent of our population have such common clinical allergies as asthma,
hay fever, allergic rhinitis, atopic eczema, urticaria, angioneurotic edema and
gastro-intestinal allergy. These are usually caused by non-infectious antigens
of environmental or extrinsic origin. However, the pathologic changes of chronic
infection often may be caused, in large part, by an allergic response of the host
to the invading micro-organism. Furthermore, the morphologic and physiologic
changes which characterize the so-called "collagen diseases", glomerulonephritis,
rheumatic fever and encephalomyelitis, are thought by some to result from auto-
antibody production to antigens present in the individual's own tissues. In erythro-
blastosis fetalis, antibodies derived from the mother pass through the placenta
to combine with antigens on the erythrocytes of the fetus. The degeneration
of homologous skin and other tissue grafts may be also attributed to the formation
by the recipient of antibodies to the grafted tissue. Many physicians are not
aware, however, that some clinical symptoms and pathological changes in the
urogenital tract may be manifestations of allergic reactions. This may be due,
in part, to the fact that the symptoms of genito-urinary hypersensitivity are
much like those of the more common urologic diseases and an adequate allergic
study to establish definitely the diagnosis of allergy has not been made. Several
tests used in the diagnosis of various diseases are based on allergic reactions.
A knowledge of allergic reactions to different diagnostic and therapeutic agents
such as various sera, diodrast and other contrast media, sulfonamides, penicillin
and streptomycin, as well as the antisyphilitic arsenicals used routinely by all
urologists, is very important to prevent severe and, at times, fatal consequences.
Allergy is therefore an ever broadening field with a profoundly important relation
to pathology and clinical medicine.

# II. Definition
## 1. Allergy

The word allergy was suggested by v. PIRQUET in 1906 as a term to cover all changes induced in the state of reactivity in consequence of contact with any living thing or inanimate substance. This definition of the term allergy, that is, an altered capacity to react, as judged from previous experiences of the same organisms or from the experience of other individuals of the species, is still used more or less widely in its original sense. It is an alteration which is specific, usually reflecting prior contact with the same material or one closely related to it chemically. v. PIRQUET described the quantitative variations of the anamnestic reaction rather than the qualitative changes which result from an existing sensitization and for which the word has been appropriated. In this article we intend to use allergy in its widest possible sense, meaning a reaction of the organism that is different from the normal reaction observed in the majority of individuals of a given population. This definition must exclude reactions which constitute instances of unduly high response to physiologically active materials when the response differs solely in intensity from the pharmacologic effects produced in other individuals, such as the hypersensitivity to the normal pharmacologic or side reactions of drugs. The terms hypersensitivity, hypersensitiveness and sensitization, will be used as synonyms. Allergy is primarily a defensive reaction in which the normal physiology has been disturbed, representing a response to an environmental maladjustment. No physician can expect to apply allergy successfully to his practice without a knowledge of some of its terms, principles, mechanisms, and reactions. Only the briefest and most simple discussion of the principles of allergy can be given here, and for more complete information, the reader is referred to the many fine textbooks and articles on the subject (URBACH and GOTTLIEB 1947; COOKE 1947; CHASE 1952).

A long held fundamental concept is that the allergic response is due to altered tissue reactivity produced by an antigen-antibody reaction which is specific. Many manifestations are encountered with varied etiology, pathology, immunology and symptomatology, affecting the cells of many tissues and organs and having no apparent relationship. There is, however, a common denominator to be found in the fact that the tissue responses are based upon the proved or reasonably assumed existence of a cellular antibody that has a specific affinity for an antigen which, when present, becomes linked to the sensitized cell. This causes a cellular response that is varied depending upon the character, function or type of cell, the chemical nature of the antigen, the type of contact and the immunologic mechanism. The fact remains, however, that the resultant reaction is always "altered" from that of the same substance in contact with non-sensitized cells. There is, however, a trend of thought to consider certain reactions of specific hypersensitiveness as not being based on an antigen-antibody reaction since proof is lacking in some instances of such an interaction. Despite a vast amount of work on the problem, the nature and mechanism of the allergic state is still not clear.

## 2. Antigen

Admitting controversy about its presence and mechanisms, the concept of the antigen-antibody reaction is still widely held and some description of its components is necessary. Antigens, the sensitizing substances, are large molecules, colloidal in nature. They are either proteins or polysaccharides, although lipoids and nucleic acids may occur in complexes with the former. Complete antigens are defined as substances which elicit the formation of antibodies as well as react with them. Partial antigens are called haptens. A hapten is a non-protein substance usually of low molecular weight which, when combined with protein material, forms a new antigen. Haptens may be simple drugs, chemicals, or complex compounds like specific polysaccharides which, when combined with protein to form a new protein, are specifically antigenic. The sulfonamides and penicillin may act as haptens (DAVIS 1942). Once sensitization has been brought about by injections of this combined hapten-protein, the hapten alone may produce an allergic reaction. Much of our knowledge that a non-protein substance can induce highly specific hypersensitivity if it possesses a chemical constitution that permits it, under favorable conditions, to attach itself to a normal protein of the body thus forming in effect a new foreign protein which stimulates the production of an antibody specific for the chemical substance that attached itself to the protein, is due to the brillant work of Landsteiner and his associates (LANDSTEINER and CHASE 1940—1941; LANDSTEINER 1945).

## 3. Antibody

Antibodies are specific proteins which appear in the serum or tissues from the introduction of an antigen and which are capable of reacting with or neutralizing the antigen. An outstanding feature is their specificity which means that an antibody is capable of reacting only with a specific substance which, with few exceptions, is that which originally called forth the antibody. After the first injection of antigen, appreciable amounts of antibody do not appear in the circulation for several days, the maximum being reached generally after seven to even ten days. Repeated injections of antigen raise the antibody level and the peak of antibody production is reached about two weeks after the last injection of antigen. Thus, an incubation period is necessary for the development of sensitization. The newly formed antibodies appear to reside in the gamma fraction of the serum globulin and with active immunization or infection, there is considerable increase in the content of serum globulin. The site of antibody-globulin formation has not been finally determined. It was felt that the whole reticulo-endothelial system participates. The latest evidence is that lymphocytes and plasma cells probably manufacture antibody (HARRIS and HARRIS). Contact of the specific antibody with the antigen produces a reaction causing irritation or injury to sensitized cells. Antigen-antibody interactions may result in different phenomena. These interactions may depend upon the following factors: the soluble or particulate nature of the antigen, toxicity or enzyme activity associated with the antigen, the presence of an associated biological property of the antigen, or the availability of one or more than one combining sites on the antibody. Consequently, the end result of a reaction between antigen and antibody may be precipitation, agglutination, lysis, complement fixation and hemolysis, toxin or enzyme neutralization, immediate wheal reactions in human skin or inhibition of these effects, or anaphylaxis or an Arthus reaction (KUHNS). Synonyms for antibodies include lysins, precipitins, opsonins, agglutinins, reagins, or antitoxins depending upon the exact nature of the reaction in question. Reagins are antibodies of the class of skin sensitizing antibodies. They can sensitize passively not only human skin but the nasal, ophthalmic and intestinal mucous membranes. Reagins are usually encountered in association with spontaneous allergic states such as seasonal coryza, asthma, and some kinds of eczema.

The manifestations of allergy are multiple and are so various that the reactions clearly belong in different classes. A given antigen will exert its effects on different tissues and in different ways in different individuals sensitized to it. Thus, different individuals sensitized to the same antigen may develop, on contact with the antigen, such different and separate reactions as urticaria, asthma, purpura, eczema, rhinitis, gastro-intestinal upsets, pneumonitis, arthritis vesical irritability or renal colic.

## 4. The mechanism of allergic reaction

While it is generally accepted that the actual symptoms of allergic diseases are the result of a cellular interaction of antigen and antibodies causing tissue injury, the exact mechanism of the allergic reaction is not known. The basic mechanisms, whatever their nature, operate in a milieu of tissues and wandering cells. The tissue or organ affected may be variously normal or abnormal, and it is often given the term "shock organ", in an attempt to distinguish the site of predilection for allergic reactions seen in different individuals as the bronchial muco us membrane (asthma), epidermal cells (contact dermatitis), endothelium of vessels in the skin (urticaria), and smooth muscle of the ureter or bladder (ureteral colic or vesical spasm). As an example, certain cells in the body become sensitized by contact with a substance, for example, ragweed antigen, and in some manner develop specific cellular antibodies for ragweed antigen. With subsequent contact between ragweed antigen and the cellular antibodies, the cell is injured resulting in liberation from the injured cell of histamine or histamine-like substances (H-substance) and undoubtedly, other substances which are less important and less understood in the part they play in the resulting allergic reaction and symptomatology (DALE; DRAGSTEDT). The close approximation of the physiologic effects of histamine on the one hand and manifestations of anaphylaxis on the other was pointed out by Dale long ago. The actual release of histamine (H-su bstance) by the antigen body reaction is thought to be mediated by stimulation of parasympathetic nerves. This would explain, at least in part, the beneficial effect of epinephrine in counteracting allergic reactions.

### Role of histamine in allergic reactions

The importance of the liberation of histamine during the allergic reaction is well recognized. The subcutaneous injection of histamine will induce the same symptoms of acute allergic shock that occasionally result from the in-advertent subcutaneous injection of a large dose of an allergen such as pollen extract. Many, but not all, of the symptoms encountered in clinical allergy may be reproduced by injecting histamine into persons.

Histamine has three major physiologic actions. It acts (1) on smooth muscle to produce contractions such as the bronchospasm of asthma or the contractions of the gut or the bladder, (2) on capillaries to produce dilatation and increased permeability which may lead to the formation of edema as in urticaria or to the swollen nasal membranes of hay fever and allergic rhinitis and (3) on the secretory glands as a secretagogue, of which lacrimation in hay fever is an example. The elevated concentration of histamine in the blood following an allergic or an-aphylactic reaction is very transient, existing for only a matter of minutes; yet, the resulting symptoms may persist for a long time owing perhaps to some change in the damaged cells which remain after the release of histamine, or to some stimulation of or effect on the immune mechanism of the body.

Histamine alone cannot completely explain all of the manifestations of anaphylactic shock or clinical allergy. Some observers feel that acetylcholine or a similar substance (cholingeric ester) acts as the mediator of parasympathetic impulses and exerts its action on contiguous cells but not on remote tissues (ROSENBLUETH; NACHMANSOHN). The choline bodies produce effects similar to those of vagal stimulation (intestinal contraction, lowering of blood pressure, cardiac slowing and increased glandular activity). There is some evidence that other substances may be liberated during hypersensitive shock. Heparin released from the liver may account for the defect in the coagulability of the blood during anaphylactic shock though a deficiency of blood platelets may account for this. Serotonin may play a role. Adenosine derivatives and potassium ions may also be freed into the circulation.

The symptoms of the allergic reaction in man are extremely variable, owing to the fact that the shock organ or the site of the reaction is not constant, even in the same individual or even in response to the same antigen. The shock tissues or sensitized cells in man appear to be confined chiefly to the skin and mucous membranes. The manner by which the foreign substance or antigen reaches the shock tissue is relatively unimportant; it must occur either by direct contact or through the blood or lymph. Allergic manifestations are rarely static. A shifting of reactions from one shock organ to another is frequently encountered. The eczema of infancy and childhood may clear up and be superseded by asthma or allergic rhinitis. The excitant may remain the same or a new sensitivity may develop.

The basic fact in all cases is the primary response of the body to an antigenic substance with the formation of antibodies. When these subsequently react with the same antigen, again in the body, the union effects certain tissues, chiefly smooth muscle, blood vessels and collagen, and one or a combination of manifestations occur. Under any given set of conditions (i.e., kind and dose of antigen, route by which the sensitizing and reactive doses enter the body and species of animal) a particular kind of reaction usually follows. Thus, the parenteral injection of a sufficient dose of protein will sensitize the organism so that a subsequent inoculation given into the skin about ten days later will cause severe inflammation and necrosis, while an injection into the blood stream is apt to result in anaphylactic shock. When certain of these conditions are varied, the end result may also differ; e.g., the spontaneous sensitization of the human being by air-borne or ingested antigens results in attacks of asthma or hay fever or urticaria on subsequent exposure to the antigen by the same or a parenteral route.

# B. Types of allergic responses

Allergic reactions fall into two chief categories which are not always sharply separable — the "immediate" and the "delayed" types. In both types the development of sensitization usually requires ten days to two weeks following infection or contact, a time consistent with that usually necessary for the formation of antibody to known antigens. Thus, following the initial injection there must be an incubation period after exposure to an antigen before active sensitization from a second and subsequent injection develops.

## I. Definition of immediate and delayed hypersensitivity

### 1. Immediate

The reactions of the "immediate" type become well developed soon after contact — within seconds or minutes — or after adequate absorption of the corresponding allergenic substance (asthma, hay fever, "hives", certain unusual cases of drug sensitivity, gastro-intestinal disturbances). In many instances of sensitivity of this sort, circulating antibodies are demonstrable, and there is some accompanying skin reactivity which assists in recognition of the allergen by means of a "wheal and erythema" response in the skin where the allergen is applied. In certain allergic manifestations, however, such as gastrointestinal allergy, in which the reaction type can be of the "early" sort, there may be no parallel skin reactivity or demonstrable circulating antibody. The hypersensitivity may be transferred by means of serum to normal recipients who thereby become temporarily sensitized themselves. Finally, the various manifestations of this state depend largely upon changes which occur in blood vessels, smooth muscle and collagen. The responses of these tissues result in the following manifestations: smooth muscle contraction may cause pulmonary difficulties, arterial constrictions, ureteral and vesical spasms; injury to blood vessels may lead to leakage of fluid into tissue, or edema of the external genitalia as well as to damage to the tissues supplied by occluded vessels; degeneration of collagen with cellular infiltration and scarring may interfere with functions of vital structures such as heart valves, or prostate gland (granulomatous prostatitis). Although different manifestations may become evident, the immediate hypersensitive states have in common a good deal that is basic including (a) rapidity of response, (b) relationship of reactivity to a demonstrable antibody of the blood which can transmit the hypersensitive state to normal recipient, and (c) non-participation of the tissue cells per se in the reaction with antigen, but only secondarily as a result of combination of antigen with antibody (CHASE 1952).

## 2. Delayed

The delayed type reactions, on the other hand require at least several hours after introduction of the allergen before an effect is manifest (reactions to poison oak or poison ivy, most drug sensitivities, reactions to products of micro-organisms-tuberculin, mallein, histoplasmin), and show progressive changes for two to three days or longer (LAWRENCE). In these cases, circulating antibodies are but rarely found, and the hypersensitive reaction is not restricted to certain types of tissue; any cells of the body may undergo injury or destruction following exposure to antigen. There are no specific shock tissues in the nature of smooth muscle, blood vessels and collagen found in this type of reaction. The transfer of the hypersensitive state to normal recipients cannot be demonstrated by humoral antibody but can be carried out by cells of the leukocyte series, particulary lymphocytes (CHASE 1951). We can assume that the cells of the animal with delayed hypersensitivity are directly vulnerable to antigen without the intermediation of humoral antibody or of any histamine-like substance. In addition, the independence of the two forms of response is indicated by the fact that one (anaphylactic) can be abolished while the other (delayed) remains intact. However, anaphylactic as well as delayed responsiveness may be simultaneously induced by the use of proper antigens and conditions, and it is possible to desensitize to anaphylaxis while leaving delayed hypersensitivity still active.

# II. Types of immediate hypersensitiveness
## 1. Atopic hypersensitivity

While most individuals are considered normally non-allergic, but may be sensitized under certain circumstances, there is a large group of individuals whose ancestors have been allergic. The term "atopy" was introduced by COCA to characterize certain hypersensitive states which he considered to be heritable and to be limited in occurrence to human beings. This group does not inherit allergic diseases as such, but merely the predisposition or capacity to become sensitized. It is very doubtful that any specific hypersensitive state in itself is inheritable but, the inheritance of a predisposition to become sensitized on the other hand seems unequivocal. This point has been repeatedly affirmed by various observers and is exemplified by the early statistics of Cooke and van der Veer which reveal that almost half of a group of 504 patients studied had one or both parents with sensitivity in contrast to about 15 per cent positive antecedents among non-sensitive individuals questioned. It is not surprising that a genetic determinant should be found to play a part here. We know that inheritance plays a role in all biologic characteristics, and in relation to immunologic phenomena, it has been shown to influence the level of native resistance to infectious diseases, the ability to acquire resistance, and the readiness with which experimental animals become sensitized to injections of antigens. About ten per cent of the population as a whole shows some clinically manifest form of atopic hypersensitivity. Most clinical forms of hypersensitivity are considered to be in the atopic class. These are the so-called spontaneous clinical allergies which develop upon natural exposure to airborne and ingested allergens. They include such conditions as hay fever, asthma, allergic rhinitis, allergic dermatitis, urticaria, gastro-intestinal allergy and natural sensitivity to serum.

There is a special nature to the antibody involved in the atopic reaction. The circulating antibodies related to atopic hypersensitivity cannot, with certainty, be demonstrated by any in vitro serologic test. That antibodies are present, however, is usually revealed by the ability of the serum from an allergic individual to sensitize passively the skin of a normal recipient. If a small amount of such serum is injected into a skin site of a normal subject, injection of antigen into the same area 24 hours later will result in a local hive. This is the so-called Prausnitz-Küstner reaction.

## 2. Evanescent cutaneous reaction

Another type of immediate hypersensitivity is the evanescent cutaneous reaction, which may be elicited in sensitized individuals by local injection of antigen into the skin. These responses are evidenced by dilatation of the capillaries and unusual permeability of the vessel walls terminating in a wheal and flare reaction. They appear to be the result of histamine liberation and differ from the Arthus reaction in becoming visible earlier, within three to four hours, and never progressing to necrosis.

The occurrence of the early type of local reaction, both in animals and in man, often coincides with the presence in the serum of antibodies that are capable of transferring corresponding sensitivities to normal subjects. This has been shown following blood transfusions or bulk injections of serum, procedures that result in a sensitivity of the entire skin, and also following intracutaneous deposition of serum, a method that chiefly sensitizes the skin in a local area. Some degree of sensitivity then persists for a variable period, according to the species and the concentration and type of antibody in the serum employed. Such a site will react when antigen is brought to it (by local injection or by conveyance in tissue fluids), and it is then desensitized. The reactions in such prepared sites are of the evanescent type, and reproduce the sensitivity of the serum donor even if not always his disease, which may demand in addition the peculiarities of his "shock tissue".

## 3. Arthus phenomenon

The Arthus phenomenon, which was first described by ARTHUS in 1903 as occurring in properly conditioned rabbits, is a severe antigen-antibody reaction. This reaction apparently stems directly from the precipitative union of antigen with antibody, presumably because the precipitate has some irritative effect upon vascular tissues. Histamine release may take part in this reaction but the classic severe response does not occur except in the presence of adequate doses of precipitating antibody and relatively high doses of antigen. Another basic element for the occurrence of the Arthus reaction is the presence of blood vessels in the tissue where the combination takes place, since the particular hypersensitive manifestation depends chiefly upon injury to blood vessels, though other effects, such as swelling and degeneration of collagenous fibers also occur. Further secondary damage to surrounding tissue may eventuate if the tissues are sufficiently injured. The reaction does not occur in avascular tissue. RICH has considered periarteritis nodosa, rheumatic fever and rheumatoid arthritis as examples of diseases probably resulting from focal anaphylactic reactions of the Arthus type of immune mechanism (RICH).

## 4. Anaphylaxis

Anaphylaxis is generally regarded as the prototype of hypersensitivities of the immediate type. It is manifested as a severe systemic reaction to the parenteral administration of antigen, particularly intravenously, ending in shock and often fatally. Anaphylaxis proper, then may be defined primarily as an acute systemic reaction, species-characteristic, that is exhibited by animals in the hypersensitive state upon re-injection with the same material. Anaphylaxis is noted most frequently in the laboratory animals but may occur in human beings. A central event in acute shock is contraction of smooth muscle which occurs throughout the body. Other events include edema, decreased coagulability of the blood, fall in blood pressure and temperature, thrombocytopenia, general leukopenia with aggregation of white cells in the pulmonary bed and often pulmonary eosinophilia. The manifestations of shock depend upon the species of animal involved. Intense contraction of the bladder often occurs. Acute anaphylactic shock in human beings is fortunately a rare occurrence and most often follows an injection of horse serum to people having a pre-existing clinical sensitivity to horse dander. It has also been caused by secondary injections of liver extracts, tetanus toxoid and viral vaccines produced in egg yolk.

That sensitivity has developed may be demonstrated in several ways: (1) by anaphylactic shock, (2) by the precipitin test, an in vitro test of precipitation and complement fixation in the presence of an antigen, (3) by the SCHULTZ-DALE reaction, the in vitro contraction of smooth muscle of the uterine or intestinal strip on addition of antigen and (4) by the injection of sensitive serum (human, guinea pig or rabbit) into the skin of normal men (passive transfer). Such a site tested after a few hours with the antigen may show a typical urticarial wheal. Desensitization of the state can be accomplished by repeated small injections of antigen into a sensitive animal; one explanation for this effect is supposed to be due to saturation of antibody by injected antigen.

### a) Serum sickness

Serum sickness is a form of the anaphylactic type of hypersensitivity which occurs in over a half the previously normal human beings who receive horse or rabbit antiserum (and less frequently other antigenic substances such as penicillin, sulfonamides, and other drugs) for prophylactic or therapeutic purposes. This disease is marked by the occurrence of hives, angioedema, painful joints, lymphadenopathy and fever, usually coming on about eight to ten days after the initial administration of the antigen, and persisting for several days (LONGCOPE 1943).

### b) Diseases probably related to the anaphylactic type of hypersensitivity

α) **Periarteritis nodosa.** It has been established, both by experimental and by clinico-pathological observations, largely due to the work of RICH, et al., that periarteritis nodosa can be an expression of hypersensitivity to a variety of agents. It has been produced in animals by subjecting them to a protracted hypersensitive reaction of the anaphylactic type by repeated foreign protein injections. Clinically, cases have been reported as developing following hypersensitivity to the sulfonamides, iodine, aspirin, penicillin, phenobarbital, dilantin, thiourea, and arsenicals. It is a necrotizing, inflammatory lesion involving particularly the walls of the medium and small arteries and arterioles with a perivascular accumulation of cells often including many eosinophiles. Almost any organ or tissue of the body may be affected. As would be expected, the symptoms are diverse, depending upon the organ or group of organs involved. Kidney symptoms include hematuria, lumbar pain and hypertension. There may be albumin and casts in the urine and kidney function tests exhibit a decrease in renal efficiency. Death from uremia is not unusual. There is nothing distinctive about the renal symptoms of periarteritis nodosa as compared to other renal vascular diseases.

β) **The relationship of allergy to human and experimental nephritis.** It has long been suspected that hypersensitivity may be an important determining mechanism in the pathogenesis of many of the instances of human glomerulonephritis. Particularly suggestive in this regard have always been post-scarlatinal nephritis, and the nephritis that is associated with tonsillitis, both of which, as is well known, do not appear during the height of the infection when the streptococci and their products are present in great abundance, but only after a lapse of time, sufficient to permit the development of antibody and of hypersensitivity. Since LONGCOPE in 1913 reported the presence of renal lesions in animals that had been subjected to repeated injections of small amounts of foreign protein, several other reports of the production of glomerulonephritis by repeated injections of foreign protein have been presented. In 1934 MASUGI and SATO described glomerular alterations in several rabbits given repeated intravenous injections of foreign protein after the removal of one kidney, but the alterations were very different from those characteristic of ordinary glomerulonephritis.

In 1943, RICH and GREGORY, in a course of study on an experimental production of periarteritis nodosa by means of anaphylactic sensitivity, observed that glomerulonephritis, with glomerular alterations characteristic of those in human glomerulonephritis, occurred in rabbits that were sensitized by the intravenous injection of non-bacterial, non-toxic foreign protein (horse serum). Nephritis occurred in animals that had received several intravenous injections of antigen but it was found by RICH, and later confirmed by others (MORE and WAUGH 1952; GERMUTH 1953), that glomerular lesions will occur in animals given only a single injection of foreign protein. Evidence has also accumulated that all the types of glomerular lesions that characterize human acute glomerulonephritis, together with the associated urinary abnormalities, can be produced in the experimental animal by hypersensitivity to non-toxic foreign proteins, and that when the experimental lesions are severe enough, death in uremia occurs. The experimental production of glomerular lesions as a result of hypersensitivity does not prove that hypersensitivity is a mechanism responsible for the injury in human glomerulonephritis. Final proof or disproof of its role in humans must rest upon further studies of the problem in man.

According to RICH (1956) much remains to be learned regarding the mechanism by which the experimental glomerulonephritis produced by hypersensitivity operates. It is reasonable to believe that renal lesions like those of the cardiovascular system can be the result of a tissue injury produced by an antigen-antibody reaction. There appears to be strong supported evidence for this view now. First, all the experimental animals developing nephritis have been made hypersensitive. Second, focal reactions of hypersensitivity can produce in other parts of the body capillary lesions (endothelial proliferation) of the same type as those seen in the glomerular experimental nephritis. Thirdly, there is a latent period between the injection of the antigen and the appearance of the glomerular lesions — a period that corresponds to that during which a sufficient amount of antibody is being formed to clear the excess of injected antigen rapidly from the circulation. Further support comes from the report of GERMUTH that in animals that have been sensitized previous to the injection of a nephritis-producing dose of antigen, the antigen was cleared from the blood stream earlier and free antibody appeared earlier in the serum than in normal animals given the same dose, and the time of occurrence of the renal lesions was correspondingly accelerated. Additionally suggestive evidence is a demonstration by SCHWAB and his co-workers and MOLL and HAWN that a decrease in serum complement occurs during the period when the renal lesions begin to appear, i.e., the period during which antigen is rapidly disappearing from the circulation because of active antibody production. A decrease in the complement titer of the serum in human glomerulonephritis has been reported by numerous investigators (LANGE et al. 1951). In the human being or in the experimental animal, widespread periarteritis nodosa resulting from hypersensitivity to drugs, for example, often occurs in the complete absence of glomerular lesions, while in other individuals sensitized to the same drug, both occur together. This may be due to the influence of local factors.

It is highly likely that in addition to the well known individual differences in the ability to produce antibody, and apart from local tissue factors, other more generalized, non-specific bodily conditions may also influence the occurrence or severity of lesions produced by antigen-antibody reactions, and so play an important role in determining the familiar differences in the reaction of different individuals. Pertinent in this regard, it was shown in RICH's laboratory, and amply confirmed by others, that cortisone and ACTH can markedly inhibit the development of anaphylactic nephritis and periarteritis nodosa.

GERMUTH regarded his studies as indicating that the vascular damage in hypersensitive reactions is suppressed by cortisone as a result of the hormone's inhibition of antibody formation, rather than by its non-specific effect which, as is well known decreases vascular reactivity to other types of injurious agents.

Similar lesions, simulating human glomerulonephritis and nephritis in animals produced by repeated foreign protein injections, also can be produced by anti-kidney anti-sera (often called "nephrotoxic" sera). This involves the injection of renal tissue suspensions from one species of animal into another. The kidney antibody containing serum from the second species is then injected back into the first species. SMADEL, MASUGI, and others have shown that the resulting nephritis physiologically and anatomically closely resembles human glomerulotubular nephritis. CAVELTI reports producing nephritis of this type in rats by injecting them with kidney tissue suspensions of the same species mixed with killed streptococci. Circulating kidney tissue antibodies were detected in the sera of many of these animals.

MASUGI injected anti-rabbit kidney serum, the so-called nephrotoxin (obtained by allergizing ducks to rabbit kidney), into the ear veins of rabbits, and produced thereby a diffuse glomerulonephritis with albuminuria, cylindruria, increased blood pressure, nitrogen retention, edema, and finally, death due to renal insufficiency. Histologic examination revealed diffuse involvement of the glomeruli. This experimental glomerulonephritis was the result, therefore, of the action of immune bodies directed against kidney protein, or in other words, of an antigen-antibody reaction. Needless to say, it cannot be assumed that glomerulonephritis in man is attributable to the action of a nephrotoxin, as in these animals; however, these experiments do suggest the possibility that allergic mechanisms may play a role in the development of glomerulonephritis in human beings.

As several other investigators have demonstrated, the so-called nephrotoxic nephritis (Masugi nephritis) is easily obtained by injection of an antikidney serum prepared by immunization of animals of a foreign species with kidney substance of the recipient species (EHRICH et al.; FOUTS et al.; SARRE 1939). The pathologic and clinical features of this renal disease have also been thought to resemble human glomerulonephritis rather closely, particularly when the lesions are produced in rabbits. When rabbit anti-rat-kidney serum is given to rats or when other mammals receive antikidney serum produced in a foreign mammalian species, the renal lesions have been found to develop immediately, that is, from within hours to a day or so. Therefore, these renal changes must be due to the direct effect of the antikidney antibodies. On the other hand, when anti-kidney serum against mammalian kidney (rabbit, dog) produced in an avian species (duck, chicken) is used, there is usually a time interval of about a week between the serum injection and the onset of the renal disease. The reason for this is not clear, but it seems that an active immunologic response on the part of the recipient animal occurs. KAY has suggested that the localization of anti-kidney antibody in the kidney does not suffice to produce nephritis, but that the renal lesions develop only after the recipient animal has formed precipitins against the foreign anti-kidney serum which react with the anti-kidney antibody already bound in the kidney. Although apparently the avian anti-kidney serum is, per se, incapable of producing renal lesions, the anti-kidney antibodies localize in the kidney immediately after injection, regardless of whether avian or mammalian nephrotoxic serum is used. This is evidenced by the prevention of renal disease in one kidney if its arterial blood supply is shut off for fifteen to thirty minutes following intravenous injection of antikidney serum and especially also by PRESSMAN'S demonstration of localization in the glomeruli of anti-kidney antibodies labelled with radioactive iodine.

EHRICH and his co-workers have suggested that two different renal lesions may be evoked by anti-kidney serum, the one type which follows immediately upon the injection of nephrotoxin being characterized mainly by alteration with thickening of the glomerular basement membrane with but little inflammatory or proliferative changes (that is, a nephrotic lesion), while the other type which develops after an interval of one week closely resembles acute human glomerulonephritis. According to EHRICH, the same rabbit anti-rat-kidney serum can produce either type of lesion in rats, a large dose resulting immediately in the nephrotic type and a small dose leading, after an interval, to the nephritic type. Others also have pointed out that there is a considerable variability to the effects of individual anti-kidney serums, even when produced in the same species. Different duck anti-rat-kidney serums have been found to exert either the immediate or the delayed nephrotoxoid effect. PRESSMAN and his associates have called attention to the fact that duck anti-rabbit-kidney antibody, when combining with rabbit kidney, does not fix complement, thus perhaps explaining the usual lack of direct nephrotoxicity of this serum.

The kidney antigen responsible for nephrotoxic nephritis appears to be species specific and located in the glomerulus (GREENSPAN and KRAKOWER 1950). Nephrotoxic sera are produced only by immunization with renal cortex, not with medulla (HEYMAN 1950). Absorption of anti-kidney serum with a suspension of isolated glomeruli removes the nephrotoxic antibody. On the other hand, substances closely related to the glomerulus antigen appear to be present in vascular endothelium or at least in the vascular bed elsewhere. In PRESSMAN'S experiments, labelled antikidney serum having a predilection for the glomeruli also localized to a small extent in the vascular bed of liver and lung. Elution and re-injection of the localized antibody resulted in a predilection for the organ of original localization, but again with some cross reacting with other locations, indicating close immunologic relationship of the vascular bed of various organs but not identity.

Autoantibodies reacting in vitro with extracts of human kidney have been found in the serum of patients with glomerulonephritis by several independent workers. LANGE and associates (1949), using the collodion particle technique, obtained positive results in 59 per cent of the cases of acute glomerulonephritis and in 100 per cent of those with chronic glomerulonephritis. PFEIFFER and BRUCH (1953), by means of the same method, found anti-kidney antibodies to be present in the blood of 72 per cent of their patients with acute glomerulo-nephritis and 83 per cent of their patients with chronic glomerulonephritis. Both groups of workers found considerably higher titers in chronic than in acute nephritis. LANGE and his co-workers (1951), in confirmation of previous reports, have shown that there is a pronounced drop of complement in the blood in acute nephritis, indicating the occurrence of a massive antigen antibody reaction, presumably of anti-kidney antibody with kidney substance.

According to PREZIOZI (1941), diffuse human glomerulonephritis can be explained in this way: a small streptococcal infection attacks the kidney and sensitizes it to the germ's toxins, and on the next revivification of the focus by one or another reason, the sensitized kidney reacts violently, with outbreak of the disease; successive onsets (relapses) of the nephropathies without apparent causes can thus be easily explained. While the majority of the nephropathies are infective ones, other causes also could determine a nephropathic relapse; introduction into the body of products toxic to the kidney, which in small doses are usually well tolerated (mercury, bismuth, pyramidon), or substances which usually are clinically and experimentally unable to cause renal lesions, aspirin, sera, vaccines, or fungi, aliments like horse meat, mollusca, etc. According to PREZIOZI, in these cases, nephritis presents these particular symptoms: pain in the lumbar region, disappearing after introduction of the sensitizing substance, frequent hematuria and the presence of other signs of allergy such as angio-neurotic edema, urticaria, etc., and purpura.

Thus as RICH says the combined evidence that experimental nephritis is the result of an antigen-antibody reaction is therefore very strong. There is lacking only the demonstration that the lesions can be promptly produced by the passive transfer of antibody in the presence of antigen. Final proof or disproof of the role of hypersensitivity in human glomerulonephritis must rest upon further studies of the problem in man.

## 5. Relationship of eosinophilia to immediate hypersensitive reactions

It has been known for many years that eosinophils characteristically put in an appearance in many of the hypersensitive states with which we have been dealing. These cells may occur about local sites of reaction or they may be found in increased numbers in the blood stream, or both. They appear to be related to the hypersensitive reaction rather than to the existence of the hypersensitive state itself. Thus, while they are not seen in abnormal numbers in sensitive guinea pigs, eosinophilia in the lungs and the blood occurs in animals which have survived an anaphylactic shock. Analogous findings are made in human beings; during the period of development of serum sickness, eosinophilia is not met with, but once the reaction has gotten under way, these cells appear in the tissues at sites of activity. Eosinophils are found in local hives, and they occur in the membranes of the respiratory tract and in the local secretions as well as in the blood of asthmatics, often only during or immediately after attacks. They may be found in the urine or tissue of the bladder, urethra, prostate or kidney. Atopic dermatitis is commonly associated with a significant blood eosinophilia. The lesions of periarteritis nodosa and, of course, rheumatic fever often contain these cells. Their occurrence is so commonly related to hypersensitive reactions of the immediate type that their presence in abnormal numbers in any disease of unknown etiology makes the factor of allergy suspect. A point of interest is the fact that cortisone, which has a certain modifying influence upon diseases of hypersensitivity, causes also a decrease of circulating eosinophils in the blood. It appears that these may take refuge in the spleen, though by what means this is not yet evident.

## III. Delayed hypersensitivity
### 1. Delayed hypersensitivity in infectious processes

Delayed allergy is a characteristic response of the body in various infections from a wide variety of micro-organisms which include bacteria, viruses, fungi and spirochetes as well as following exposure to certain plants and chemical substances, i.e., contact dermatitis where the manifestation is usually of the eczematous type. Delayed allergy plays a prominent role in conditioning the host's response in those bacterial infections characterized by a chronic course and a granulomatous type of response. Tuberculosis is pre-eminent in this regard in that the sensitive state is not only easily demonstrable by appropriate skin tests with antigenic material, but also because the tissue injury and destruction which ensues from this reactivity play a considerable part in the pathogenesis of the disease. Delayed hypersensitivity is also demonstrable in brucellosis, typhoid fever, tularemia, glanders, chancroid and whooping cough, among the bacterial diseases. Although it is not ordinarily considered in relation to the more acute infectious disease, this allergic state can be demonstrated following infections with the pneumococcus, the streptococcus and other bacteria by means of skin tests with the respective proteins of these organism. It is perhaps safe to say that a study of any bacterial infection from this standpoint would disclose a very general existence of this form of hypersensitive response. Interestingly, in all those cases where the chemical nature of the bacterial component responsible for this reactive state has been revealed, this has been protein. Whenever attempts have been made to sensitize by means of soluble components of bacteria, the sensitivity achieved has been of the Arthus type. We may say that microbial allergy plays a part in the onset of infection, in the clinical manifestations of the disease, in the course of the infection and lastly, in its outcome.

## a) Bacterial

The hypersensitivity of infection is commonly referred to as the "tuberculin type sensitivity" for its prototype is the hypersensitivity to tuberculo-protein that develops during tuberculous infection. The local inflammatory response to the antigen is delayed and prolonged. Chase has shown that though passive transfer of this type of sensitivity cannot be accomplished with serum of the sensitized body, it can readily be accomplished by transferring washed, living mononuclear cells (lymphocytes) isolated from peritoneal exudates, spleen, lymph nodes or blood of sensitized animals into a normal one. This fundamental contribution provides the most direct evidence to date that tuberculin sensitivity is probably mediated by an immune mechanism intimately bound to cells and is not the result of some non-specific response. In other words, the reaction is an allergy. A further important discovery is that of RAFFEL who found that the induction of bacterial sensitivity in tuberculosis depends upon both the wax (a fatty acid ester) about the tubercle bacillus and the antigenic protein in the bacillus (RAFFEL 1948). The essential component of the waxy substance was found to be a lipopolysaccharide. When deprived of this lipoid wax by chloroform, sensitivity did not develop. He also noted that lipoid factors serve to direct sensitivity to antigens unrelated to tubercle bacillus, as for example, egg albumin and picryl chloride. Thus, CHASE has demonstrated conclusively that the mechanism for the tuberculin reaction involves a specific antibody that is strictly cellular, in other words, the reaction is an allergy (antigen-sensitized cell reaction). So far as is known, all bacteria are capable of producing the same specific sensitivity, hence the use of the modifying term "tuberculin type". A similar skin test may be employed, therefore, as a diagnostic procedure in such other diseases as typhoid fever, brucellosis, tularemia, glanders, syphilis, certain fungus infections and in the viral infections such as the one causing lymphogranuloma venereum.

## b) Virus

Viral infections which have been shown to induce delayed allergy include vaccinia, lymphogranuloma venereum and mumps. The diagnostic Frei test, indicative of the presence of lymphogranuloma venereum is a demonstration of skin sensitivity to the intradermal injection of a small amount of inactivated virus. In lymphogranuloma venereum a high degree of delayed hypersensitivity develops, and in its more advanced state, this infection is accompanied by considerable tissue destruction. Among its more common clinical expressions are: ulceration of the vulva, pudendal elephantiasis, stricture of the rectum and inguinal buboes.

MARSHALL and ENDICOTT have used the Frei test in a clinical study of obscure bladder disease for evidence of lymphogranuloma venereum. They reported a group of nine patients, 7 women and 2 men, with "cystitis" of indeterminate origin. Although the cystoscopic picture varied, they all had positive Frei reactions or complement fixation tests, or both. GRAY has reported 23 instances of urethritis in women considered due to the disease. While routine Frei testing on a urological service does not seem indicated, patients with inflammatory lesions of the external genitalia and rectum, and those with obscure diseases of the urethra and bladder are worth testing.

### c) Fungus

Fungus infections evoking an allergic response of the delayed type include coccidioidomycosis, histoplasmosis and epidermatophytosis, as well as sporo-trichosis, blastomyocosis and aspergillosis. Some of these diseases involve organs of the urogenital tract such as the kidneys and occasionally the prostate and external genital tract through dissemination of the infection in the blood stream. The allergic skin reaction tests are valuable diagnostic procedures in differen-tiating the lesions produced by these diseases from those of tuberculosis which they may often resemble closely clinically and pathologically (ROLNICK and BAUMBRUCKER 1958).

## 2. Diseases in which the role of delayed allergy has been demonstrated

### a) Infectious diseases: Tuberculosis

Of the infectious diseases, tuberculosis is an outstanding example of the effect of delayed allergy on the response of the host to the infectious process. Considerations in this regard are of significance to any physician dealing with tuberculosis in the urogenital tract. In addition to the subtle primary effect of virulent bacilli on the normal physiologic activity of phagocytes, there develops, during infection, an allergic hypersensitivity to tubercular proteins and to other components of the bacteria. The early appearance of hypersensitivity modifies the host-parasite relationship in very complex fashion and is an inseparable part of natural tuberculous infections. The clinical symptoms of general toxicity in this disease are probably, in large part, a consequence of acquired systemic hypersensitiveness to metabolic products of the parasite. As KOCH demonstrated, the guinea pig does not react to the local injection of tubercle bacilli until two to three weeks have elapsed. At this time, co-incident with the development of the delayed allergy, there is a focal reaction around the injection site. Sub-sequent injections of tubercle bacilli also evoke a delayed inflammatory response which tends to inhibit dissemination of the bacilli. A parallel situation in human infection is the acquisition of the "Ghon complex" as a result of the first meeting with tubercle bacilli as compared to the caseating, necrotizing type of inflamma-tory response in the lung (and which may also later occur in kidney) which occurs in the adult re-infection type of tuberculosis. Thus, the early exudative lesion of tuberculosis may heal by resolution, i.e., multiplication of bacilli is inhibited and they may be destroyed and tissue healing may take place without a scar. It may undergo necrosis and lead to massive cavity formation or it may develop into a productive (proliferative) type of lesion, the most frequently observed lesion in tuberculosis because of its chronic character. The development of the chronic lesion depends upon a large number of bacilli or their rapid multi-plication in a host of low resistance, or a high degree of hypersensitivity of the host, and leads to early and widespread necrosis, even at sites where, presumably, the typical tubercle hardly has an opportunity to form (caseous and gelatinous pneumonia). Tuberculin sensitivity once developed is usually lasting.

The tuberculin test which is based on hypersensitivity of the skin to tuberculin indicates infection, but not necessarily disease. A negative test usually rules out disease. Systemic symptoms evoked by relatively small amounts of tuber-culin are seen following the diagnostic skin test performed on sensitive subjects.

Larger amounts of tuberculin inhaled by laboratory workers preparing this material have caused more serious symptoms. There is also recorded observations of flaring up of quiescent lung lesions following the administration of large amounts of tuberculin. The caseation necrosis of adult tuberculosis in addition to favoring a protracted course and impeding spontaneous eradication of the bacillus probably also inhibits antimicrobic therapy in this disease. MacLeod has suggested that the development of resistance to antimicrobic therapy is favored by the impediment to diffusion of the drug which the tuberculous lesion, a granuloma, presents. This is conducive to the growth of strains of tubercle bacilli exposed to low concentrations of drug within the lesion — an excellent means of selecting resistant strains. Similar factors may be operative in conditioning the manifestations to other bacterial, fungus and virus infections where granulomatous lesions form, such as, brucellosis, coccidioidomycosis, blastomycosis, chancroid and lymphogranuloma venereum which at times infect the urogenital tract.

The significance of the role of allergy in immunity against tuberculosis has long been a subject of intense controversy. Several viewpoints are held but it is not our purpose to discuss this aspect here since we feel that judgement should be reserved on this subject until further data are available. However, there seems little doubt that the amount of caseation necrosis which can be produced by any specific number of tubercle bacilli is determined in large measure by the degree of hypersensitivity of the host (RICH 1951; KOURILSKY 1952).

## b) Non-infectious processes: Dermatitis venenata

A contact type of delayed allergy may result from exposure to poison ivy, poison oak, sumac, or to a great variety of simple chemical compounds such as arsenic, nickel and mercury. The induction of sensitivity occurs ordinarily through the skin and subsequent contact with the inciting agent is followed by skin lesions. In the sensitized individual, the dermatitis resulting from contact may begin to appear within a day, evolving as papular and vesicular lesions with later oozing, crusting and desquamation, all during a period of a week or ten days.

The catechol derivative of the poison ivy plant, urushiol, causes the allergy known as poison ivy dermatitis. Acute nephritis following severe poison oak dermatitis has been described by RYTAND in seven patients, while in two others, he found periarteritis nodosa as a sequel. The writer has noted a case of acute nephritis occurring in a ten year old boy following poison oak dermatitis.

Many drugs and chemical substances, including such elements as nickel or mercury, may produce similar contact forms of hypersensitivity. Although sensitization to drugs injected or ingested may take an immediate form, this is very infrequently the case when sensitivity has been incurred through skin contact. Subsequent exposure to the drug by contact, sometimes by ingestion, then generally results in a dermatitis with the characteristics of the delayed reaction. An interesting example of this is seen following the application of penicillin and other chemotherapeutic and antibiotic agents to the skin and mucous membranes. The incidence of sensitization to penicillin as the result of this form of therapy has been reported to be as high as 10 to 15 per cent. The delayed contact sensitivity which results from topical application of penicillin shows manifestations very similar to those seen in poison oak or ivy dermatitis.

The manifestations of allergy to drugs are manifold, and can duplicate all the aspects of allergic reactions that we have been considering — anaphylaxis, immediate type reactions and delayed reactions. More commonly encountered, by far, is the delayed type reaction. Various forms of drug allergy include serum sickness, arthralagia, scarlatiniform and morbilliform rashes, asthma, flare and wheal reactions, urticaria, exfoliative dermatitis and many others. It should be understood that we are dealing with allergic manifestations, and not with exaggerated sensitivity to the established pharmacologic properties of the respective materials. The causative agents are, plainly enough, not antigens, but it appears that by combining with the tissues of the host (either directly or after some intermediary chemical alteration in vivo) they acquire antigenic capacity and function somewhat like the "conjugated antigens" of LANDSTEINER, which arise when hapten structures become attached to indifferent foreign protein. Thus, it is supposed that repeated contact with a given chemical, such as formalin, leads eventually to the formation of an antigen constructed from a combination of the chemical with the body proteins of the individual. After this has taken place, an allergic reaction results from intimate contact with the chemical.

Plant and chemical contact allergies are ordinarily acquired via the skin rather than by a parenteral route. As an illustration, the application of penicillin preparations to skin or mucuous membranes in general results in contact sensitivity to the drug. In contrast, parenteral injections of penicillin are apt to induce the serum sickness type of sensitivity with no reactivity to subsequent contact but responsiveness to subsequent injection. The lesion in contact sensitivity is usually a papular indurated one which later becomes vesicular. There is an independence of delayed hypersentitivity from humoral antibody and specific shock tissues. Congenital transmission of delayed hypersentitivity of either the infectious or contact type does not take place in man or animals.

# C. Pathologic anatomy and physiology

KLEMPERER has said "allergy is a dynamic process which provides certain tissue changes which in themselves are not characteristic. To try to prove the existence of a dynamic process from purely morphologic observations may lead to sterile speculation." While none of the histologic lesions in allergic states can be said to be pathognomonic, several of them are highly characteristic. The allergic reaction results in injury to the tissues which is followed by that wide variety of changes placed under the general title of inflammatory reactions. Death may ensue so rapidly, either because the stimulus is very strong or because the reactivity of the subject is so violent that no anatomic changes are demonstrable; or the duration of the stimulus and the response may be so brief and restitution to normal so rapid that again no anatomic changes as yet have been found. One may correlate the histologic classes of change and the clinical and immunologic phenomena in allergic diseases (BOHROD 1947).

The elementary morphologic changes which occur may be placed in four groups: (1) evidence of injury, (2) exudation, (3) proliferation and (4) repair. Evidence of injury includes necrosis and accumulation of abnormal substances in cells (degeneration). Necrosis is present in some degree, usually slight or moderate, in almost all of the histologic lesions of allergy. In certain of them, however, necrosis dominates the whole picture, or may even be the sole anatomic feature. The ARTHUS and SHWARTZMAN phenomena of experimental allergy are such lesions and they have their counterpart in human diseases such as periarteritis nodosa. Anatomically, the lesions are characterized by diffuse necrosis involving parenchymal cells, interstitial tissue, vascular structure and anything else in the area. There is often a sharp boundary betweeen areas of necrosis and normal tissue. Nuclear debris may be a striking feature in the necrotic zone. Around the area there is a variable amount of infiltration with inflammatory cells usually neutrophilic leukocytes. Eosinophils are rare. As examples of some human pathologic states which fall into this group, we can consider renal carbuncle and diffuse cortical necrosis of the kidney. Characteristically, these are preceded by renal infections of some kind (local sensitization) followed by very sudden, widespread necrosis of renal substance. They usually follow two types of renal infection, with staphylococcus and pyocyaneus. There is a sudden onset, diffuse necrotization and little or no inflammation at the onset. It may be seen in drug sensitivity where a phenonema of note is organ sensitivity. It can also occur as a result of protein hypersensitization. Thrombocytopenic purpura can result from sensitivity to chemical substances; and leukopenic states may be the result of either drug or protein hypersensitivity. As we have indicated, the anaphylactoid allergic diseases are characterized clinically by quick onset, relatively short course and often equally rapid regression, that is, by the immediate reactions of allergy. They are characterized pathologically predominately by exudative changes; edema, swelling of collagen and fibers, and in some cases, degeneration and fibrinoid necrosis of collagen. The diseases which make up the bulk of an allergist's practice fall into this group as well as some interesting conditions whose position as allergic is equivocal such as periarteritis nodosa and glomerulonephritis. Since many of the anaphylactoid lesions are at a quick tempo and short in duration, there is not time for anatomic change other than edema and the tissues are soon restored to a normal state. However, if the allergic insult is repeated often enough, restitution may not be entirely to normal and anatomic changes may be encountered which are the beginning of secondary phenomena observed in the allergic states such as smooth muscle hypertrophy, polyposis of mucous membranes and thickening of basement membranes. Cellular exudation varies in degree and kind. In very acute lesions, the only cells present may be neutrophile leukocytes; in other more chronic lesions, large phagocytic cells may be numerous or even predominate. There is a tendency for all of these lesions to contain a large number of eosinophils. Tissue eosinophilia is a highly characteristic finding in allergic lesions of the anaphylactoid type but is not pathognomonic. The necrosis which occurs in the anaphylactoid lesions differs from that of both predominately necrotizing and granulomatous lesions. In most instances it affects collagen and exhibits staining reactions resembling that of fibrin, hence, the term "fibrinoid necrosis". This is a characteristic finding in periarteritis nodosa so the latter is often called necrotizing arteritis. The latter may also be seen in glomerulonephritis.

Granulomatous lesions made up of inflammatory cells which have proliferated locally may be seen in allergic reactions. The essential structure consists of an essential area of necrosis surrounded by a proliferation of reticulo-endothelial cells which often assume a radial, palisaded arrangement. Other features are variable. Giant cells may or may not be present. They may be absent in tubercular and may be very numerous in non-tuberculous granulomas. In some of the allergic granulomas the central area of necrosis is in the proliferative and inflammatory tissue and is called caseation necrosis. The anatomic difference delimits two groups of granulomatous allergic lesions, the tuberculoid and rheumatoid. The work of RICH has shown that the anaphylactic type of hypersensitivity reaction to soluble antigen is capable of producing not only the banal types of inflammatory lesions, but also lesions of a distinctly tuberculoid character, i.e., accumulations of epitheloid giant cells which may closely simulate tuberculous lesions.

Tuberculoid allergic lesions are seen in such infections as brucellosis, tularemia, sporotrichosis, lymphopathia venereum and coccidioidomycosis. With allergic inflammation, all of the elements that constitute an inflammatory exudate, namely, serum, fibrin, granulocytes, including eosinophilic leukocytes, and histiocytes, accumulate with greater rapidity and in greater number than in the normal animal; antibodies, if present in the blood, are brought to the site of inflammation in increased quantity. These processes fix both foreign proteins, including doubtless those derived from micro-organisms, and micro-organisms themselves, at the site of inflammation so that passage from the site of inoculation into the blood stream is prevented. Intensified inflammation at the site of entrance of the injurious agent protects internal organs and in consequence, anaphylactic shock is unlikely to occur under normal conditions. In this process of local fixation it is not possible to estimate the relative importance of antibodies or phagocytes and of the inflammatory reaction itself. In the sensitized animal, both fixation and destruction of bacteria occur locally and in the regional lymph nodes.

Aside from the inflammatory changes and necrosis of tissue, we may say that some of the characteristic physiologic responses in allergic diseases are: (1) increased capillary permeability with resulting loss of fluid into the tissue, (2) increased secretion from mucous glands, (3) eosinophilia in tissue, blood and secretions, and (4) smooth muscle spasm. No matter which tissue is the site of reaction, the response is similar with one or another of these changes predominating. As has been intimated, it is readily understood that these reactions are functional and reversible. Obviously, if the reactions are long continued, secondary changes may occur. Smooth muscle spasm may lead to hypertrophy, mucous membranes may become polypoid and increased mucous secretion may be so marked and so viscid that obstruction to an organ, such as a small bronchus or the urethra, may occur.

The histopathologic physiology of allergic anaphylactic reactions, according to CHASE is characterized principally by an attachment of leukocytes and platelets to endothelium of small vessels for a time, with resulting leukopenia, liberation of histamine, liberation of heparin and decrease in blood coagulability, probably an increase in blood proteose, arteriolar and venous spasm, often followed by vasodilatation, rapid development of edema, indicative of injury to vascular endothelium, and a decrease in "complement". These changes are not listed in the order of their occurrence.

The presence of blood eosinophilia has been considered a characteristic sign of allergic diseases but this manifestation is found in numerous other conditions, so we cannot consider blood or tissue eosinophilia, per se, as conclusive evidence of the existence of an allergy. It appears that the eosinophilia is less important than fluctuations in the eosinophilic curve. Remarkably few changes in the blood are to be found even in severe allergic manifestations except acute anaphylactic shock. There may be a fall in the total leukocyte count, a decrease in the number of neutrophils with a relative increase of the mononuclear cells and a lowering of the refractive index of the serum. In anaphylactic shock there is a drop in the body temperature and prolongation of the blood coagulation time. The latter is said to be due to the release of heparin from the liver. Both of these symptoms are absent in histamine shock. While observations in animals have demonstrated an increase in the histamine contents of the blood in allergic reactions and it is recognized that histamine plays a role in clinical allergy, its fundamental significance is still under dispute. The changes in blood chemistry of allergic patients are so inconsistent that they must be designated as non-characteristic.

The physiologic response to hypersensitivity in the urinary tract usually expresses itself in the form of edema of the capillary epithelium of the urethra, bladder or ureter or spasm of the smooth muscle of the bladder, ureter or renal pelvis. At times there may be necrosis of tissue, particularly in the kidney. It has been demonstrated experimentally that smooth muscle spasm occurs in the bladder and uterus when specific allergens are injected into previously sensitized animals. MANWARING and MARINO presented proof that bladder allergy does exist and substantiated their evidence by the production of an allergic reaction in rabbits. MANWARING and others have demonstrated definite uterine and bladder contractions produced by injecting horse serum into previously sensitized dogs.

By means of a direct immunologic technique, BARETZ, HARTEN and WALZER have demonstrated that traces of unaltered protein are rapidly absorbed from the urinary bladder in Rhesus monkey and in humans. This organ must, therefore, be considered as a possible site of absorption of allergenic substances introduced into the bladder for therapeutic or diagnostic purposes. From the allergic point of view, such traces of absorbed protein are more than sufficient to produce severe reactions in individuals who are sensitive to the allergen employed.

Bacterial sensitization occurs in various organs of the urogenital tract, especially the kidney. LONG and FINNER perfused kidneys of tuberculous swine with tuberculin and found that a diffuse inflammation of the kidneys was produced which they felt was very similar to acute glomerulonephritis with severe glomerular injury, including hemorrhage and proliferation of tuft and capsular epithelium. In addition, they noted an acute, non-suppurative interstitial nephritis and all the tubular damage that goes with glomerular injury. Casts were numerous and the urine contained protein. This effect did not occur following the perfusion of the kidney of non-tuberculous swine with tuberculin. LONG has also noted that when a small amount of tuberculin is introduced into the testis of a tuberculous guinea pig, an initial, acute, exudative reaction occurs, with active hyperemia and escape of plasma and leukocytes into the interstitial tissue, and at the same time, with severe injury to the cells of the seminiferous tubules, the spermatocytes are particularly affected. This reaction, which takes place within twenty-four hours, is followed by a period of absorption of the exudate and degenerated parenchymatous cells. At the end of the month, the germinal cells, with the exception of the spermatogonia, are entirely absorbed and the interstitial tissue is increased. The reaction is specific for the hypersensitive state, the introduction of the tuberculin into the testis of the normal animal being without effect (G. VOISIN, A. DELAUNAY and M. BARBER 1951).

In connection with the above experiment, it is well to note that infection with tubercle bacilli enhances the ability of the host to respond to antigens not related to tubercle bacilli. Antibody formation is non-specifically increased and sensitization is altered (FREUND 1947).

FREUND and associates have presented experiments to show that the injection of a suspension of homologous or autologous testicular material, combined with paraffin oil and killed mycobacteria, into guinea pigs, produces aspermatogenesis without inflammation and also the formation of specific antibodies. Control experiments of various kinds seem to indicate that the aspermatogenesis so induced is organ-and-species-specific; that is, of immunologic nature (FREUND 1953).

# D. Predisposing and contributory factors in allergy

## I. Hereditary factors

For many years, hereditary predisposition has been respected as constituting one of the basic factors in the development of atopic hypersensitivity in an individual. As indicated in the discussion on the atopic type of allergy, it has been recognized that what is inherited is not the allergic disease, that is the clinical type of reaction, but merely the allergic tendency or a capacity for a pathologically increased physiologic reactivity. At times, heredity predisposes to specific manifestations such as asthma, hay fever, migraine or angioneurotic edema affecting special tissues, and may even tend to the development of sensitization to specific allergies. Thus, ROWE says that he has noted milk and egg sensitization in two or three generations. The theory of heredity has found support in statistics showing that more than 50 per cent of allergic patients gave positive allergic family histories, while the general population reported family histories of allergy in only about 10 per cent of the cases. We have found no mention or record of the inheritance of urogenital allergy in the literature (SPAIN and COOKE 1924).

It is felt, if allergy is inherited, it is done so as a dominant characteristic in accordance with mendelian law and also by active as well as passive sensitization in utero. WIENER, ZIEVE and FRIES have proposed that the heredity of atopy depends on a single pair of alleles, H and h, where gene h determines the atopic constitution, and gene H, the normal. According to them, the expressivity of the gentotype is irregular in that about $1/_6$ of the heterozygotes are atopic. The homozygous atopic genotype is expressed before puberty. This hypothesis is widely accepted today.

## II. Climatic influences

Clinically, it is well known fact that seasonal, meterologic and climatic influences are important factors in the production of allergic diseases and also in the elicitation of individual attacks. In the spring and autumn, sensitivities appear to be increased or organism resistance lessened. There is a seasonal dependency of allergic dermatitides and prurigo, a spring peak in sensitivity to tuberculin, and connections between the weather and asthma and hay fever. There is some importance of meterologic and atmospheric conditions such as barometric pressure, air motion, temperature, high humidity, and degree and duration of sunshine. Geographic influences are important. Damp areas favor development of asthma and rhinopathy, whereas dry regions (desert) are better for patients with asthma. The type and quantity of vegetation in a given region are of importance.

## III. Infections

It can be assumed that bacteria or their toxins lower the threshold of tolerance to antigens. Both acute infectious diseases and chronic foci of infection are to be considered in this regard. Important sites for foci of infection are to be sought in the urogenital tract: kidney, bladder, urethra, prostate, endometrium and endocervix, as well as in the teeth, sinuses, ears, bronchi, bone and joints, skin and gastro-intestinal tract.

## IV. Endocrine glands and autonomic nervous system

The endocrine glands and their products have an effect on allergies. Hyperthyroidism, menstruation, and the menopause have an enhancing effect, while myxedema, pregnancy, epinephrine, pituitrin and parathyroid extract have an inhibiting effect on human allergies. It is a well known fact that drugs that stimulate the parasympathetics favor allergization or tend to prolong an existing hypersensitiveness. In most allergic patients, one is impressed by the high incidence of vasomotor instability or irritability. Some of the most characteristic manifestations of allergic disease, including increased smooth muscle tonus, vasodilatation of the blood vessels and the increased secretory activity of the mucous membranes appear to be causally related to a heightened parasympathetic or cholingeric activity.

## V. Social and environmental factors

Allergic diseases are definitely diseases of civilization — what is responsible for this is not known. Factors to be considered are faulty diet, tension and excitement of city life, central heating and air conditioning, pollution or dust and social factors predisposing to allergy. The intellectually and socially superior classes appear to have a considerably higher incidence of allergies. The rural population has a lower incidence of hay fever than urban. Among environmental factors, exposure to allergen is by far the most important. Allergization depends as much on quantitative as on qualitative factors. The factor of exposure is important in predisposition to dermatitides, asthma and rhinopathies due to increased contact with chemicals in industry and the home and exposure to pollens, molds and smuts.

## VI. Psychosomatic

There is a steadily accumulating body of evidence indicating the importance of psychic factors in predisposing to, precipitating, aggravating and maintaining allergic diseases. They may be an eliciting factor or trigger mechanism in an already established allergic disease — essentially a conditioned reflex. The explanation of the manner in which psychic factors predisposes to allergy is not easy. They may do so by bringing on alterations in excitability of the automonic nervous system, or an increase in blood supply of peripheral tissue. The personality of the allergically susceptible individual is commonly characterized by emotional immaturity, relative passivity and need for dependence upon some authoritative, yet kindly person (SAUL 1941).

# E. Classification of etiologic agents of allergic disease (allergens)

Most of the etiologic factors in human allergy are found in our environment. There are a great variety and number of allergens or exciting agents, some of which have been noted to affect the urogenital system. Any physician who wishes to treat allergic conditions should be cognizant of the totality of the environment of his patients. Many substances are capable of exerting an allergenic influence by way of more than one route of entry. For example, penicillin may produce manifestations of hypersensitiveness after injection, ingestion, or contact with the skin. A knowledge of the distribution of allergens in nature, food, fabrics and other ways in the environment is essential both in properly evaluating the patient's exposure as a first step in establishing the etiologic diagnosis and in planning an effective therapeutic regimen. The following classification is made on a more or less arbitrary category with some unavoidable overlapping.

# I. Inhalants

Considered in this class of allergens are those epidermal substances inhaled into the body, such as pollens, house dust, rusts, molds or volatile oils. Their allergic expression is usually in the clinical form of asthma or rhinopathy, but occasional cases of urticaria, angioneurotic edema, neurodermatitis, and migraine may develop from them. Dust is the most important of the inhalant allergens. While it has not been possible to demonstrate the existence of a single characteristic antigenic entity in house dust and so little is known about its nature, house dust must be considered a specific antigen, unrelated to other recognized inhalants. The group of epidermal allergens includes animal and human dander, hair, hides, sheep's wool and feathers. Allergy due to inhalation of air borne insect fragments or mites is comparatively rare.

Plant pollen are principle causes of the symptom complex called hay fever. Inhalation of certain chemicals may cause asthma and other sensitivity. The author has had three cases in his experience where exposure to walnut pollens caused symptoms of marked bladder irritability — frequency, urgency and tenesmus — all relieved when the patient avoided contact with the pollen.

# II. Ingestants

One large class of allergens are the ingestants, i.e., substances taken by mouth such as food and drugs. Foods can evoke almost all, including the most unusual, allergic manifestations. In principle, there is no food or drug, whether of animal, vegetable or inorganic origin, that cannot be an allergen. They are of predominant importance in causing allergic diseases of the gastro-intestinal tract, but they are also of great significance in allergic disorders of the skin, of the nervous system and of the urinary tract. Some of the possible clinical manifestations of food allergy in the urinary system are enuresis, bladder irritability, renal colic, hematuria and albuminuria. The existence of an underlying food allergy requires unequivocal proof in every case. This is best done by elimination diets, trial diets or protein diets in connection with careful food diaries. It must be noted that some forms of hypersensitivity in man, particularly to foods, can occur without evidence for circulating antibody and without positive cutaneous reactivity to the offending allergen. Young babies are said to have been sensitized by substances or foods in the maternal diet.

Drugs may produce their effects through ingestion, injection, inhalation, contact with, or injection into the skin and very rarely, through absorption by the mucous membranes of the mouth, rectum, urethra and vagina. In this section, we are considering drugs as ingestants. A distinction must be made between drug intolerance consisting in an exaggeration of the physiological actions of the drug, which are manifestations of the toxicity to the drug and not allergy, and true allergic hypersensitivity, in which the type of reactive manifestation is entirely independent of the chemical and pharmacodynamic properties of the drug, and depends only on which tissue has been allergized. The diagnosis of drug allergy can be established with certainty by appropriate avoidance and re-exposure tests. Other tests are placing minute amounts of the drug on the tongue or on conjunctiva, as in testing for diodrast sensitivity, and occasionally intradermal tests. An accurate and comprehensive history is important.

Drugs can evoke every type of skin manifestation, and the same drug may elicit the most varied responses in the same patient. Aside from the skin eruptions, the following are among the reactions most frequently encountered: asthma, rhinitis, nausea, malaise, attacks of abdominal cramps and diarrhea, bleeding from the urogenital tract, lymphadenopathy, granulocytopenia, swelling of the joints, fever, pain in the extremities and finally, anaphylactic death.

## III. Injectants

This group comprises all the antigenic substances that allergize the organism by way of the parenteral route, and which when re-injected, elicit manifestations of hypersensitivity. It includes drugs, foreign sera, hormones and vitamins. The allergic manifestations of injected drugs are similar to the responses from the same drugs administered orally except that, as a rule, they are more severe and of longer duration. The chief drugs of primary interest to urologists are the antibiotics such as penicillin, the arsenicals, diodrast and other iodine containing pyelographic media, and local anesthetic agents. The effect of horse serum in producing anaphylaxis has been noted above.

## IV. Contactants

The allergens which elicit manifestations of hypersensitiveness by means of direct contact with the skin or the mucosa are manifold. This group is probably the largest and most heterogenous of all allergens, embracing not only thousands of various chemicals, including cosmetics and drugs, but also innumerable plants and animal products that are capable of allergenic action. The clinical manifestations vary considerably. They include many types and degrees of inflammation of the skin and mucosa, such as dermatitis, urticaria, chelitis and occasionally, stomatitis. It would be impossible to submit here a complete list of the agents that have been found to act as contactants or to innumerate the various trades and professions with respect to the dermatitis-producing substances peculiar to each. There is probably no organic or inorganic substance that cannot, under appropriate circumstances, become an allergic contactant. A frequent manifestation of contact hypersensitivity is a dermatitis due to poison ivy. Contact sensitivities are usually of the delayed type. Sensitization is accomplished by repeated applications made on or into the skin. The sensitivity arises in 5 to 20 days and is often seen first on the 7th or 8th day, as a flare in old sites, owing to a reaction with remaining traces of the sensitizing complex. To affect the sensitization, chemicals combine with proteins to make derivative or partial antigens. In man, immediate type, flare and wheal reactions, to drugs have been found in several instances (salvarsan, formaldehyde, chloramine-T, sulfathiazole, sulfadiazine) and are accompanied by demonstrable reagins. Manifestations of contact dermatitis in the urogenital system usually find expression in dermatitis of the penis from condom rubber, chemicals, contact with irritative allergens in the patient's occupation or from the clothes he is wearing, which also usually give rise to dermatitis of the scrotum and surrounding perineum. Patients sensitive to fungus often have an outbreak of dermatitis on the scrotum after the administration of penicillin and other antibiotics which the writer has seen on several occasions. Poison ivy or poison oak may involve the genitalia and produce severe dermatitis.

## V. Infectants

Bacteria, viruses and fungi can act as allergic agents as indicated under the discussion on delayed hypersensitivity. It is felt that with bacteria, an allergic response can be elicited by two entirely different mechanisms, one mediated by toxins, and the other, by the bacterial proteins or carbohydrates. As was noted, microbial allergy plays a part in the onset of infection, in the clinical manifestation of the disease, in the course of infection, and lastly, in its outcome. In patients suffering from or recovered from an infection, bacterial antigen used for skin testing reacts with the cellular antibodies as manifested most commonly by delayed inflammatory and only occasionally, by immediate wheal responses. Such is the situation in using bacterial extracts such as tuberculin mallein, brucellergen and trichophton, which indicate the presence of a specific hypersensitiveness in the infected organism by a delayed inflammatory reaction. Of particular interest to urologists are diagnostic tests for chancroid and lympho-granuloma venereum. As shown by Frei test, the presence of the latter can be demonstrated by a specific allergic skin reaction to sterilized pus aspirated from an unruptured inguinal bubo. Once a Frei test is positive, it remains so for life. By means of intra-cutaneous reactions to Ducrey's bacillus vaccine, it is possible to demonstrate that the reactivity of the skin of the chancroid patient has been specifically altered. This altered activity of the skin persists for decades after the disease has been cured and possibly, for a lifetime.

## VI. Physical agents

By the term "physical allergy" is implied the type of reaction—nasal, bronchial, cutaneous—which simulates, in general character, the inherited human allergies commonly classed as pollen disease and food and drug hypersensitivities but which is caused by physical agents such as light, heat, cold, mechanical irritation, freezing, burns and mental or physical effort. The manifestations resulting from exposure to such agents have become well recognized, but the nature of their cause continues to be questioned. In order to identify an immunologic mechanism in their causation, there has been repeated search for specific skin—transferable antibodies in the serum of affected patients or the production of anaphylaxis in experimental animals. Positive-passive transfer has been demonstrated in a significant number but not all cases of cold and light urticaria. Passive transfer never has been demonstrated in patients with generalized heat sensitivity. On the other hand, evidence has been presented to show that the symptoms of physical allergy may be mediated through a non-allergic mechanism involving excitation of peripheral nerves with the release of acetylcholine or involving the direct release of histamine, or possibly involving the generation of toxic substances in the tissue as a direct effect of the physical agents involved. In some instances, antihistamines have been helpful in controlling the symptoms of cold, heat and light urticaria (SACK 1957).

## VII. Common allergens affecting the genitourinary tract

While most of the above mentioned substances or physical agents could act as allergens and produce manifestations of hypersensitivity in the urogenital system, there are certain substances which are the most frequent offenders. As will be noted later, these include the more common foods: the cereal grains, especially wheat, eggs, milk, sea foods, meat, beans, nuts, tomatoes, potato, and citrus fruits; drugs such as phenolphthalein, ephedrine, iodine—containing contrast media, foreign sera, sulfonamides, penicillin and streptomycin; certain inhalants such as various pollens and dust; alcoholic beverages; coffee, tea and soft drinks; surface anesthetic agents and miscellaneous therapeutic chemical agents and other substances coming in contact with the external genitalia of both sexes. Bacterial, viral and fungal agents are important causes of expressions of delayed hypersensitivity, as noted above.

# F. Criteria for considering a condition allergic

In coming to consideration whether or not a given urogenital condition is a manifestation of hypersensitivity, it is well to keep in mind certain criteria. DOERR (1929) has outlined four criteria which must be fulfilled before a condition may be properly accepted as being of truly allergic origin: (1) Aberrance from the norm, as evidenced by comparison between an individual's present and previous behavior, or in a congenital case, between the given individual's behavior and that of others. (2) Specificity: either mono-or polyvalent, to one or many agents of the same class. (3) The symptomatology of the allergic reaction must be totally unrelated to the pharmacodynamic properties of the given allergen. One must differentiate toxic and allergic reactions to drugs. (4) There should be proof of the organic basis of the allergic manifestation by demonstration of specific antisubstances (antibodies). This can be accomplished in any of several ways, namely: by passive transfer of the reactivity by means of blood serum or of blister fluid (Prausnitz-Kuestner method), by testing the reactivity of isolated organs or tissues by means of the Schultz-Dale experiment, or by specific hyposensitization. Unfortunately, the demonstration of antibodies is by no means practical in every case. It will suffice in principle that the demonstration of the antigen-antibody mechanism can be made in a sufficient number of cases of a given type or during certain phases of these cases. There must be previous exposure, since no allergic reactions occur on initial exposure. The symptoms must disappear when contact with the suspected substance is avoided or prevented. The original reaction or symptoms must be capable of artificial induction at will on resumption of contact with the allergen. True allergic reactions are consistent. One is not sensitive to milk one day and not again the next day under equivalent circumstances.

# G. Diagnosis

## I. History

The most important factor in diagnosis of an allergic disorder is a complete and detailed history. This must be taken in a careful and painstaking manner and often requires two or more consultations before all the pertinent facts can be marshalled for a proper workup. The patient as a whole must be thoroughly evaluated. The challenge of proper differential diagnosis exists in every patient. When an initial history is made it is often wise to have the patient keep a written diary of the exact times his symptoms occur in relation to his daily activities such as food intake, work, recreation, and sleep. One begins by taking an allergy history in the same manner as an ordinary medical history is obtained. It is best at first to allow the patient, in his own words, to outline his symptoms. Thus, one can often make certain that some non-allergic condition is not the most probable cause for the patient's complaints. Although allergic symptoms may be continuous, most often they are intermittent and occur in paroxysms. Allergic diseases are usually generalized and unilateral lesions suggest a non-allergic state. Probably the most important part of the allergic history is a detailed account of the course of the disease. The physician should know if the symptoms are continuous or intermittent in character and the date of onset of the first symptom. He should inquire about the frequency and duration of the episodes of symptoms. Next, seasonal variations and symptomatology should be determined. Find out the time, then the place the symptoms occur.

Is he better on vacations or trips to distant places? Is he worse or better off at work or home? Is he better outdoors than indoors? Inquire of any environmental agents which seem to precipitate or aggravate his symptoms. Ask about the relationship of symptoms to infection, emotional upsets and endocrine factors such as pregnancy and menstruation. After the patient has related his own story, it is necessary to find out about any previous diagnostic studies or therapy. This inquiry has a fourfold purpose: (1) It is of interest to see if the person studied has responded previously to drugs and other symptomatic measures usually effective in allergic disease. A good response tends to substantiate an allergic basis for the complaints, while failure to obtain relief would tend to make one reconsider other causes for the illness. (2) Previously prescribed measures of therapy may have perpetrated the patient's disease. The excessive use of nose drops, sensitivity to ointments that are being applied to the skin, and allergy to drugs are examples of this. (3) Inquiry about previous tests and treatment may save the needless repetition of procedures which have proved to be of no value. The physician should be certain that such previous measures really were properly carried out for an adequate length of time before considering them to have failed. (4) The patient may be taking medications which alter the physical findings and skin tests. It may be necessary to defer the latter until such medications have been discontinued.

A complete systemic history should be taken on every patient examined for allergy. In this way, the physician is likely to unveil important symptoms which may point to other diseases. For purposes of our discussion, particular attention must be paid to the genitourinary system. In Table 1 is a suggested history outline for allergic patients.

Since heredity is considered to play a rather important part in predisposing a patient to an allergic disease, the existence of allergy on the maternal and/or paternal side of the patient's family should be recorded. Often it is helpful to ask of either parent or any relatives had "catarrh", sinus trouble, periodic headaches, attacks of shortness of breath and coughing, skin trouble or hives. It is also well to ask if there is any family history of tuberculosis, heart disease, cancer or diabetes.

## II. Symptomatology

### 1. General

In addition to the presenting symptoms, there may be elicited a history of urticaria, skin eruptions, itching, headaches, sneezing, rhinitis, joint pains, eye symptoms, gastro-intestinal upsets, wheezing, dyspnea or cough. It is not uncommon to encounter multiple symptoms in one patient. More than one allergic disease may be present in the same patient, as asthma and vesical spasm or irritability. Thus, we can have collateral allergy.

### 2. Urogenital

The symptoms of genito-urinary hypersensitivity are much like those of the more common urologic diseases. These include renal colic, frequency of, and burning or pain on urination, nocturia, suprapubic distress, tenesmus, enuresis, hematuria, difficulty with urination, itching and edema of the genitalia.

Table 1. *History outline for allergic patients*

| Chief complaints | Chief complaints of patient |
|---|---|
| History of Present Illness | 1. Initial attack:<br>Character, time of onset and place of symptoms, precipitating factors and duration.<br>2. History of succeeding attacks:<br>Frequency and time of occurrence.<br>3. History of last attack:<br>Date, time and place of occurrence.<br>Duration of attack.<br>Relation to meals, time of day and to sleep.<br>Initial and later symptoms, e.g., lacrimation, itching of eyes or nose, sneezing, rhinorrhea, cough, expectoration, dyspnea or wheezing, frequency, urgency, burning on urination, ureteral colic, hematuria. Effect of following factors upon attack: Changes in climate, wind, dust, exertion, meals, inhalation of such irritants as house dust, powders, tobacco smoke, camphor, tar, etc. Occupation, changes in residence, environmental changes (vacation, visits), changes in temperature or humidity, chilling, cold baths, etc.; also, effect of menses.<br>4. General health of patient at time of examination, occurrence of headaches, vertigo, chest pain, gastro-intestinal complaints, menstrual difficulties or cutaneous disorders like hives, etc. |
| Past Medical History | 1. Diseases of infancy and childhood:<br>Eczema, cyclic vomiting, "colds", bronchitis, feeding problem, broncho-pneumonia, urticaria, skin lesions, migraine.<br>2. Vaccination or immunization (reactions from). Smallpox, typhoid, tetanus, diptheria, and scarlatina, influenza.<br>3. Previous treatment for present condition, successful or not.<br>4. Operations, injuries, hospitalizations.<br>5. Diseases of greatest medical importance: Rheumatic fever, tuberculosis, diabetes, heart disease, hypertension and kidney disease.<br>6. Review of systems: Cardiovascular, genito-urinary, gastro-intestinal and neuromuscular. |
| Family History | 1. History of allergic diseases:<br>Asthma, hay fever, migraine eczema, and epilepsy in immediate family or relatives (including grandparents, uncles, aunts or cousins) on maternal and paternal sides. |
| Social History and Environmental History | Occupation and residence (whether private or store). Character of bedding (pillows, mattresses and blankets). Presence of dust-containing articles (like rugs, curtains). Contact with animals (horse, dog, cat, etc). Exposure to dust, plants, cosmetics, tobacco, insecticides, etc. Character of patient's diet, nature, type of foods eaten and food dislikes (detailed). Ingestion of drugs and determination of possible idiosyncrasy. |
| Habits | Use of tobacco, alcohol, tea, coffee, cola, etc., and amounts. |
| Hobbies | Aviation, botany, cooking, gardening, painting, photography, swimming, etc. |
| Psychosomatic | Investigation of possible psychic or emotional problems when indicated: marriage (adjustment), fatigue, tension, worry, etc. |
| Physical Agents | Heat, cold, weather change, sunlight, exercise, drafts. |

# III. Physical examination

A complete physical examination is necessary for every patient suspected of having an allergic disease. Whether this is done by the urologist or the referring doctor is not so important as the fact it is done to determine the status of the patient's health and to be sure that no disease accompanying the allergic problem has been overlooked. Of course, particular attention should be paid to the usual allergic shock organs, the skin, lungs and nose. Foci of infection and evidence of frank systemic disease should be recorded carefully. Special attention should be given, of course, to the region of chief complaints which, in our discussion, is the urogenital system. Urologically, careful inspection and palpation of the abdomen, external genitalia, and prostate gland are very necessary to note any abnormalities. Those of most allergic significance will be inflammation or edema of the skin (dermatitis or urticaria) of the penis or scrotum, inflammation or edema of the urethra, tenderness over the kidneys, muscle spasm in the flank and abdomen and the size and consistency of the prostate gland and seminal vesicles. Marked congestion of the prostate gland in the absence of severe infection may be suggestive of an allergic reaction.

## IV. Laboratory examinations

After a complete history and careful physical examination, certain laboratory tests should be made to help confirm the diagnosis as they are indicated. Many of these are special examinations and should be made by an allergist or a physician versed in the technique and interpretation of the reactions rather than by the urologist who is usually not prepared or competent to perform them.

### 1. Urinalysis

A complete urinalysis should be made in every case to help rule out non-allergic disease and to detect certain suggestive findings of allergic disease such as eosinophils and mononuclear cells in the stained urinary sediment. Urinalysis may have to be repeated several times. In chronic cases, bacteria and polymorpho-nuclear leukocytes may be found as well as mononuclear cells and eosinophils (KINDALL and NICKELS). Hematuria may be of any degree from the finding of a few red blood cells in the urine to a frank red or port wine urine. In some cases of abacterial bladder or urethral inflammation considered to be on an allergic basis, the writer has found large clusters or clumps of desquamated cells of transitional epithelium as the only finding in the urinary sediment.

### 2. Blood

A complete blood count with particular study of the stained smear for eosinophilic cells should be made in every case of suspected allergy. At times, it may have to be repeated to discover possible allergy. The peripheral blood in the allergic patient usually is not altered except for possible presence of eosinophilia. More than 3 eosinophils per 100 white cells is regarded as significant. If the eosinophilia ranges from 3 to 7 per cent, extrinsic protein sensitivity (pollen or food allergy) is suggested. Remarkably few changes in the blood are to be found even in severe allergic manifestations except anaphylactic shock. There may be a fall in the polyleukocyte count, a decrease in the number of neutrophils with a relative increase of the mononuclear cells and a lowering of the refractive index of the serum. In anaphylactic shock, there is a prolongation of the blood coagulation time. As previously indicated the changes in blood chemistry of allergic patients are so inconsistent that they must be designated as non-characteristic.

## 3. Microscopic examination of removed tissue

A careful microscopic examination of tissue removed by biopsy, cystoscopy, or surgery from the external genitalia, urethra, bladder, prostate or kidney, in cases of suspected allergic lesions should be made to help detect any signs or evidence of allergic inflammation such as eosinophilia in large amounts, granulomata or fibrinoid necrosis.

# V. Special examinations

## 1. Skin tests

Skin tests help to confirm the diagnosis of sensitivity on an objective basis. They should be done only after taking a careful history and are not necessary or advisable in every case. They should be performed by an allergist or physician acquainted with the techniques and the interpretation of the reactions which at times may be rather violent and even fatal. The two main groups of allergens for which skin tests are carried out are foods and inhalants. Skin testing for foods is often not very reliable as relatively few of the positive reactions are correlated with clinical sensitivity. A trial or elimination diet followed by individual food additions is the most reliable method for determining clinical sensitivity to foods. On the other hand, one can place considerable reliance for clinical purposes upon the results obtained from skin testing for sensitivity to inhalants (ROWE 1937; RINKEL 1944).

*Types of skin tests. Scratch test:* These are made on the back. Drops of antigen are placed on the patient's back, then a sharp darning needle is taken and a prick or scratch about 2 millimeters in length is made in the patient's skin through the drop of antigen. This is done with several antigens and after 20 minutes, the erythema or wheal reaction is interpreted and recorded. Controls are done with saline. *Intracutaneous tests:* These are a more sensitive technique than scratch tests. They are only done when the latter are negative for a certain antigen. The diluted antigen is injected as superficially as possible into the skin and the results are read after twenty minutes. *Passive transfer:* (PRAUSNITZ-KÜSTNER test) This is used where direct skin tests cannot be performed satisfactorily. The serum of the sensitized individual is injected into the skin of another (normal) person. Then 24–48 hours later, the testing antigen is injected into the same site and the reaction is noted. *Patch tests:* This is the specific diagnostic procedure for establishing the etiologic agent or agents responsible for contact dermatitis. There is no reason for performing scratch or intradermal tests in contact dermatitis patients. Patch testing induces a delayed skin response which is not maximal until 24 hours or more after the material is applied. The technique involves placing patches of antigenic material on the back (usually 25 tests are done at a time) then gauze is placed over the material and on top of this a piece of ordinary bond paper is placed and this is covered by adhesive tape. The patient returns in 24 hours for reading of the tests.

## 2. Ophthalmic tests

In this test, antigen is placed in direct contact with the mucous membrane of the eye which is watched for response. When the patient gives an excellent history for sensitivity to a particular antigen but demonstrates a negative reaction to skin tests for that antigen, it may be helpful in establishing the diagnosis to perform an ophthalmic test. If redness of the conjunctiva or sclera occurs, the reaction is regarded as positive. Frequently this is associated with lacrimation, itching and rhinitis. At the end of the test, the eye should be washed out with saline or boric acid and it is often advisable to give an antihistamine by mouth if the reaction is a strong one. Urologists at times use this test for sensitivity to diodrast or other contrast media before injecting for pyelograms.

### 3. Other tests

At times one may use buccal or nasal mucosal tests in certain cases for sensitivities.

## VI. Complete urological survey

A complete urological investigation should be performed to rule out any organic disease in the genito-urinary tract and to discover any evidence of possible allergic inflammation such as marked edema or redness of the tissues, muscle spasm or polypoid and granulomatous lesions. Aside from careful inspection and palpation of the abdomen, the external genitalia, the female pelvic organs and the prostate gland, it is necessary to calibrate the urethra to detect the presence of stricture or spasm, estimate the bladder capacity and make tests for residual urine. Cultures should be made of any urethral discharge and when no bacteria are found, study of the secretion for eosinophils is indicated. In certain instances of congestive prostatitis it may be advantageous to culture the expressed secretion and if no organisms are found, to make stained smears for eosinophils. Besides a complete urinalysis, cultures of the urine from the bladder and both kidneys may have to be obtained as well as differential studies of renal function by the more common tests such as the indigo-carmine, phenolsulfonphthalein and urea clearance tests. This will involve cystoscopy at which time careful inspection of the entire urethra, as well as the neck of the bladder and the bladder, should be made thoroughly, looking particularly for evidence of edema of the tissues, cysts, polyps and other signs of inflammation of the mucosa of the entire lower urinary tract. Visualization of the urinary tract by cysto-urethrograms, intravenous and retrograde pyelography should be performed to detect any anatomic or physiologic abnormalities. In certain cases, these studies may have to be repeated 2 or more times. It is particularly advantageous to investigate the patient during an acute attack of the disease or symptoms, since allergic manifestations are transitory.

## VII. Therapeutic or clinical trial

Therapeutic or clinical trial is a very helpful procedure which often has to be employed to detect the offending agent, most frequently a food or drug. It involves the use of elimination, provocative or restricted diets with subsequent resumption of individual food items until the causative agent is discovered. Some form of dietary diary is essential in this work. One with a column giving the hour of symptom onset is especially valuable. A careful scrutiny of this diary, which can also be used in patients taking drugs or other non-food substances, and repeated testing for the possible incriminating deleterious factors it suggests, will usually sooner or later reveal the inciting agent, secondary unsuspected sensitivity or minor sensitivities that are delaying clearing of the condition.

For detailed information, the reader should consult ROWE's book on allergy in which several types of diet are presented to aid in diagnosis and treatment. Briefly, the following is the usual procedure. In testing for food sensitivity, one should consider first the common offenders which are the staple articles of diet, such as milk, wheat or other cereal-grains, eggs, citrus fruits, etc. The first trial diet is made upon the basis of a history of known or suspected foods, together with those giving positive skin reactions. This diet is changed from time to time by adding or omitting certain foods, according to clinical response. If no improvement is evident within a reasonable period of time, the elimination diet is indicated. It is a more restricted diet and includes comparatively few foods that are not commonly used by the patient. When improvement is noted, then each food is added singularly and its allergenic status is evaluated. The causative food is sometimes easily determined, or it may require a more detailed and persistent procedure. There is no set rule; each patient is an individual clinical problem and must be treated as such. Abstinence from the offending food for a varying time, depending on clinical sensitivity, is the best treatment. The trial response to such drugs as epinephrine, ephedrin, antihistamines or cortico-steroids may offer additional evidence in support of a diagnosis of allergy.

# H. Differential diagnosis

*Allergic versus common urogenital diseases.* Since the symptoms of allergic and non-allergic diseases in the urogenital tract are identical or very similar, the diagnosis of allergy can be entertained only after a complete urological study has excluded all other pathological changes and the previously mentioned criteria for considering a condition allergic fulfilled. There are no general diagnostic measures or tests for the differential diagnosis of allergic diseases. Certain features, such as periodicity, familial incidence, a history of other definite allergies in the patient and eosinophilia of the blood, tissue and secretions are common to enough of the various diseases of allergy to be helpful, but none is pathognomonic of allergy, and the differential diagnosis depends primarily on knowledge of the clinical features of each disease entity. Tumors and tuberculosis of the urogenital tract should be very carefully ruled out as they are great mimics of many diseases. Urinary infections may co-exist with allergy and their role in the disease picture must be properly evaluated. This is of particular significance when deciding whether or not symptoms of cystitis are of allergic origin.

Allergic reactions in the genitourinary system may mimic most of the common complaints usually referrable to this system except those due to gross anatomic changes. The possibility of allergic etiology is further enchanced when the symptoms co-exist with other more definitely allergic conditions such as asthma, nasal allergy and urticaria. At times, definite proof will still be in doubt until adequate allergy management, including dietary variation, specific hyposensi, tization programs, or therapeutic trial with drugs, completes the diagnostic picture. The physician should always be allergy conscious and remember that tissues and organs comprising this system are not immune to participation in the specific pattern of allergic disease.

Since allergic conditions involving this system are relatively uncommon, it is incumbent upon the physician suspecting them to establish the diagnosis most carefully, by means of a thorough personal and family history, physical examination, search for associated allergic states, roentgenologic and urologic studies, and clinical pathologic tests, in addition to the indicated allergic approach. The commonest allergenic offenders appear to be foods, particularly wheat, eggs, citrus fruits, sea foods and milk; but inhalant, bacterial, fungus, drug and other allergens must be considered.

# I. Manifestations of allergy in specific organs of the urogenital tract

Manifestations of an allergic reaction in the urogenital system may be the only expression of allergy in a patient, i.e., they represent an isolated locale, or they may be part of a general systematic allergic response, such as hematuria occurring as one symptom of purpura or of periarteritis nodosa. Allergy may effect the kidney, its pelvis, the ureter and urethra causing congestion, edema, spasm and even colic similar to that due to kidney or ureteral stone. The kidneys may be involved by an allergic reaction as seen in serum sickness, drug allergy, purpura and periarteritis nodosa. The symptoms of urinary allergy as reported involve the lower urinary tract with irritative symptoms and the upper urinary tract with ureteral or renal colic, hematuria, or albuminuria. The external genitalia may be involved in contact dermatitis from various substances or expressions of angioneurotic edema. Vaginitis, leukorrhea, dysmenorrhea and vaginal irritation on urination have occasionally been found to be of allergic origin. Renal damage is frequently seen in visceral angiitis of which periarteritis nodosa is a clinical example. ENGEL and MCCORMACK have reported a case of acute necrotizing angiitis of the bladder considered to be due to a hypersensitivity reaction to a sulfonamide (Gantrisin). The symptoms were abdominal pain and hematuria and at surgery a dusky, red, edematous lesion was noted on the right side of the bladder which disappeared on suprapubic drainage.

## I. Kidney

Renal disturbances may be suspected of being allergic in origin when they occur simultaneously or alternately with manifestations that are usually of allergic nature such as asthma, urticaria, angioneurotic edema or migraine. The assumpton of an underlying allergy is further supported when the usual antispasmodic measures fail to bring relief, while an injection of epinephrine is, on the other hand, properly beneficial and furthermore, when there are no calculi or gravel in the urine after the attack of renal colic, but eosinophils instead. These renal disturbances manifest themselves, not only by pain in the kidney area, sometimes of a colicky nature, but also, frequently, by albuminuria, as often occurs in serum reactions, severe prolonged attacks of asthma or following an acute anaphylactic reaction and occasionally also by hematuria.

The upper urinary tract symptom of hematuria, often painless, has been ascribed to allergy to various substances in several cases. An interesting case was published by RHODES. A man of 21 injured his thumb and was given 1,500 units of tetanus antitoxic prophylactically. Two days later he reported with hematuria. His urine showed gross hematuria, contained no casts, and was sterile on culture. A guinea-pig inoculation was negative for tuberculosis. At cystoscopy the bladder was found to be normal, a clear efflux was seen from the left ureteric orifice, a bloody one from the right. A pyelogram was normal. A diagnosis of renal purpura due to hypersensitivity was made with the appearance four days later of petechiae in the skin around the site of injection. Five weeks later the urine was clear and the patient remained well. There was no past history of an allergic diathesis, and no serum sickness. Nine years later he was seen again. He had had no further hematuria and was well. MILLER and UHLE have reported a case of painless bleeding for 12 days following the ingestion of codfish in a 29 year old white male who had a past history of recurrent attacks of urticaria. On avoidance of fish, the urine became free of blood within 7 days. KITTREDGE and JOHNSON have described a case of hematuria produced by the ingestion of unboiled milk in an 8 year old boy in whom the diagnosis was made by an elimination diet. All urological and other studies for organic diseases were negative. Withdrawal or boiling milk caused the urine to clear, re-introduction into the diet produced it. TZANK and COTTET have reported hematuria following administration of tetanus and diphtheria antitoxin. They also noted renal intolerances to mercury, bismuth, gold, arsenic, aspirin, quinine, blood transfusions, typhoid and other vaccinations evidenced by albuminuria to nephritis with urea retention. Other allergic manifestations were often present. RICHET, TZANCK and COUDER also described the onset of albuminuria, hypertension, nitrogen retention and edema, together with severe asthma and purpura, in a patient sensitive to horse serum, whose symptoms arose with the eating of horse meat. The rapid disappearance of the albuminuria, hypertension and edema with the control of the asthma suggested allergic reactions in the kidney. Two other cases of hypersensitiveness to arsenic presented similar symptoms. In 1930, COCA reported two cases of essential hematuria in individuals with associated allergic symptoms. He considered the hematuria allergic in origin but this fact was not established by adequate studies. Cooke has described a patient with asthma who had attacks of hematuria following the use of iodides. Cystoscopic examination during an attack showed the bladder mucosa studded with purpuric areas. KOEHLER noted hematuria in a 43 year old woman with asthma from the use of aspirin.

Hematuria in association with abdominal pain or renal colic has been noted by several men. ADELSBERGER observed it following an injection of house dust extract in an asthmatic patient. EISENSTAEDT has observed it following the ingestion of roquefort cheese, milk and codeine. THOMAS and WICKSTEN have reported hematuria of 15 months' duration associated with attacks of severe pain in both flanks in a 52 year old male. Repeated urologic investigations failed to explain the hematuria which was found on cystoscopy to be caused by bleeding from both ureteral orifices. Pyelograms were normal. Sensitization studies showed significant reactions to a number of the common inhalants and molds and to certain foods, including mushroom, squash, pumpkin, cantaloupe, cucumber and watermelon. Elimination of the offending foods, and an inhalant avoidance regimen and hyposensitization with an extract of house dust, feathers, orris root and mixed molds abolished the patient's symptoms.

In the present state of our knowledge, anaphylactoid purpura (HENOCH-SCHÖNLEIN) is considered to be related to a hypersensitivity reaction due either to bacterial infections, drugs, or foods and occurring in the endothelium of certain small blood vessels. This leads to increased capillary permeability permitting the extravasation of unusual quantities of plasma and blood elements into the tissues. Histologically, in renal purpura, MARTIN has noted subepithelial hemorrhage containing a high proportion of esosinophils, edema of the connective tissue, and in some of the small vessels, eccentric local edema immediately surrounding the capillary wall.

Hematuria during the course of Henoch-Schonlein purpura has been reported as due to food sensitivity (milk, egg, wheat, potato, chicken, beans) by ALEXANDER and EYERMAN and LAZARUS. Allergic purpura may cause abdominal pain simulating renal colic or hemorrhages into the kidney resulting in hematuria and renal colic. Nephritis somewhat similar to glomerulonephritis has been noted as a complication along with anuria and uremia (BROWN 1946). MARTIN has reported a case of renal, ureteric and vesical purpura associated with a fully developed Henoch-Schonlein syndrome in a 63 year old male presumably from taking an excess of sulfonamides. The patient died in uremia and at autopsy many isolated, and in places, confluent submucous hemorrhages of the renal pelvis, ureters and bladder were seen. Kern observed renal manifestations with hematuria and nitrogen retention together with the classic symptoms of anaphylactoid purpura all due to allergy to onions. Thomas and Wicksten found acute hematuria associated with allergic purpura to be precipitated by the inhalation of tar fumes in a 16 year old boy in whom sensitization had presumably taken place some years before from repeated chewing of tar.

Gairdner, in a study of 12 cases of the Henoch-Schonlein syndrome, found microscopic red cells in all his cases, and gross hematuria in four. Over half the cases were associated with a hemolytic streptococcal respiratory tract infection. A precisely similar syndrome was produced in a patient with a hypersensitivity to tomatoes. Gross hematuria occurred in four cases, one of which died in renal failure with subacute glomerulonephritis. Though 2 cases were left with chronic nephritis, and 2 with a "latent nephritis", 7 made a good recovery with no evidence of any renal impairment. His conclusion was that an antigen-antibody reaction provides a pathological link between this condition and acute nephritis.

Lazarus describes the case of a young man of 18 who, after four episodes of painless hematuria, developed the Schonlein manifestation and bilateral subconjunctival hemorrhages. Urological investigation revealed sterile urine from the bladder and both kidneys. At cystoscopy, a few petechiae were seen around the right ureteric orifice. He was found to be sensitive to various foods (rice-wheat, veal, chocolate, nuts, raw vegetables and fruit).

Renal colic from allergy to foods such as meat, fruit and milk has been noted by Duke, Rowe, Litzner and others. Gutman felt it was caused in a patient from drinking beer. Vaughn and Hawke have reported a case of angioneurotic edema and renal colic in a 25 year old male from eating tomato and egg and relieved by adrenalin.

Blaustein attributed angioneurotic edema of the penis, bladder and scrotum and vesical orifice with anuria for 18 hours from drinking goats milk in a 36 year old white male. Cystoscopy revealed a gelatinous edema present throughout the bladder with no bladder capacity. There was also marked, pale, shining, pitting edema of the penis, scrotum and perineum. The symptoms disappeared spontaneously 36 hours after onset.

Hemoglobinuria: Paroxysmal hemoglobinuria represents an allergy to malaria protozoan products according to Fernan-Nunez, who studied 52 cases in Colombia. He found 16 positive skin tests to malaria protein in 410 persons tested. Moving these 16 persons to other stations eliminated blackwater fever from the area. Autopsies of 11 other patients dying with blackwater fever showed eosinophilia of the tissues. No other reports of studies confirming or amplifying this work have been found. It is possible that blackwater fever may be due to quinine etiology.

The effects of hemoglobin and products of tissue breakdown on the kidney have been described in an excellent review by Ross, in which he points out that sensitivity of the kidney to hemoglobin may be the mechanism operating in paroxysmal cold hemoglobinuria, paroxysmal nocturnal hemoglobinuria, and the very rare "Haff" disease.

Hutton has reported a case of "favism" in which a man of 21 years showed signs of sensitivity to the Vice-fava bean. His history contained a familial predisposition. His symptoms were those of an acute systemic reaction, including the presence of hemoglobinuria.

## II. Ureter

The ureter may be the shock organ for allergic responses. Because of its smooth muscle and mucous membrane structure, the symptoms may be due to spasm or edema of the muscle or to edema of the mucous membrane. The symptoms will largely be in the nature of pain, dull or colicky, in the flank, or side of the abdomen, and there may be associated frequency and urgency of urination. Adrenalin is often efficacious for the relief of immediate symptoms until the offending allergen can be detected. LITZNER has described edema about the ureteral orifice and trigone in a nurse suffering from urticaria and renal colic considered to be a manifestation of allergy to meat. FINEGOLD has noted anuria resulting from allergic edema involving the ureters and bladder following the administration of a small amount of sulfadiazine in a patient with asthma. Prompt resumption of excretion of urine in adequate amounts occurred within one hour after the administration of adrenalin and aminophyllin.

## III. Bladder

Probably the most frequent manifestations of hypersensitivity in the urogenital tract occur in the bladder. The symptoms are those of cystitis, or vesical irritability, such as frequency, pain or burning on urination, urgency, tenesmus, difficulty with urination in the form of slowness or weakness in the urinary stream, and suprapubic distress. The occurrence of bladder symptoms as a result of allergic reactions to foods was first suggested by DUKE in 1922, who noted bladder pain in a patient from the ingestion of tomato or the subcutaneous injection of an extract of tomato. He believed that food allergy was a common cause of such symptoms as frequent and painful urination, vesical tenesmus, and bladder pain or polyps, in patients with little or no evidence of organic bladder pathology upon repeated examinations. ROWE has recorded case reports of bladder irritability with such symptoms as frequency of and burning on urination, with suprapubic distress, not relieved by medical or urological treatment in women due to hypersensitivity to cantaloupe, wheat, cabbage, cauliflower, tomato, onion, potato, eggs, milk, fruits and nuts. He has seen two women who developed severe bladder pain and tenesmus, together with aching in various joints, due to allergy to quinidine. THOMAS and WICKSTEN reported such symptoms as urinary frequency, burning, dysuria, or tenesmus in patients found allergic to various foods such as eggs, beer, corn, chocolate, and acid fruits and to tar and paint fumes. Most of these patients also had other co-existent allergic manifestations. FEIN has reported a case of a 52 year old white female with symptoms of cystitis and painful bladder spasms from eating shrimp or chocolate. She also suffered from hay fever due to ragweed and allergic rhinitis due to inhalants, pollens and foods. Hyposensitization treatments given with endodust, mixed molds, mesquite and grasses yielded marked improvement in the bladder symptoms. FEIN also noticed bladder irritability in a 39 year old white female relieved by an antihistamine in whom urinalysis and cystoscopy were negative. She was found sensitive to house dust, ragweed, mountain cedar, grasses, mesquite and trees. She also had marked vaginal irritation and secondary urticaria from penicillin. She was treated by hyposensitization with endodust and the prevalent pollens and the use of long acting antihistamines. She became greatly improved and lost her bladder symptoms and obtained increased bladder capacity. The writer has noticed symptoms of bladder irritability or spasm from sensitivity to the following substances: *Foods:* citrus fruits, tomatoes, chocolate, wheat, eggs, shell fish, nuts, spices and condiments; *Beverages:* coffee, tea, cocoa, soft drinks such as coca cola and alcohol, particularly gin and beer; and walnut pollen. The symptoms of severe frequency and burning on urination and suprapubic distress have been found due to hypersensitivity to walnut pollen in 3 women. They all had an accompanying blood eosinophilia and occasionally eosinophils were found in the urinary sediment. The symptoms in all cases were eliminated by the avoidance of the pollen in season and hyposensitization by an allergist (BURKLAND 1951).

The anatomy and pathological physiology at work in this condition has been well described by KINDALL and NICKELS in their excellent paper on "Allergy of the Pelvic Urinary Tract in the Female". As they explain, the symptoms of dysuria and frequency are due to irritability of the mucous membrane of the trigone of the bladder, superimposed on the longitudinal muscles. The latter arising from the outer coats of the ureters spread out in a fan shaped arrangement decussating with those from the opposite side and from the trigone and some of them extend through the vesical orifice fibers into the urethra. Thus, it is understandable that from this arrangement of fibers, increased ureteral irritability and activity is usually associated with irritability of the bladder, resulting in symptoms of urinary urgency and frequency. They also point out that the symptoms of pain are due to an allergic edema of the mucous membrane of the ureter or urethra, interfering with free drainage of urine into or from the bladder. In chronic cases, they have found that there may be narrowing of the urethra at any point due to a stricture or to a submucosal infiltration of mononuclear cells associated with hypertrophy of the underlying muscle layers.

KINDALL and NICKELS point out that in the urinary sediment in mild cases, one may find only an occasional white cell which in many cases turns out to be a mononuclear leukocyte or eosinophil. In chronic cases, one may find polymorphic nuclear leukocytes and bacteria, as well as eosinophils and mononuclear leukocytes. In a few of my personal cases, I have at times found large clusters of transitional epithelial cells.

On cystourethroscopic examination, one frequently encounters a reddened, pouting urethra. The mucous membrane of the urethra often appears edematous and bright red in color. At the vesical orifice one frequently sees a hypertrophied mucous membrane which may hang in folds causing obstruction or a number of injected polyps or cysts. The mucous membrane of the bladder may appear normal, slightly pink, deeply vascularized or markedly hyperemic with occasional areas of questionable ulceration. The ureteral orifices are frequently swollen and edematous with areas of increased vascularity at their margins. The ureter appears to be in spasm as it resents the passage of a catheter, which, at times, is quite difficult. KINDALL and NICKELS report a case of a 43 year old woman complaining of dysuria, frequency and pain in the right lower quadrant within two hours of drinking gin punches. The symptoms all cleared after several hours but as a therapeutic test, when she again took gin punches, there was prompt recurrence of her symptoms. Cystoscopic examination revealed many hyperemic areas in the mucous membrane of the bladder and around the right ureteral opening the mucous membrane was edematous. Urine spurts from this opening averaged two per minute. She was given a small amount of epinephrine and in 12 minutes the hyperemic areas in the bladder and the edema about the ureteral opening disappeared and urine spurted at greater frequency. All her pain disappeared. They also report a case of renal colic with vomiting in a 44 year old woman with normal urinalysis who was relieved by the administration of ephedrine for her acute symptoms and the elimination of several foods to which she was found sensitive caused disappearance of hyperemia and edema of the vesical mucosa and her urinary symptoms.

Some of the polypoid, cystic and fibrotic changes seen around the vesical orifice and in the posterior urethra in women with so-called chronic urethritis have been considered due to allergy. POWELL and POWELL studied 154 private female patients with cysto-urethritis in whom their symptoms were felt to be on an allergic basis. They divided them into the three following classifications: *Group A:* 40 patients with a clinical diagnosis of vesical allergy not operated upon since their symptoms could be controlled by antihistamine and local treatment. *Group B:* 42 patients with a clinical diagnosis of vesical allergy upon whom transurethral bladder neck resection was done since their obstructive symptoms did not respond to local treatment, medication and antihistamines; *Group C:* 72 patients without a clinical diagnosis of vesical allergy upon whom transurethral bladder neck resection was done since their symptoms of bladder neck obstruction could not be relieved by conservative measures.

They considered the 82 patients making up Groups A and B as having allergy of the bladder and urethra since they satisfied the criteria they set up for the diagnosis. They found that usually these patients had more than one food that caused the attacks, there being 163 "proved" allergies in the 82 patients, the commonest offenders being the citrus fruits, tomatoes and tomato products, condiments and seasonings, chocolate, fresh fruits in season, nuts and sea foods. On the 114 patients comprising Group B & C, they performed transurethral bladder neck resections since they had obstructive changes and could not be cured by office procedures. All tissues removed from the bladder, bladder neck and posterior urethra were sectioned. Using high-dry-power of the microscope, they counted the eosinophils in each piece of tissue on every slide without any knowledge of the clinical histories. The presence of eosinophils in these sections was considered the criteria for the final diagnosis of the allergic reaction since such conditions as parasitic infestations, leukemia, malignant disease, x-ray reaction and periarteritis nodosa were ruled out in each case. In Group B, 24 cases with clinically proved allergies had no, or such a rare eosinophil that they were considered well controlled from an allergic standpoint; 17 cases had slight evidence of an allergic reaction while only one case had definite microscopic evidence of extreme eosinophil concentration in the tissue study. All these patients, except the one, had been relieved of their bladder symptoms by omitting the suspected allergen from their diet and antihistamine as indicated. In Group C, there were 49 cases without any appreciable allergic reaction, while 18 cases showed slight evidence. But 5 cases revealed a high eosinophil count, over 50, in the resected tissue which they took as their criteria of definite allergy. They felt that this showed that the evidence of tissue allergy in a group in which they had not suspected it was five times higher than in the allergic series where diet was controlled and antihistamines were given. On the basis of the total of 6 cases with very high eosinophil counts, they conclude that the occurrence of vesical allergy is definitely proven, and that when suspected clinically, the simple combination of omitting the allergen from the diet and protecting neutralization with antihistamines will prevent allergic responses in the great majority of cases.

Of considerable clinical interest are the observations of RANDOLPH, ROLLINS and WALTER, who find that it is not generally appreciated that the dextrose employed intravenously is derived from the simple hydrolysis of corn starch, that the ingestion or intravenous injection of corn sugars commonly results in the productions of allergic symptoms in at least some persons highly sensitive to corn and, lastly, that this phenomenon is not neglibible in view of the fact that allergy to corn is currently a leading cause of chronic sensitivity to food. They cite an example in a 30 year old woman who had several reactions to the administration of 5 per cent dextrose intravenously on different occasions. Shortly after a glucose injection, the patient developed severe dysuria and tenesmus along with intense nausea and vomiting. Four months later, she was given more intravenous dextrose therapy as a nutritional measure and her urinary frequency, burning and urgency promptly reappeared. All corn products were excluded from her diet and in 2 days she began to improve and in a week, felt fairly comfortable. A month later she was given 25.0 c.c. of five per cent dextrose intravenously and in 30 minutes, urgency, frequency, and burning in the region of the bladder recurred. Symptoms failed to develop several days later with an injection of 25 c.c. of isotonic sodium chloride solution. They felt that these clinical reactions to the administration of glucose or dextrose were not all to be interpreted on the basis of pyrogen contamination or speed shock.

BRAY, who has made a thorough study of a large number of cases of enuresis, reports the successful relief of enuresis in at least 100 cases by treatment based on allergic principles. One group of patients had enuresis in association with such other allergic manifestations as asthma, hay fever, eczema, etc., and produced by the same allergen as that causing the associated allergic conditions; a second group of patients had enuresis along with conditions which proved to be allergic and disappeared upon the removal of the offending allergen; while a third group included patients in which the enuresis was the only manifestation of allergy. In the latter group, determination of the specific excitants and their removal were followed by complete relief of the enuresis in patients in whom the usual routine procedures had failed. KITTREDGE and BROWN have found ephedrine sulfate a very effective agent in the symptomatic treatment of enuresis. The writer has noticed several patients with enuresis, including a few young adults, who have responded to the elimination of an offending food or to the administration of ephedrine or an antihistamine and a bland diet when other means have failed. These observations emphasize the necessity of studying, from an allergic standpoint, every case of enuresis that does not respond to the routine means of fluid restriction, belladonna and training and in whom no gross urological abnormality has been found.

Interstitial cystitis, a condition of obscure etiology, may prove to be a manifestation of hypersensitivity. A few of my patients suffering from this lesion have benefitted from elimination diets and the use of antihistamines. THOMAS and WICKSTEN have described one patient with interstitial cystitis, whose symptoms were aggravated by foods (chocolate and grapefruit juice) and who improved in six weeks after desensitization and an elimination diet was started. HAND has discussed the relation of allergy to interstitial cystitis in a survey of 223 cases. He found that 33 of these patients or 15 per cent also had allergic disorders. In 223 consecutive general clinic admissions he found only 19 patients with allergy. He considers an incidence of allergy of 15 per cent in interstitial cystitis as more than coincidental, and as one which warrants further investigation. Further evidence that interstitial cystitis may have an allergic component is the reports of successful treatment in a few instances with ACTH or cortisone. More study of this condition as a possible collagen disease and the effect of cortisone upon it will be needed before we can obtain the proper perspective of its nature and treatment (DEES 1953).

# IV. Suspected urogenital allergies from miscellaneous substances

## 1. Beverages

### a) Alcohol

Alcoholic beverages may sometimes produce expressions of hypersensitivity in the urinary tract in the form of frequency, urgency, or burning on urination with or without gross hematuria. At times, there may occur such marked edema or congestion of the urethral mucosa or swelling or congestion of the prostate gland that urinary retention occurs. This has been noted several times by the writer, particularly in patients after they have been drinking beer, gin or straight whiskey. GUTMANN (1933) has discussed allergic reactions to various beverages and noted the common conclusion that alcohol exacerbates allergic symptoms but probably does not cause them. The patient may be allergic to one of the constituents or the substance from which the beverage is made, such as yeast and hops in beer, barley, wheat or other grains in whiskey, or grapes used in making wine. One beer will agree at times and another will not. The methods of manufacture must be investigated in susceptible patients. Systematic elimination of various forms of alcoholic beverages, one at a time, thus becomes necessary in order to identify the offender. A survey of the literature on the immunologic properties of alcohol has been made by ROBINSON (1950) who concludes that the status of alcohol as an allergen needs further detailed studies for possible confirmation.

### b) Coffee, tea and cocoa

These beverages may also be a cause of allergic reactions. Marked frequency of urination, burning, strangury, and distress in the bladder, prostatic and urethral regions have been noted in many sensitive patients by the writer and others. Tea and coffee sensitization has been noted by ROWE in a few patients. Notably in one who had a peculiar irritation — a mild, cramping, throbbing distress in the perineum — together with a burning at the end of the penis when he drank tea. It is hard to differentiate clinically those urinary symptoms due to the stimulating and diuretic effect of caffeine and other substances in these beverages and those due to hypersensitivity. GUTMANN has suggested that the various allergic manifestations arising from coffee are due in part to the stimulating effect of caffeine and other substances such as aldehyde, furfural, acetone, pyridine and ammonia. This is not especially apparent. Certain impurities in these beverages may be a cause of hypersensitivity. The various adulterants of coffee include chickory, carrots, parsnip, turnip, dandeline, various seeds, acorns, figs, sugar and molasses. Postum and similar coffee substitutes are made of roasted cereal and dried fruits.

### c) Soft drinks

Likewise, sensitization to soft drinks which may cause bladder irritability necessitates a knowledge of their ingredients. Coca cola is said to contain caffeine, caramel, essential oils, lime juice, phosphoric acid, extract of coca leaves or Kola nuts. Ginger ale contains ginger, lemon juice and at times, catsicum. Root beer contains a variety of substances including cologne, sarsaparilla, orange, sassafras, wintergreen, etc.

Regardless of the mechanism, alcohol and these other beverages seem to enhance any existing allergies, probably through increasing capillary permeability, and their use in any proven allergy, particularly of the urogenital tract, should be strictly forbidden.

## 2. Spices and condiments

Sensitization to pepper as revealed by skin tests is quite common. Paprika, green, red or black pepper act alike. Mustard and vinegar disturb many people. Various spices may produce allergic reactions in the urinary tract. These include cinnamon, sage, nutmeg and dill herb.

## 3. Other

Allergic reactions may occur to artificial dyes and flavors in food such as vanilla and peppermint. ROWE has noted marked burning on urination from taking of peppermint. Honey allergy is frequent and DUKE has described two cases of severe abdominal allergy due to this food. Urticaria may occur and there may be specific allergy to bee protein in honey itself.

## V. Urethra

REITER'S syndrome has been considered an allergic reaction but recent studies indicate that a pleuropneumonia organism is present in a large number of patients. Angioneurotic edema on an allergic basis and involving the urethra has been noted in which the swelling has caused urinary retention. Personal communications from several allergists state that urethral discharge and itching are frequently noted during the pollen season in many of their patients who are free when the hay fever season is over. There are reports of sensitivity to certain chemicals, often in self-administered solutions, that have caused persistent urethritis in males. Of particular significance is the ever present possibility of sensitivity to local anesthetics used in the urethra. A case has been reported by RATTNER in which a non-specific urethritis with a concomitant dermatitis of the penis resulted from sensitization to the rubber used in condoms. A patch test was positive to the rubber. Both conditions disappeared upon substitution of other methods. GRILLO has reported the case of a 59 year old male who was given an injection of antitetanus serum following injury with fishing equipment. Six days later he developed fever, joint symptoms, itching, burning on urination and a muco-purulent secretion which contained a 40 per cent eosinophilia but no bacteria. Treatment with antihistamine cleared the urethral symptoms in 3 days and skin symptoms in 6 days. Symptoms of burning in the urethra, vesical irritability, urethral discharge, scrotal itching, urticaria and other general manifestations have been attributed to ascaridal antigen or products of oxyurias infection in patients suffering from intestinal ascaridiasis and oxyuriasis by GRILLO and BURKERT. A large number of eosinophils have been noted in the blood, urine and urethral discharge of these patients. They have been relieved of their urinary and urethral distress by the administration of antihistamine and anti-parasitic treatment. GRILLO feels that the diagnosis of urethral disturbances due to allergy to specific antigens is helped by the characteristic course, the clinical parallelism with co-existent allergic expression, the presence of local eosinophilia and the absence or scarcity of germs in the bacterial discharge. HABER has described a fixed eruption and urethritis due to phenolphthalein occurring in a 25 year old male. A rash on the penis and a urethral discharge with pain on micturition occurred in several attacks from taking laxatives containing phenophthalein by the patient.

LECA has reported a few cases of urethritis which he felt were of allergic origin which responded well to treatment with antihistamines and irrigations of silver nitrate. One 25 year old student developed urethritis every time he took a sedative solution (Thiocal).

# VI. Prostate gland

Some inflammations of the prostate gland, particularly so-called granulomatous prostatitis may be manifestations of allergy in this organ. MELICOW has presented the first report of allergic granuloma of the prostate gland. The patient was a 63 year old man with a history of frequent attacks of asthma for several months, who suddenly developed urinary distress, and rectal examination revealed a considerably enlarged and firm prostate gland. Examination of the blood smear revealed an eosinophilia of 15 per cent. Urinalysis revealed albumin, 2-plus, and numerous red and white cells. A suprapubic prostatectomy was done. Microscopic study of the excised tissue revealed, in addition to the picture of benign prostatic hypertrophy, sections showing scattered, irregular, deeply pink staining areas that were granulomatous in appearance. A few giant cells were seen but stigmata of tuberculosis were lacking. High power study revealed that the reddish areas were composed of disintegrated connective tissue fibers surrounded by an intense eosinophilic infiltration. Some round cells, plasma cells and lymphocytes were also present. A pronounced eosinophilic perivascular infiltration was also present in the tortuous wall of a blood vessel. Postoperatively, the patient developed a cough, rise in eosinophilia to 37 per cent, and x-rays of the chest revealed lesions suggestive of Loeffler syndrome. He left the hospital shortly thereafter, suffered exacerbation of his asthma, developed abdominal cramps and diarrhea and finally expired. Post-mortem examination revealed, among other lesions, organizing and necrotizing pneumonia of the left lung, allergic granulomata in the prostate, bladder, rectum, seminal vesicles, esophagus and heart. Because of the clinical course, laboratory and pathological findings, it was felt that the patient suffered from a diffuse vascular "allergic syndrome" which involved the urogenital tract as well as other organs.

THOMPSON and ALBERS analyzed a series of 36 cases of non-tuberculous, chronic granulomatous lesions of the prostate, but described only six in detail. In two of these, the prostatic tissue removed by transurethral resection was the seat of extensive eosinophilic infiltration and in both instances the patients were asthmatics.

In the first case, a 46 year old man, blood studies revealed an eosinophilia of 50 per cent. In both patients, the prostate gland felt quite hard, leading to the suspicion of carcinoma. In the second case, a 55 year old man, a severe attack of asthma with severe urticaria, facial edema and urinary difficulty developed three months after prostatectomy and cystotomy disclosed extensive edema of the base of the bladder.

STEWART, WRAY and HALL have reported on two patients, both asthmatics, in whom prostatectomy and prostatic biopsy respectively disclosed a striking and unusual lesion consisting of focal granulomata with central fibrinoid necrosis of the type usually associated with various allergic diseases, in one case, with focal and diffuse eosinophilic cell infiltration of great intensity. They state that inasmuch as one of their cases showed eosinophilic pus in considerable amounts within many of the prostatic glands, they would suggest that in any asthmatic who develops prostatic symptoms, and indeed in those who do not, the urine should be examined microscopically for eosinophil cells, both before and after prostatic massage.

HARRISON and NEANDER have reported another case of allergic granuloma of the prostate in a 74 year old man who suffered from asthma for 5 months. The patient died 6 weeks after prostatectomy because of severe bronchial asthma.

The autopsy specimen of the prostate showed intense eosinophilic infiltration in granulomatous tissue.

Urinary symptoms may come on suddenly in asthmatics and suggest that the acute urinary distress that may occur in young men following the ingestion of alcohol, even in small amounts, and causing great swelling of the prostate gland may be on an allergic basis. The allergy is probably not due to the alcohol but probably to hypersensitivity to products such as corn, barley, rye, etc., from which the alcohol is made. This matter deserves much further study for demonstration of proof of the allergic basis.

IDIOPOE-GOMEZ has described 7 cases in which he felt allergic syndromes originated through the existence of microbic foci in the prostate. By treatment of the infected prostate and elimination of the infection, he states that he has cleared up such varied conditions as bronchitis, asthma, chronic eczema, urticaria, blenorrhagia and neuralgias. In all of these cases, the only treatment was that of prostatitis with autovaccines or with polyvalent gonococcic vaccines followed by diathermy treatment of the prostatic lesion along with two courses of sulfa-thiazole. He believes a chronic infection of the prostate can be the point of departure of various allergic syndromes.

## VII. External genitalia

Cutaneous eruptions from the use of various therapeutic chemical agents on the external genitalia of either sex can produce an intense allergic response. Poison ivy may involve the genitalia. Dermatitis involving the external genitalia and perineum may occur from different articles of clothing. It is not necessarily due to the original cloth material but may be due to dyes or to chemicals employed in finishing the goods. Drug eruptions may resemble almost every known type of dermatitis and must always be considered in the differential diagnosis of every obscure cutaneous lesion. While many drugs cause skin rashes which are identical in appearance, certain substances evoke characteristic lesions which suggest the responsible agent. The term "fixed drug eruption" indicates that the locus of a skin lesion is fixed and has a tendency to recur in the same skin areas with the subsequent use of a specific drug. Fixed drug eruptions may persist when the offending agent is used repeatedly. The lesions are often circumscribed, edematous plaques, usually bright red or salmon colored. Often the involved areas remain pigmented after gradual clearing occurs. Infrequently, the eruptions may be papular or vesicular. Fixed eruptions vary in size and distribution, often involving the face, hands and genitalia. Among the medications which cause fixed drug reactions are: phenolphthalein, quinine, barbituric acid derivatives, heavy metals, iodides, and bromides. An eczematous or seborrheic type of skin eruption in the groins, perineum and involving the scrotum may occur from allergy to penicillin, either as a localized expression or as a part of generalized allergic response. HOLLANDER has reported dermatitis of the penis in a pollinosis case occurring when the patient neglected to wash his hands after using an ephedrine nasal spray prior to urination. Direct application of a spray to the penis caused intense contact dermatitis. FORD reports a case of contact dermatitis due to quinine, confirmed by positive patch test to the drug. The patient had a dermatitis involving the penis, scrotum, eyes, cheeks, ears, and sides of neck. It first started on the genitalia. The etiologic agent was found to be a contraceptive vaginal suppository containing quinine, bisulphite, and boric acid in a cocoa butter base. VAUGHN and FOLKES have described dermatitis of the penis in a man allergic to cocoa whose wife used a contraceptive suppository with a base of oil of theobroma. In an analysis of 125 cases of eruption proved to be caused by sensitization by rubber articles, LEIDER, FURMAN and FISHER found 6 cases in which sensitivity to condom rubber was the cause of dermatitis of the penis.

Balanitis has been noted to occur to sensitivity to certain chemicals in contraceptive creams and jellies. Edema of the foreskin has been noted by the writer from hypersensitivity to shrimp and other shell fish.

Vaginitis and vulvar itching due to sensitivity to pollen, solutions used for douching and various contraceptive creams have been noticed. MITCHELL has reported 8 cases of vulvo-vaginal pruritis associated with hay fever, all involving girls under 12 years of age. They were all seasonal, occurring during the ragweed pollinating season. The vulvar itching responded as readily as the hay fever to specific immunization against or avoidance of the offending pollen. Preseasonal pollen therapy prevents vulvar itching in most cases. FEINBERG has also noticed vaginitis and vaginal itching occurring during the hay fever season in ragweed sensitive patients. FOX has described a situation in a 35 year old white woman with a history of grass pollinosis of 5 years duration in which vaginal pruritis and dysuria resulted from pollen injections given in an attempt to hyposensitize the patient. The patient also noticed that crab and lobster caused vulvar and vaginal itching after eating them.

Leukorrhea may result from allergy and is most commonly seen in the pollen season in susceptible women. ADELSBERGER and MUNTER have reported instances of leukorrhea with numbers of eosinophils during the hay fever season in women suffering from pollinosis. JOACHIMOVITZ reported a case in which the allergic menorrhagia was aggravated by topical application of the allergen to the cervix, and the menstrual fluid contained large numbers of eosinophils. THOMAS and WICKSTEN have reported leukorrhea associated with allergic rhinitis in a 39 year old school teacher found sensitive to many inhalants and to eggs and wheat. There was a 6 per cent eosinophilia. Examination of the vaginal secretion revealed numerous eosinophils. The nasal symptoms and leukorrhea responded favorably to dietary restrictions, to the avoidance of inhalants, and hyposensitization. They also recorded a case of seasonal leukorrhea associated with ragweed, hay fever, and asthma in a 50 year old woman who was absolutely free of leukorrhea except during the ragweed season. ROWE states that leukorrhea may not infrequently be due to food allergy, and is relieved by food elimination. He says that one of his patients had had leukorrhea, swelling of her face and other parts of her body, together with a general toxemia for many years, due to milk and he has noticed the disappearance of leukorrhea in 2 children from the elimination of allergy producing foods.

# VIII. Internal genitalia

The uterus is probably susceptible to allergic reactivity the same as other body tissues. ROWE feels that spasm in the musculature with edema of the mucosa might explain some cases of dysmenorrhea. KAHN has reported a case of uterine spasm complicating a pollen anaphylactic action. The possibility of allergic reaction in the genito-urinary tract must be considered in the treatment of pregnant women. Reactions to serum or ragweed hyposensitization may cause abortions or premature labor. SMITH has reported 12 patients with essential dysmenorrhea, leukorrhea, and irregular periods who were relieved by the elimination of specific foods. DUTTA recorded 3 cases of dysmenorrhea from allergy, eosinophils being found in the secretions in one case.

# IX. Urological conditions suspected of having an allergic basis

In a critical analysis, DEES and SIMMONS state that although urinary tract allergy may occur, there are few reports in which an organic basis has been completely excluded and an allergic basis incontrovertibly proved. An analysis of 613 cases by them, with 6 urological conditions, selected because they resemble types reported as due to allergy and because the etiology was either unknown or not fully explained, confirmed allergy in only 12 per cent. The urologic conditions were essential hematuria, orthostatic albuminuria, enuresis, ureteral spasm, chronic trigonitis and chronic urethritis and interstitial cystitis. They felt that since this percentage is so similar to the accepted incidence of allergy in the general population, that it is not justifiable to suspect that allergy played any major role in these disorders. In none of the patients who underwent complete urologic and allergic study did the allergy appear etiologically significant. The consensus of clinicians in an official poll conducted by the authors was that urinary allergy is rare.

## 1. Essential hematuria

Essential hematuria in 32 patients who received complete urologic study was accompanied by personal allergy in five. Of these, only one had major allergy, this person was skin tested and allergic management did not influence the bleeding.

## 2. Orthostatic albuminuria

They analyzed 82 cases of orthostatic albuminuria and found personal or family allergies in 18 per cent. Major allergy was present in 5 cases, minor allergy in 9, all of whom were skin tested. Four patients had positive family histories, but were not skin tested. Three of the patients with major allergy had both complete allergic and urologic studies. In none of these patients did allergic treatment seem to have any effect on orthostatic albuminuria.

## 3. Chronic non-specific cystitis, trigonitis, urethritis

Three hundred patients with chronic cystitis, trigonitis, and urethritis studied by DEES and SIMMONS had no demonstrable infection in the urine with the diagnosis confirmed by cystoscopy in all. Thirty-eight per cent, or 114 cases, had intravenous urograms, retrograde pyelograms, and kidney function tests when there was any suggestion of upper urinary tract disease. The cases were divided into 2 groups: Group I, consisting of all 300 cases without exclusion for co-existing gynecological or urologic findings; Group II, 210 patients, had no co-existing disease. Ninety cases were excluded for the following in order of frequency: cystocele, stricture of urethra, chronic cervicitis and vaginitis, rectocele, cystourethrocele, fibromyomata, and ovarian cysts. Co-existing allergy was found in 11 per cent of the entire group of 300 patients.

## 4. Ureteral spasm

Of 14 patients with ureteral spasm, 2 patients had a personal history of allergy, all had intravenous urograms, x-ray of the abdomen and cystoscopy with calibration of ureters. The allergy in one patient consisted of skin rash from a sulfonamide, and the other had chronic asthma. No allergy investigation was recorded in the latter.

## 5. Interstitial cystitis

Their 31 patients with interstitial cystitis had an incidence of personal allergy in five (16 per cent). One patient was sensitive to aspirin and had positive passive transfer tests to foods. A second patient had no frank allergy, but was skin tested directly and by passive transfer technique with positive reactions to foods. In neither of these patients was any allergic regimen carried out, so the significance of these tests is not known. The other 3 patients were not studied with skin tests.

## 6. Enuresis

They reviewed 185 cases of enuresis. Seventeen cases of the total gave a personal history of allergy, 12 with major allergies and 5 with minor allergies. Fifteen patients were studied urologically. Six patients of those studied were found to have urologic conditions which might have explained the enuresis. When those cases who gave a family history of allergy, with or without personal history of allergy were included, there was a total of 26 cases. One of the enuretics with a personal history of allergy was cystoscoped, and in this case, stricture of the urethra was established.

DEES and SIMMONS also made a critical review of the literature and analyzed reports of urinary allergy, comparing allergic and urologic studies up to 1950. It was their conclusion that in most of the reports there had been either an incomplete allergic study or an inadequate urological study, or both, to establish the diagnosis of allergy as a cause of the patient's genitourinary disturbance. In many instances, urinalysis, cystoscopy and x-ray studies of the urinary tract had not been made as well as inadequate allergy tests for identification of any specific allergen. They felt that most reports contain too scanty information for a definite diagnosis as witnessed by the fact that not all organic causes for bleeding of the urinary tract had been eliminated, cultures for acid fast organisms had not been made, nor was retrograde pyelography done in any great number of cases to rule out tumor of the bladder, ureter, kidney, as causes of hematuria.

## X. Reports of miscellaneous cases of genitourinary allergy

Since there are relatively few reports of allergy of the urogenital tract cited in the literature, a questionnaire was sent to the members of the International Correspondence Society of Allergists asking if any of them had noted reactions of hypersensitivity in the genitourinary system. The following is a summation of their replies:

Hematuria was noted following ingestion of orange juice, milk, codeine, turkey meat, eggs and aspirin in different patients by different observers. Several episodes of profuse bleeding from the urinary tract occurred in a nurse in whom it was finally determined, on repeated exposures, that the hematuria was due to codeine administered for the relief of menstrual cramps. Cystoscopy revealed the blood to come from both kidneys but x-rays revealed no organic pathology. It was found in her case that other opiates, such as morphine and dilaudid, would cause bleeding but not pantopon. Hematuria was noted due to aspirin in a 7 year old girl with a background of allergy in the form of eczema and rhinitis. She was noted to bleed from her kidneys whenever intentionally or inadvertently given aspirin. Retrograde studies of the bladder and kidneys on two occasions revealed no evidence of organic pathology. A two and half year old male child was noted to have blood in urine at stool and diarrhea from eating eggs. There was prompt resumption of symptoms upon taking eggs in any form or a few drops of egg albumin in water. Three bouts of abdominal pain and hematuria were observed in a 4 year old boy each time he ate walnuts. Asthma and hematuria, with an edematous and inflammatory lesion in the bladder observed on cystoscopy, was noted in a 17 year old girl found sensitive by passive transfer tests to egg, milk, orange and tomato. Renal colic occurred in a nurse sensitive to wheat, cystoscopic and x-ray studies were all negative. Symptoms of cystitis and severe bladder irritability were noted by different observers from sensitivity to milk, orange juice, peas, eggs, fig, raisins, carrot, lettuce, spinach, tuna and pork. One patient was the wife of a physician who had severe symptoms for several years due to drinking orange juice. She had been seen by several urologists for observation and treatment without relief since none of them recognized the condition to be allergic in origin. Symptoms of cystitis were noted from sensitivity to tomatoes, pineapple, chocolate and canta-loupe. A 19 year old girl developed considerable bladder irritability when she ate fish and her urine contained many eosinophils. Dysuria and incontinence occurred within two hours from the use of pepper by a 56 year old woman. The patient was followed intermittently for 5 years and had no bladder symptoms as long as pepper was avoided. Scratch tests with this substance showed a tremendous wheal. The concomitant presence of hay fever and urethral dis-charge, refractory to antibiotics during the pollen season, was commented upon by several men. Recurrent abacterial urethral discharge was noted over a period of 15 years in an adult male from drinking too much gin. There was no discharge from drinking other forms of alcohol. Several allergists felt that a certain percentage of enuresis was due to allergic causes, some cases occurring only in the pollen season and others due to foods and clearing up by elimination diet. In a 14 year old boy, enuresis was found to be definitely due to milk. Urinary retention was noted from the use of ephedrine for asthma or rhinitis in elderly patients and when given in high doses it also caused urinary retention in children. Fixed drug eruptions on the genitalia were noted by several observers from the use of phenolphthalein or coal tar derivatives. Vaginal pruritis was noted in female patients under treatment for pollinosis due to grasses or ragweed. Two cases of impotence were reported following the use of antihistamines.

# J. Allergy to diagnostic and therapeutic agents used in urology

## I. Diagnostic agents

There are numerous reports in the literature of reactions, many of them fatal, to various contrast media containing iodine used for diagnostic pyelo-graphy, usually by the intravenous route. Generalized reactions of the ana-phylactic type, as reported in the literature, have included urticaria, rhinitis, lacrimation, salivation, syncopy, and shock. Such reactions have been reported following the injection of diodrast, skiodan, uro-selectan, neoiopax, hippuran, and miokon. Replies to an inquiry by PENDERGRASS and his associates elicited the information that 26 deaths were attributed to injections of urographic contrast media in 661,800 examinations and 132 instances of anaphylactic shock. Urticarial and erythematous eruptions and numerous other reactions have been noted. Before their report in 1942, 11 fatalities had previously been reported from the use of pyelographic contrast media. There has recently been reported a case of fatal anaphylactic reaction to 1 c.c. of 50 per cent mikon, a new urographic media, occurring in a 65 year old patient with a negative history of allergy (PAYNE et al 1956). Hypersensitivity reactions may also occur from these compounds when used for aortography. Physicians using these agents should be very careful to question their patients in regard to a history of any allergy and to ask particularly, if they have ever had the media used on them previously. Tests for sensitivity to these compounds have not been uniformly trustworthy and the most practical procedure is to inject 1 c.c. of the contrast media very slowly, then wait 2 or 3 minutes, and if the patient does not have any reaction, to inject the rest of the dose. A few urologists feel that it is a worthwhile practice to give an antihistamine before the injection of any contrast media, as a prophylactic measure to prevent a reaction (WINTER; SANGER and EHRLICH).

## II. Therapeutic agents

Hypersensitivity with marked reactions, occasionally fatal, have been noted to many of the therapeutic agents that are widely used in urology and medicine in general. Many clinical and experimental studies have established the fact that sulfonamides frequently cause hypersensitivity reactions. They are aften serious and may be fatal. Necrotizing arterial lesions, resembling those of peri-arteritis nodosa, are not an infrequent manifestation. Dermatitis, agranulo-cytosis, acute hemolytic anemia, hepatitis, necrosis, severe bronchial asthma, purpura and a syndrome similar to serum sickness are major clinical expressions of the hypersensitivity reaction (KUTSCHER et al 1954; LOWELL 1955). ROLLING-HOFF has reported anuria with interstitial nephritis occurring after the use of sulfathiazole as an allergic manifestation. The fact that patients can be sensitized to sulfonamides so that later use of these drugs evokes serious anaphylactic responses and widespread tissue injury is the strongest possible argument against their indiscriminate use.

A number of allergic reactions have occurred from the administration of penicillin which has been used widely (KERN and WIMBERLY 1953; WELCH et al. 1953). Both immediate, anaphylactic type, and delayed reactions (serum sickness type) may take place although the delayed reaction appears most common. Urticaria is the most single manifestation but various bullous, pur-puric, and exfoliative skin eruptions have been seen as well as renal and myo-cardial involvement. One may have serum sickness with a typical triad of the skin eruption, fever and joint pains. Contact dermatitis is common, being due to topical application or occupational exposure in such persons as doctors, nurses, drug-gists and workers in the manufacture of the drug. A great number of fatal anaphylactic reactions from penicillin have been reported in the literature, the majority occurring in a few seconds to 10 minutes (ROSENTHAL 1954).

Aside from the toxicity for the auditory and vestibular mechanism, the streptomycins evoke a variety of hypersensitivity reactions such as skin rashes, eosinophilia, drug fever, and blood dyscrasias. Rarely, angioneurotic edema and bronchial asthma may be caused by these drugs. Di-hydrostreptomycin is less likely to cause hypersensitivity reactions than streptomycin. Contact dermatitis in the case of nurses, doctors, pharmacists, and others who habitually come in contact with the drug, is fairly frequent on the hands, forearms, and occasionally, the face and conjunctiva (COHEN and GLINSKY 1951).

Reactions of hypersensitivity to the tetracycline drugs, erythromycin, neo-mycin, chloramphenicol and polymixin-B are rare but one may have rather severe toxic reactions from the use of these drugs.

It is important for all physicians to realize that sensitivity to these drugs can occur, and they should always question a patient about previous administration and tolerance to the drugs before prescribing them for a new infection. They should be administered, penicillin in particular, only when there are clearcut indications for their use. If a patient has had a reaction from penicillin, streptomycin, the sulfa or other drugs, another drug should substituted for the one causing a reaction. When reactions do occur, they may require the administration of epinephrine, ephedrine, or an antihistamine and in the case of severe serum sickness, it may be necessary to use ACTH or one of the cortisone derivatives. In case of an immediate anaphylactic shock reaction, the first thought should be to administer 0.5 c.c. to 1 c.c. of 1:1,000 aqueous of solution of epinephrine.

It is not uncommon to see allergic reactions to local anesthetics such as procaine, cocaine, pontocaine, butacaine and similar preparations frequently used by urologists for urethral instillation or local injection. They may manifest themselves as an eczematous allergic reaction, typical asthmatic attacks or a fatal anaphylactic reaction. An allergist has informed the writer of an unreported rapid death after instillation of pontocaine into the urethra prior to cystoscopy. THOMAS and FENTON have reported 7 constitutional reactions and 3 deaths associated with the use of pontocaine. CRIEP and RIBEIRO have reported on 3 fatalities from allergy to procaine.

# K. Treatment of urogenital allergy

## I. Preventive measures

The best treatment is prophylaxis when it is possible. Since the underlying cause of human hypersensitiveness is unknown, no complete prophylaxis based on fundamental etiology is as yet possible (GLASER 1955). Nevertheless, there are a few ways of achieving a certain amount of prevention. In the non-allergic group, chronic foci of infection that are a source of continuous absorption of bacteria or their products should be eradicated, for they act not only as sensitizers, but as the underlying cause of many of the inflammatory or degenerative diseases in man. Their discovery and proper management may be a means of avoiding allergic disease. Considerable care must be used in giving drugs with high sensitizing capacity such as the sulfonamides and penicillin, those giving dangerous clinical reactions such as aspirin, and injections of foreign serums. Watch the child for inhalants around the home and protect them against infection. This can be aided by giving them inoculations against diptheria, tetanus, measles, and protection against ordinary acute respiratory infections. Thus, the control of environmental excesses, highly antigenic food excesses, promiscuous and thoughtless use of sera and drugs, as well as the management of diseases which tend to increase the permeability and dysfunction of our protecting membranes, all tend to reduce the incidence of allergy.

## II. General principles of treatment

We might say that there are 3 general principles of treatment which are applicable to the treatment of urogenital allergy as well as allergic disease in general. First, is separating the patient from the offending allergens, i. e., avoidance; second, is increasing the patient's tolerance to the causative allergens by means of hyposensitization. The third is symptomatic relief by the means of various drugs.

# 1. Elimination of offending allergens

The avoidance or elimination of the offending allergens from the environment offers the patient the best chance of relief of his disease or symptoms. During the pollination season of plants involved, if the patient leaves his customary environment and goes to a place that has no such vegetation, such as the mountains, seashore or desert, his symptoms will be relieved. If dust causes trouble, he should sleep in a dust free room. Various foods and drinks are the commonest cause of hypersensitivity in the urogenital tract, and when they are discovered, elimination from the diet often gives prompt relief. The only certain and successful method of prevention of drug allergy is that of absolute avoidance of possible excitants. Thus, treatment is simplest and most effective when the causative factors are eliminated, avoided, or completely controlled as soon as they are determined. Elimination of inhalant allergens such as dust, pollen, mold, animal dander and fumes is the treatment of choice but if this is impossible, hyposensitization must be attempted.

# 2. Hyposensitization

Hyposensitization consists essentially in administering by injection, ingestion, application or spray, a dilution of the antigen just sufficient to elicit a minute reaction in the shock organ and in then repeating administration when these manifestations of the antigen-antibody reaction have disappeared (in about 3—7 days). The most common procedure is to inject increasing increments of diluted allergen in a course as tolerance of the patient permits, either intra- or subcutaneously, to develop an excess of specific antibodies in the patient's blood. When this antigen is encountered later, it is so completely bound by the antibodies circulating in the blood that it cannot enter into contact with the tissue antibody, which, of course, are the only antibodies leading to the elicitation of allergic manifestations. Hyposensitization works best in the case of the inhalant class of allergens, such as pollen, house dust, animal danders and feathers. It is also of help in molds and bee venom. Hyposensitization can be carried out in some cases of sensitivity to food protein by the use of propetans. Propetans are preparations derived from the individual proteins by digestion with hydrochloric acid, pepsin, and trypsin. Their use may help the patient develop tolerance towards a natural food. Hyposensitization is rarely necessary in the treatment of genitourinary allergy. The various procedures connected with it are best carried out by an allergist who is familiar with the technique, interpretation of the results and management of any reaction.

# 3. Symptomatic relief by means of varios drugs

Medications, including antihistamines, are entirely palliative and should not replace the well established procedures of cause and effect investigations, or isolation of the trigger allergen and its removal, or hyposensitization when removal is impossible. We might say that the drugs used in the treatment of allergy fall into certain classifications.

First are drugs which act by stimulating the sympathetic nervous system. One of the most important drugs in the symptomatic treatment of allergic diseases is epinephrine, which by stimulating the endings of the sympathetic nerves, produces vasoconstriction and thereby counteracts the anaphylactic dilatation of of blood vessels. In a dose of 0.5 to 1 c.c. of a 1:1,000 solution, given subcutaneously, it is an important remedy for anaphylactic shock. Smaller doses will relieve the pruritis of acute urticaria, the swelling of angioneurotic edema and numerous other allergic manifestations such as renal colic or ureteral spasm on an allergic basis. In minor cases, one may use ephedrine sulfate, orally or by injection. It has been of help in the treatment of enuresis and bladder irritability. The oral dose is $^3/_8$ to $^3/_4$ of a grain, 3 times a day in adults with correspondingly lower doses in children. A precaution to be observed is that it may cause urinary retention, particularly in the older prostatic patients, and it also may give rise to tenesmus or dysuria in younger patients (BALYEAT and RINKEL).

Second are drugs which act primarily through inhibition of parasympathetic activity such as atropine, belladonna and hyoscyamus which are very helpful in the treatment of bladder spasms and irritability.

A third class are the sedatives such as phenobarbital and chloral hydrate which may be helpful in allaying nervous tension and emotional disturbances which frequently accompany allergic conditions. There should be an infrequent use of opiates.

A fourth class are the antihistaminics which belong to the broad classification of blocking agents which apparently prevent the combination of histamine with cellular receptives. They exhibit a valued palliative action for the symptomatic relief of a variety of allergic disorders which presumably result from the release of histamine. In addition, certain members of the series manifest central actions which have therapeutic application. They have a number of side reactions, the chief of which is on the central nervous system causing depression leading to a sedative effect. They may occasionally cause restlessness, nervousness and insomnia, dizziness, tinnitus and incoordination. Gastrointestinal symptoms such as loss of appetite, nausea, vomiting, epigastric distress, constipation or diarrhea may occur (McGAVACH et al. 1951). They have a local anesthetic action and are very effective antipruritic agents. There are other miscellaneous reactions which include impotence, urinary retention and hematuria. They are most efficacious in the treatment of urticaria, angioneurotic edema and allergic dermatitis. They are of help in serum sickness, some drug reactions and physical allergy. They may afford valuable adjuvant action when used with epinephrine.

There is a large number of antihistaminic drugs and little distinction can be made between them on the basis of efficacy as histamine antagonists. They vary somewhat with respect to potency, dosage, relative incidence of side reactions and types of preparation available. The adult dose of antihistaminic drugs is usually one tablet given 3 or 4 times daily as needed. The individual dose ranges from 4 mg. to 100 mg., depending on the compound being used. In the treatment of severe serum reactions, or allergic shock, 50 to 100 mg. of Benadryl given intravenously may be effective. Children should be given proportionately smaller doses than adults. Some of the preparations have a short acting effect and others, long acting. Some of the very efficient antihistamines are Benadryl, Decapryn, Neohetramine, Pyribenzamine and Phenergan. The latter is very effective in a large number of allergic disorders but because of the side reaction of drowsiness, it is best administered at bed time. Chlor-Trimeton, Pyronal and Perazil are very effective and have less side effects than other preparations. The writer likes to use Perazil because the duration of the effect is long. In cases of bladder irritability suspected of an allergy basis, he has had good results with oral administration of 1 tablet, 50 mg. at bedtime for a week or 10 days. In urology the antihistamines are helpful in the symptomatic treatment of bladder irritability and spasm and ureteral spasm which are presumably due to edema of the bladder neck or urethra or ureter on an allergic basis and in the treatment of urticaria, dermatitis, pruritis, and edema of allergic origin affecting the external genitalia. CRAIG et al. have used antihistamines in the treatment of acute nephritis, particularly in children, and felt that they cut down the duration of the disease as measured by the severity of symptoms.

There are certain endocrine preparations such as ACTH and cortisone and its derivatives which are useful adjuncts in the therapy of various aspects of allergic manifestations (FEINBERG et al. 1951). The explanation of their marked effect is not definitely known. Their use is not advocated in the routine management of patients with allergic disease because of the high rate of relapse after treatment is discontinued, the potential hazards involved from deleterious side effects and the fact that satisfactory results can be obtained in most patients by the use of treatment with well established methods of elimination or hyposensitization or the use of simpler drugs. They are to be used in the more desperate situations such as status asthmatics, severe serum sickness, severe drug reaction and in the acute phases of severe exfoliative dermatitis. In urogenital diseases, there should be little need for them except as indicated above in the marked manifestations of a severe allergic reaction, in anaphylactoid purpura causing hematuria or nephritis (STEFANNI et al. 1950), or in periarteritis nodosa. The proper dosage of either ACTH or cortisone and its newer derivatives is the smallest amount which will produce the desired therapeutic effect. This will vary from one patient to another. A dosage of 100 to 200 mg. daily of cortisone and of 50 to 100 mg. of ACTH may be given for 4—5 days and then tapering off the dosage as the condition of the patient improves.

In some cases a combination of therapeutic measures may have to be employed and pending the detection of the offending allergen, the use of antihistaminic therapy is often very beneficial, particularly in many cases of bladder and urethral irritability.

## 4. General constitutional measures in treatment

General measures of a hygienic nature include proper elimination, rest, elimination of foci of infection, psychotherapeutic procedures and correction of co-existent pathology. The physician should insist on good hygienic measures of living for his patients. They should eat a proper well-balanced diet and take vitamins if necessary to build up their constitution and general body resistance. They should secure rest and peace from emotional upsets and physical overexertion. Relaxation and diversion, vacations, engagement in sports and hobbies should be advocated. Sun baths and fresh air are of help to strengthen the patient. They should drink plenty of water daily and have adequate natural bowel evacuations. Since many irritants, such as spices, condiments, alcohol, coffee and tea tend to support and maintain allerization, their physician should recommend a diet that is poor in these substances, rich in fruit and vegetables, and somewhat restricted as to proteins.

The use of a sympathetic, reassuring attitude and minor psychotherapy are very often helpful and can often be carried out by the urologist. This may require several interviews to determine what nervous, emotional or mental factors or tensions in the patient's environment are tending to cause him stress so that they may be either avoided or eliminated. This will help prevent the precipitation or minimize the aggravation of many allergic conditions. Even if a patient is psychoneurotic and suffering from considerable emotional stress, his symptoms must still be evaluated from the allergic or immunologic standpoint. The treatment, therefore, depends upon individual evaluation of the allergic and psychological features of each case (BURDEN 1955).

## 5. Specific urological treatment

Urological treatment of allergic genitourinary disease may involve the elimination of any co-existing infections, obstructions, calculi, or tumors in the urogenital tract. Infection tends to enhance allergic symptoms and vice versa. The patient should drink large amounts of water daily (3—4 quarts) to flush out the urinary passages and to dilute the urine for a soothing effect. Appropriate chemotherapeutic or antibiotic agents may have to be prescribed for infection, depending upon the etiologic agent. The physician must, at all times, keep, in mind the possible sensitizing factors in any of these drugs. Dilatations of the urethra are frequently helpful in cases of female cystourethritis to provide free drainage from an inflamed or edematous tract. Hot sitz baths are also helpful in allaying inflammation. Occasionally, along with adrenalin or an antihistamine, dilatations of the ureter are of aid in eliminating spasm and edema to allow free drainage of urine from the kidneys. Transurethral resection or fulguration of bladder neck polyps or of those in the urethra aid in eliminating obstruction and irritation. Prostatectomy, transurethral, suprapubic, perineal or retropubic may be necessary for allergic granulomas of the prostate although most of these lesions are discovered co-incidentally. A dorsal slit, circumcision or meatotomy may be of help if acute edema of the urethra or penile foreskin fails to subside or becomes chronic and the administration of adrenalin or an antihistaminic is not efficacious.

# L. Prognosis

Since most of the spontaneous diseases of allergy are in the group in whom hereditary or familial influences are significant, it seems to be a proper deduction that in all such cases, allergy represents a constitutional defect. Individuals in this class of hereditarily sensitized state have a problem that has to be considered throughout their life, and gives point to the statement "once an allergic, always an allergic". It is therefore obvious that the prognosis as far as a loss of the spontaneously developed state of sensitization is concerned, is not favorable, and must be so recognized by both the patient and the physician. There is, however, a great difference between the allergic state and allergic disease. The patient is most concerned with the latter and the resultant symptoms. With these the prognosis will be dependent upon diagnosis and management. Allergy is often readily arrested or rendered asymptomatic and this should be particularly true in the genitourinary tract, but rarely cured. To reiterate, sensitization, once established, is liable to persist for life. If the patient is careful to avoid the offending allergen, he will, in most cases, be symptom free. If he becomes inadvertently exposed, or avoidance is impossible, hyposensitization and symptomatic treatment with drugs often gives a considerable measure of relief.

# M. Summary

Expressions of allergy, defined as altered reactivity of the organism, to many and various substances and agents have been noted for years but not understood or defined until the past 50 years. It is at present fairly widely recognized that the manifestations of allergy are due to an antigen-antibody reaction causing injury to cells with a release of certain chemical mediators from the tissues, such as histamine, or histamine-like substances. It is also well known that many of the symptoms of an allergic reaction can be produced by histamine. The exact mechanism, however, of the antigen-antibody reaction is still not clear. It is specific for a given antigen and its antibody.

Allergy may produce many types of pathologic lesions affecting many different organs of the body, including those of the urogenital tract. In individuals already sensitized by the entrance of antigens into tissues, different types of reactions may occur. The most familiar type is the immediate, reversible reaction in which local edema, vasodilatation, spasm of smooth muscle and activation of mucous glands may occur within a few minutes after contact with a specific allergen. In most cases, these lesions last a few hours and subside without leaving any residual changes. Common examples are hay fever, bronchial asthma, acute urticaria and bladder irritability or spasm on an allergic basis. The violent and sometimes fatal anaphylactic reactions to penicillin and heterologous serum are of the same type. Other allergic lesions of the anaphylactic type consist of exudation, infiltration of wandering cells, and proliferation of histiocytes which develop more gradually and last for days or weeks, but subside with slight or no scarring. Clinical examples include such lesions as purpura, erythema nodosum and the arterial lesions of serum sickness and drug allergy. There is considerable experimental and clinical evidence to indicate that periarteritis nodosa can be an expression of a hypersensitivity reaction to a variety of drugs. The evidence that human glomerulonephritis may be a manifestation of allergy is very suggestive but final proof or disproof must rest upon further studies in man. In the immediate type of allergic response, circulating antibodies are generally detectable in the plasma and the antibodies may also show the property of passively sensitizing normal human skin.

The other main type of allergic lesion is the delayed type in which necrosis of tissue is a striking feature. The chief example of this is the tuberculin reaction, but it can be produced by a variety of bacterial, viral and fungal agents in addition to certain drugs and chemicals. These lesions develop slowly and heal gradually with the formation of scar tissue. Contact dermatitis, produced by poison ivy and a variety of chemical agents, also fall into this group. In experimental animals, sensitization of the delayed type can be transferred to normal animals by injecting suspensions of lymphoid cells from the lymph nodes or spleen. Bacterial sensitization can be similarly transferred in humans by suspensions of leukocytes but attempts to transfer contact dermatitis in humans have usually failed.

The type of sensitization which develops in response to an antigenic stimulus depends on the chemical nature of the antigen, the route by which exposure takes place, the dose of the antigen, and the hereditary background of the individual. The substances producing anaphylactic or atopic sensitizations are usually typical protein antigens, while those producing contact dermatitis are more often chemicals of low molecular weight which combine with tissue proteins as haptens.

There are a number of important predisposing and contributing factors in allergy. Chief of these is heredity, which plays an important role in determining the susceptibility of certain individuals to hypersensitivity. Others are climatic influences, infections, social, environmental and psychosomatic influences and hormonal and autonomic nervous system factors.

Allergens, the sensitizing substances, may be divided into several classes according to their portal of entry such as inhalants, ingestants, injectants, contactants, infectants and physical agents. The most common allergens affecting the urogenital tract are foods, drugs and infectants.

The diagnosis of urogenital allergy depends upon a very careful and detailed history with particular attention to hereditary and environmental factors, a complete physical examination with particular emphasis on the urogenital system, laboratory examinations of the urine, blood and removed tissues, the performance of certain special tests as indicated such as skin tests and complete urological survey. The response to such drugs as epinephrine, the antihistamines and the steroids may be additional presumptive evidence in support of a diagnosis of allergy. The diagnosis of urogenital allergy is difficult because the symptoms are so much like those of the common urological conditions and can only be entertained after exhaustive study has ruled out the presence of organic disease.

The manifestations of allergy may affect the organs of the urogenital system as an isolated locale or as part of a general systemic response such as in purpura or periarteritis nodosa. The organ most commonly affected appears to be the bladder with symptoms of irritability or spasm — frequency, urgency, burning, tenesmus and suprapubic distress — but hematuria, albuminuria and dull or sharp flank pain may occur from lesions affecting the kidney and ureter. Urethritis may occur from sensitivity to substances or chemicals administered for diagnostic or therapeutic purposes. The prostate may be the seat of an allergic granuloma or congestion. The external genitalia of either sex may be involved in lesions of contact dermatitis or angioneurotic edema.

Many urological conditions such as essential hematuria, orthostatic albuminuria, non-specific urethritis and trigonitis, interstitial cystitis, and enuresis have been suspected of having an allergic basis but this has as yet not been proven. Nevertheless, the empirical treatment of some of these conditions on allergic principles often affords marked symptomatic relief. This involves the avoidance or elimination of possible offenders and the use of certain drugs such as epinephrine, ephedrine, the antihistamines or the steroids as adjuvants.

A consideration of allergy to diagnostic and therapeutic agents which are widely used in urology is important in the prevention of serious and, at times, fatal consequences. This involves discrimination in the use of iodine-containing contrast media, local anesthetics of the procaine group, chemotherapeutic agents such as the sulfonamides, and the antibiotics, particularly penicillin and streptomycin.

The treatment of urogenital allergy involves certain preventive measures such as the avoidance of incriminating substances, the elimination of the offending allergen, hyposensitization to foods and pollens when indicated, symptomatic relief by means of various drugs such as sympathemimetic and parasympatholytic drugs, sedatives, the antihistaminic and the endocrine drugs such as ACTH and cortisone or its derivatives, general constitutional measures such as the proper diet, rest and elimination, and the drinking of large amounts of water daily. Psychotherapy is often important. The avoidance of alcohol, coffee, tea and condiments should be advised either for their possible allergenic or irritant effects. Specific urological treatment is indicated to eliminate any co-existing pathology such as infections and obstruction. The dilatation of the urethra or ureter, along with the administration of epinephrine and an antihistamine, may aid in eliminating spasm and providing free drainage. Occasionally surgery, most frequently transurethral and at times open, for allergic, polypoid, edematous or granulomatous lesions is necessary. Of all these therapeutic measures, the most successful is the elimination of the offending allergen when it can be detected.

The prognosis for recovery from acute allergic lesions of the urogenital system is good but to prevent a recurrence the patient must be very careful to avoid the offending allergen. It is possible, in time, for complete desensitization to occur but as a general rule, while allergy is frequently arrested and alleviated, it is rarely completely cured.

# References

ADELSBERGER, L.: Zum Symptomenbild und zum Krankheitsverlauf der allergischen Krankheiten. Dtsch. med. Wschr. **1931**, 585. — ALEXANDER, H. L., and C. E. EYERMANN: Food allergy in HENOCH's purpura. Arch. Derm. Syph. (Chicago) **16**, 322 (1927). — ARTHUS, N.: Injections repetees de serum du cheval chez de lapin. C. R. Soc. Biol. (Paris) **55**, 817 (1903). — BALYEAT, R. M., and H. J. RINKEL: Urinary retention due to use of ephedrine. J. Amer. med. Ass. **98**, 1545 (1932). — BARETZ, L. H., M. HARTEN and M. WALZER: The absorption of proteins from the urinary bladder. J. Urol. (Baltimore) **50**, 71 (1943). — BLAUSTEIN, N.: Angioneurotic edema of entire genito-urinary system. J. Urol. (Baltimore) **16**, 379 (1926). — BOHROD, M. G.: Classification of the histologic reactions in allergic diseases. Amer. J. Med. **3**, 511 (1947). — BRAY, G. W.: Enuresis of allergic origin. Arch. Dis. Child. **6**, 251 (1931). — Recent advances in allergy, 3. edit. Philadelphia: Blakiston Son & Co. 1937. — BROWN, ALEXANDER: Henoch-Schoenlein purpura and acute nephritis due to food allergy. Glasg. med. J. **27**, 84 (1946). — BURDEN, S. S.: The role of the psyche in allergic disease. Ann. intern. Med. **43**, 1283 (1955). — BURKERT, S.: Role of allergy in chronic cystitis associated with oxyuriasis. Z. Urol. **46**, 158 (1953). — BURKLAND, C. E.: Manifestations of hypersensitivity in the genito-urinary system. Urol. cutan. Rev. **55**, 290 (1951). — CASTEX, R.: Allergic manifestations in the urinary apparatus. Pren. med. argent. **26**, 1667 (1939). — CAVELTI, P. A.: Autoimmunologic disease. J. Allergy **26**, 95 (1955). — CAVELTI, P. A., and E. S. CAVELTI: Studies on the pathogenesis of glomerulonephritis. I. Production of autoantibodies to kidney in experimental animals. Arch. Path. (Chicago) **39**, 148 (1945). — CHASE, M. W.: The cellular transfer of cutaneous hypersensitivity to tuberculin. Proc. Soc. exp. Biol. (N.Y.) **59**, 134 (1945). — Studies on the sensitization of animals with simple chemical compounds. X. Antibodies inducing immediate-type skin reactions. J. exp. Med. **86**, 489 (1947). — Development of antibody following transfer of cells taken from lymph nodes of sensitized or immunized animals. Fed. Proc. **10**, 404 (1951). — The Allergic State. In: Bacterial and Mycotic Infections of Man, pp. 168—221, 2nd Ed. edit. by R. J. DUBOS. Philadelphia: J. B. Lippincott & Co. 1952. — COCA, A. F.: Specific sensitiveness as a cause of symptoms in disease. Bull. N. Y. Acad. Med. Ser. 2 **6**, 593 (1930). — COCA, A. F., and E. F. GROVE: Studies in hypersensitiveness. XIII. A study of the atopic reagins. J. Immunol. **10**, 445 (1925). — COHEN, A. C., and G. C. GLINSKY: Hypersensitivity to streptomycin. J. Allergy **22**, 63 (1951). — COOKE, R. A.: Allergy in theory and practice. Philadelphia: W. B. Saunders Company 1947. — COOKE, R. A., and A. VAN DER VEER: Human sensitization. J. Immunol. **1**, 201 (1916). — CRAIG, J., N. S. CLARKE and J. D. CHALMERS: Antihistamine drug treatment of acute nephritis. Brit. med. J. **1949**, 6. — CRIEP, L. H., and C. RIBEIRO: Allergy to procaine hydrochloride with three fatalities. J. Amer. med. Ass. **151**, 1185 (1953). — DALE, H. H.: Adventures in physiology. London: Pergamon Press 1953. — Transmission of nervous effects by acetylcholine. Harvey Lect. **32**, 229 (1937). — DAVIS, B. D.: The binding of sulfonamide drugs by plasma proteins. Science **95**, 78 (1942). — DEES, J. E.: Use of cortisone in interstitial cystitis, preliminary report. J. Urol. (Baltimore) **69**, 496 (1953). — DEES, S. C., and E. C. SIMMONS: Allergy of the urinary tract. Ann. Allergy **9**, 714 (1951). — DOERR, R.: Unterempfindlichkeit und Überempfindlichkeit. Arch. Derm. Syph. (Berl.) **150**, 509 (1926). — Allergic phenomena. In Handbuch der normalen und pathologischen Physiologie, Bd. 13, S. 650. 1929. — DRAGSTEDT, C. A.: The significance of histamine in anaphylaxis. J. Allergy **16**, 69 (1945). — DUKE, W. W.: Food allergy as a cause of bladder pain. Ann. clin. Med. **1**, 117 (1922). — Food allergy as a cause of illness. J. Amer. med. Ass. **81**, 886 (1923). — DUTTA, P. C.: Allergy and Dysmenorrhea. J. Obstet. & Gynaec. Brit. Emp. **42**, 309 (1935). — EHRICH, W. E., C. W. FORMANN and J. SEIFTER: Diffuse glomerular nephritis and lipid nephrosis. Arch. Path. (Chicago) **54**, 463 (1952). — EISENSTAEDT, J. S.: Allergy and drug hypersensitivity of the urinary tract. J. Urol. (Baltimore) **65**, 154 (1951). — ENGEL, W. J., and L. J. McCORMACK: Acute necrotizing angiitis of the bladder. J. Urol. (Baltimore) **79**, 230 (1958). — FEIN, BERNARD T.: Personal communication to the author. — FEINBERG, S. M., T. B. DANNENBERG and S. MALHIEL: ACTH and cortisone in allergic manifestations. J. Allergy **22**, 195 (1951). — FINEGOLD, A. N.: Anuria resulting from allergic edema following administration of sulfadiazine in a patient with asthma. J. Urol. (Baltimore) **56**, 652 (1946). — FORD, W. K.: Drug eruption due to quinine.

Recurrence following use of contraceptives. J. Amer. med. Ass. 103, 483 (1934). — FOUTS, P. J., A. C. CORCORAN and J. H. PAGE: Observations on the clinical and functional course of nephrotoxic nephritis in dogs. Amer. J. med. Sci. 201, 313 (1941). — FOX, J. L.: Vaginal and urinary symptoms following pollen injections. Ann. Allergy 13, 187 (1955). — FREY, W.: New skin tests in inguinal lymphogranuloma. Klin. Wschr. 1925, 2148. — FREUND, J.: Some aspects of active immunization. Ann. Rev. Microbiol. 1, 291 (1947). — FREUND, J., M. M. LIPTON and G. E. THOMPSON: Aspermatogenesis in the guinea pig induced by testicular tissue and adjuvants. J. exp. Med. 97, 711 (1953). — GAIRDNER, D.: The Schoenlein-Henoch syndrome (Anaphylactoid purpura). Quart. J. Med. 17, 95 (1948). — GERMUTH jr., F. G.: A comparative histologic and immunologic study in rabbits of induced hypersensitivity of the serum sickness type. J. exp. Med. 97, 257 (1953). — GERMUTH jr., F. G., J. OYAMA and B. OTTINGER: The mechanism of action of 17-hydroxy-11-dehydrocorticosterone (compound E) and of the adrenocorticotropic hormone in experimental hypersensitivity in rabbits. J. exp. Med. 94, 139 (1951). — GERMUTH jr., F. G. and J. C. TIPPETT: The effect of sensitization to homologous and cross-reactive antigens on the rate of antigen elimination and the development of allergic lesions. J. exp. Med. 101, 135 (1955). — GLASER, J.: The prophylaxis of allergic disease with special reference to the newborn infant. N. Y. St J. Med. 55, 2599 (1955). — GRAY, L. A.: Lymphopathia venereum (lymphogranuloma inguinale) of female urethra. Surg. Gynec. Obstet. 62, 745 (1936). — GREENSPAN, S. A., and C. A. KRAKOWER: Direct evidence for the antigenicity of the glomeruli in the production of nephrotoxic serums. Arch. Path. (Chicago) 49, 291 (1950). — GRILLO, V.: Allergic urethritis; urethral manifestations of cutaneous and mucous allergies. G. ital. Derm. Sif. 91 (1), 67 (1950). — GUTMANN, M. J.: Allergische Erscheinungen durch Genußmittel und deren Beseitigung. Dtsch. med. Wschr. 1933, 1281. — GUTTMANN, J. J.: Die allergischen Erkrankungen. Med. Welt. 1930, 730. — HABER, H.: Fixed eruption and urethritis due to phenolphthalein. Brit. J. Derm. Syph. 62, 23 (1950). — HAND, J. R.: Interstitial cystitis. Report of 223 cases. J. Urol. (Baltimore) 61, 291 (1949). — HARRIS, T. W., and S. HARRIS: The genesis of antibodies. Amer. J. Med. 20, 114 (1956). — HARRISON, F. G., D. G. NEANDER: Allergic granuloma of the prostate. J. Urol. (Baltimore) 72, 218 (1954). — HEYMANN, W., C. GILKEY and M. SALCHAR: Antigenic property of renal cortex. Prox. Soc. exp. 73, 385 (1950). — HOLLANDER, L.: Dermatitis of the penis caused by ephedrine. J. Amer. med. Ass. 106, 706 (1936). — HUTTON, J. E.: Favism. J. Amer. med. Ass. 109, 1618 (1937). — IDOIPE-GOMEZ, F. J.: Prostate as a starting point of allergic syndromes. Farmacoter. act. 11 (11), 319 (1945). — JOACHIMOVITS, R.: Menstrual disturbances in hay fever; study of anaphylactic phenomenon on uterus. Med. Klin. 1926, 294. — KAHN, I. S.: Uterine spasm complicating pollen anaphylactic reaction. J. Amer. med. Ass. 90, 2101 (1938). — KAY, C. F.: The mechanism of a form of glomerulonephritis: nephrotoxic nephritis in the rabbit. Amer. J. med. Sci. 204, 483 (1942). — KERN, J.: Quoted by ADELSBERGER. — KERN, R. A., and N. A. WIMBERLY jr.: Penicillin reactions: their nature, growing importance, recognition, management and prevention. Amer. J. med. Sci. 226, 357 (1953). — KINDALL, L., and T. T. NICKELS: Allergy of the pelvic urinary tract in the female. A preliminary report. J. Urol. (Baltimore) 61, 222 (1949). — KITTREDGE, W. E., and G. BROWN: Ephedrine sulfate in the treatment of nocturnal enuresis. New Orleans med. Surg. J. 96, 512 (1944). — KITTREDGE, W. E., and C. JOHNSON: Allergic hematuria due to milk. New Orleans med. Surg. J. 101, 419 (1949). — KLEMPERER, P.: Pathologic-anatomic aspects of allergy. In R. A. COOKE, Allergy in theory and practice, 69. Philadelphia: W. B. Saunders Company 1947. — KOEHLER, H. D.: Allergic hematuria. Harefuah 43, 70 (1952). — KOURIISKY, R., G. DECROIX et P. GANTER Études sur l'allergic tuberculinique: La transmission de l'allergic. Rev. Immunol. (Paris) 16, 333 (1952). — KUHNS, W. J.: Types and distribution of antibodies. Amer. J. Med. 20, 251 (1956). — KUTSCHER, A. H., S. L. LANE and R. SEGALL: The clinical toxicity of antibodies and sulfonamides. J. Allergy 25, 135 (1954). — LANDSTEINER, K.: The specificity of serological reactions. Rev. Ed. Cambridge: Harvard University Press. 1947. — LANDSTEINER, K., and M. W. CHASE: Studies on the sensitization of animals with simple chemical compounds. J. exp. Med. 66, 337 (1937); 71, 237 (1940); 72, 431 (1941). — Experiments on transfer of cutaneous sensitivity to simple compounds. Proc. Soc. exp. Biol. 49, 688 (1942). — LANGE, K., F. CRAIG, J. OBERMAN, L. SLOBODY, G. OGUR and F. LO CASTRO: Changes in serum complement during the course and treatment of glomerulonephritis. A.M.A. Arch. intern. Med. 88, 433 (1951). — LANGE, K., M. M. A. GOLD, D. WEINER and V. SIMON: Autoantibodies in human glomerulonephritis. J. clin. Invest. 28, 50 (1949). — LANGE, K., L. SLOBODY, F. CRAIG, G. OGUR, J. OBERMAN, and F. LO CASTRO: Serum complement in acute glomerulonephritis and the nephrotic syndrome. Pediatrics 8, 814 (1951). — LAWRENCE, H. S.: The delayed type of allergic inflammatory response. Amer. J. Med. 20, 428 (1956). — LAWRENCE, H. S.: The cellular transfer of cutaneous hypersensitivity to tuberculin in man. Proc. Soc. exp. Biol. (N.Y.) 71, 516 (1949). — LAZARUS, J. A.: Idiopathic purpura associated with hematuria. J. Urol. (Baltimore) 62,

354 (1949). — LECA, J.: Allergic urethritis of various origins. J. d'Urol. 59, 383 (1953). — LEIDER, M., D. FURMAN and A. A. FISHER: Sensitivity to rubber materials. An analysis of one hundred twenty-five cases of eruptions proved to be caused by rubber articles. A.M.A. Arch. Derm. Syph. 65, 587 (1952). — LITZNER, S.: Die Bedeutung der Allergie für die Innermedizin über allergische Reaktionen der Harnorgane. Med. Klin. 1936, 523. — Allergic disease of urinary organs, further observation. Dtsch. med. Wschr. 1937, 1546. — LONG, E. R.: Allergic reaction in kidney and testes. J. Urol. (Baltimore) 20, 565 (1928). — LONG, E. R., and L. L. FINNER: Experimental glomerulonephritis produced by intra-renal tuberculin reactions. Amer. J. Path. 4, 571 (1928). — LONGCOPE, W. T.: The production of experimental nephritis by repeated protein intoxication. J. exp. Med. 18, 678 (1913). — Serum sickness and analogous reactions from certain drugs, particularly the sulfonamides. Medicine (Baltimore) 22, 251 (1943). — LOWELL, F. C.: Allergic reactions to sulfonamide and antibiotic drugs. Ann. intern. Med. 43, 333 (1955). — MAC LEOD, C. M.: Interactions of host, microbe and chemotherapeutic agents. Bull. N. Y. Acad. Med. 31, 427 (1955). — MANWARING, W. H., and H. D. MARINO: Reactions of urinary bladder in rabbit anaphylaxis. J. Immunol. 13, 69 (1927). — MANWARING, W. H.: Hepatic reactions in anaphylaxis. J. Immunol. 10, 567 (1925). — MARSHALL, V. F., and E. ENDICOTT: A clinical study of obscure bladder disease. Using Frei tests. J. Urol. (Baltimore) 50, 76 (1943). — MARTIN, K. W.: Purpura of the urogenital tract. Brit. J. Urol. 23, 233 (1951). — MASUGI, M.: Zur Pathogenese der diffusen Glomerulonephritis als allergische Erkrankung der Niere. Klin. Wschr. 1935, 373. — Die Pathogenese der diffusen Glomerulonephritis im Lichte experimenteller Erzeugung dieser Nierenerkrankung bei Tieren. Zbl. inn. Med. 56, 417 (1935). — MASUGI, M., and Y. SATO: Über die allergische Gewebsreaktion der Niere. Virchows Arch. path. Anat. 293, 615 (1934). — McGAVATH, T. H., A. M. SHERMAN, I. WEISBERG, A. M. FUCHS and P. M. SCHENKMAN: Newer antihistaminics. J. Allergy 22, 31 (1951). — MELICOW, M. M.: Allergic granulomas of the prostate gland. J. Urol. (Baltimore) 65, 288 (1951). — MILLER, M. W., and C. A. UHLE: A Survey of urinary tract allergy. Int. Clin., N. Ser. II 3, 183 (1939). — MITCHELL, W. F., I. SWAN and J. H. MITCHELL: Vulvo-vaginal pruritis associated with hay fever. Ann. Allergy 6, 144 (1948). — MOLL, F. C., and C. Z. v. HAWN: Experimental hypersensitivity. Relationship of dosage to serological and pathological responses following injection of heterologous protein. Proc. Soc. exp. Biol. (N.Y.) 80, 77 (1952). — MORE, R. H., and D. WAUGH: Diffuse glomerulonephritis produced in rabbits by massive injections of bovine serum gamma globulin. J. exp. Med. 89, 541 (1949). — NACHMANSOHN, D.: Symposium on physiology of acetylcholine. Bull. Johns Hopk. Hosp. 83, 463 (1948). — NUNEZ, M. (M. FERNAN-NUNEZ): Hemoglobinuric fever: is it an allergic phenomenon? Amer. J. trop. Med. 16, 563 (1936). — PAYNE, W. W., W. H. MOSSE and S. L. RAINES: A fatal reaction following injection of urographic medium. J. Urol. (Baltimore) 76, 661 (1956). — PENDERGRASS, E. P., G. W. CHAMBERLIN and E. W. GODFREY and E. D. BERDICK: A survey of deaths and unfavorable sequellae following the administration of contrast media. Amer. J. Roentgenol. 48, 741 (1942). — PFEIFFER, E. F., and H. E. BRUCH: Die Autoallergie in der Pathogenese der diffusen Glomerulonephritis. Ergebn. inn. Med. Kinderheilk. 4, 670 (1953). — PIRQUET, C. v.: Allergie. Münch. med. Wschr. 52, 1457 (1906). — POWELL, N. B., and E. B. POWELL: Vesical allergy in females. Sth. med. J. (Bgham. Ala.) 47, 841 (1954). — PRAUSNITZ, C., u. H. KUSTNER: Studien über die Überempfindlichkeit. Zbl. Bakt. 86, 160 (1921). — PRESSMAN, D.: The zone of localization of antibodies. IV. The in vivo disposition of anti-mouse-kidney serum and anti-mouse-plasma serum as determined by radioactive tracers. J. Immunol. 63, 375 (1949). — PRESSMAN, D., H. N. EISEN, M. SIEGEL, P. J. FITZGERALD, B. SHERMAN and A. SIVERSTEIN: The zone of localization of antibodies. X. The use of radioactive sulfur 35 as a label for antikidney serum. J. Immunol. 65, 559 (1950). — PRESSMAN, D., L. KORNGOLD and W. HEYMANN: Localizing properties of anti-rat-kidney serum prepared in ducks. Arch. Path. (Chicago) 55, 347 (1953). — PREZIOZI, P.: Allergic nephritis. Rif. med. 65 (12), 329 (1951). — RAFFEL, S.: The components of the tubercle bacillus responsible for the delayed type of "infectious allergy". J. infect. Dis. 82, 367 (1948). — Bacterial hypersensitivity. J. Allergy 27, 169 (1956). — RAFFEL, S., and J. E. FORNEY: The role of the "wax" of the tubercle bacillus in establishing delayed hypersensitivity. 1. Hypersensitivity to a simple chemical substance, picryl chloride. J. exp. Med. 88, 485 (1948). — RANDOLPH, T. G., J. P. ROLLINS and CLYDE K. WALTER: Allergic reactions following the intravenous injection of corn sugar (dextrose). Arch. Surg. (Chicago) 61, 554 (1950). — RATTNER, H.: Dermatitis of the penis from rubber. J. Amer. med. Ass. 105, 1189 (1935). — RHODES, J.: Hematuria after use of tetanus. J. Urol. (Baltimore) 38, 410 (1937). — RICH, A. R.: The role of hypersensitivity in periarteritis nodosa as indicated by seven cases developing during serum sickness and sulfonamide therapy. Bull. Johns Hopk. Hosp. 71, 123 (1942). — Additional evidence of the role of hypersensitivity in the etiology of periarteritis nodosa. Bull. Johns Hopk. Hosp. 71, 375 (1942). — Hypersensitivity to iodine as a cause of periarteritis nodosa. Bull. Johns Hopk.

170     CARL E. BURKLAND: Urogenital allergy

Hosp. **77,** 43 (1945). — Hypersensitivity in disease. Harvey Lect. **42,** 106 (1946/47). — The pathogenesis of tuberculosis, edit. 2. Springfield, Ill.: Ch. C. Thomas 1951. — The pathology and pathogenesis of experimental anaphylactic glomerulonephritis in relation to human acute glomerulonephritis. Bull. Johns Hopk. Hosp. **98,** 120 (1956). — RICH, A. R., M. BERTHRONG and I. L. BENNETT jr.: The effect of cortisone upon the experimental cardiovascular and renal lesions produced by anaphylactic hypersensitivity. Bull. Johns Hopk. Hosp. **87,** 549 (1950). — RICH, A. R., and J. E. GREGORY: The experimental demonstration that periarteritis nodosa is a manifestation of hypersensitivity. Bull. Johns Hopk. Hosp. **72,** 65 (1943). — RICHET jr., C., A. TZANCK and A. COUDER: Does anaphylactic nephritis exist? J. med. franç., **19,** 180 (1930). — RINKEL, H. J.: Food allergy. II. The technique and clinical application of individual food tests. Ann. Allergy **2,** 504 (1944). — ROBINSON, M.W.: The immunological properties of alcohol. A survey of the literature. Ann. Allergy **8,** 468 (1950). — ROLLINGHOFF, W.: Allergic renal lesion due to sulfonamide. Klin. Wschr. **27,** 553 (1949). — ROLNICK and G. U. BAUMRUCKER: Genito-urinary blastomycosis. J. Urol. (Baltimore) **79,** 315 (1958). — ROSENBLUETH, A.: The transmission of nerve impulses at neuroeffector junctions and peripheral responses. New York: John Wiley & Sons 1950. — Eight fatal anaphylactic reactions to penicillin. N. Y. J. Med. **54,** 1485 (1954). — ROSS, J. F.: Hemoglobinemia and the hemoglobinurias. N. Engl. J. Med. **233,** 691 (1945). — ROWE, ALBERT H.: Clinical allergy: Manifestations, diagnosis and treatment. Philadelphia: Lea a. Febiger 1937. — Elimination DIETS and patient's allergies. Philadelphia: Lea a. Febiger 1944. — Management of food allergy. Postgrad. Med. 8, 52 (1950). — RYTAND, D. A.: Fatal anuria, the nephrotic syndrome and glomerular nephritis as sequels of the dermatitis of poison oak. Amer. J. Med. **5,** 548 (1948). — SACK, S.: Physical allergy. N. Y. St. J. Med. **57,** 3689 (1957). — SANGER, M. D., and D. E. EHRLICH: A method of reducing reactions in intravenous pyelography with an antihistamine. Ann. Allergy **14,** 254 (1956). — SARRE, H.: Die Durchblutung der Niere bei der experimentellen diffusen Glomerulonephritis. Dtsch. Arch. klin. Med. **183,** 515 (1939). — Allergic disease of urinary tract. Münch. med. Wschr. **1954,** 515. — SAUL, L. J.: Some observations on relations of emotions and allergy. Psychosom. Med. **3,** 66 (1941). — SCHWAB, L., F. C. MOLL, T. HALL, H. BREEN, M. KINK, C. Z. v. HAWN and C. A. JANEWAY: Effect of inhibition of antibody formation by x-radiation or nitrogen mustards on the histologic and serologic sequences, and on the behavior of serum complement, following single large injections of foreign protein. J. exp. Med. **91,** 505 (1950). — SHELDON, J. M., R. G. LAVELL and K. P. MATHEWS: A survey and evaluation of the antihistamine drugs. Bull. Amer. Soc. Hosp. Pharm. **7,** 252 (1950). — SMADEL, J. E.: Experimental nephritis induced by injection of anti-kidney serum. I. Preparation and immunological studies of nephrotoxin. J. exp. Med. **64,** 921 (1936). — SMITH, D. R.: Essential dysmenorrhea and allergy. J. Mo. med. Ass. **28,** 382 (1931). — SPAIN, W. C., and R. A. COOKE: Specific hypersensitiveness: Familial occurrence of hay fever and bronchial asthma. J. Immunol. **9,** 521 (1924). — STEWART, M. J., S. WRAY and M. HALL: Allergic prostatitis in asthmatics. J. Path. Bact. **67,** 423 (1954). — THOMAS, J. W., and M. R. FENTON: Fatalities and constitutional reactions following the use of pontocaine. J. Allergy **14,** 145 (1943). — THOMAS, J. W., and V. P. WICKSTEN: Allergy in relation to the genito-urinary tract. Ann. Allergy **2,** 396 (1944). — THOMPSON, G. J., and D. D. ALBERS: Granulomatous prostatitis. J. Urol. (Baltimore) **49,** 530 (1953). — TZANK, A., and J. COTTET: Les intolerances renales. Presse méd. **42,** 415 (1934). — URBACH, E., and P. M. GOTTLIEB: Allergy, edit. 2. New York; Grune & Stratton 1946. — VEER, A., VAN DER R. A. COOKE and W. C. SPAIN: Diagnosis and treatment of seasonal hay fever. Amer. J. med. Sci. **174,** 101 (1927). — VAUGHN, W. T., and R. W. FOULKES: Allergic reactions associated with cohabitation. J. Amer. med. Ass. **105,** 955 (1935). — VAUGHN, W. T., and E. K. HAWKE: Angioneurotic edema with some unusual manifestations. J. Allergy **2,** 125 (1931). — VOISIN, G., A. DELAUNAY and M. BARBER: Lesions testiculaires provoquees chez le cobaye par injection d'extraits de testicules homologues. C. R. Acad. Sci. (Paris) **232,** 1264 (1951). — WINTER, C. C.: The value of chlor-trimeton in the prevention of immediate reactions to 70% urokon. J. Urol. (Baltimore) **74,** 416 (1955).

# Tetanie

Von

G. W. PARADE

Mit 4 Abbildungen

## A. Einleitung

Wenn der Urologe einen Fall mit Krampfzuständen im Bereich des Ureters vor sich hat, so sucht er mit Recht nach der organischen Ursache dieser Krämpfe. Die Koliken können durch verschiedenartige mechanische oder entzündliche Faktoren bedingt sein. Wenn aber alle diese auslösenden Momente auf Grund sorgfältigster Durchuntersuchung auszuschließen sind, so bleibt eine gewisse Anzahl von Fällen übrig, wo eine rein spastische Genese in Frage gezogen werden muß. Nun ist bekannt, daß es Krampfzustände an den verschiedensten glattmuskeligen Organen gibt, die ihrer Genese nach einem Krankheitsbild zuzuordnen sind, dessen Leitsymptom die Krampfneigung ist, nämlich der Tetanie. Bei dieser Erkrankung, die primär nichts mit Entzündung oder organisch-mechanischer Behinderung der Tätigkeit von Hohlorganen zu tun hat, werden schmerzhafte spastische Zustände quergestreifter und glattmuskeliger Organe, wie z. B. des Larynx, des Oesophagus, des Magens, der Gallenblase und der Gallenwege, des Uterus usw. beobachtet. Insbesondere bei der Gallenblase ist heute der Begriff der Dyskinesie wohlbekannt; sie kann, wenn sie mit schmerzhaften Spasmen einhergeht, bekanntlich zu Gallenkoliken führen. Diese können unter Umständen auf einer tetanischen Übererregbarkeit beruhen. Auch die ableitenden Harnwege, Ureteren und Blase, mit ihrem komplizierten muskulären Funktionsspiel, können in die spastischen Entäußerungen der Tetanie einbezogen werden. Diese Tatsache ist nicht genügend bekannt. Sie ist aber wichtig, weil bei völlig negativem Untersuchungsergebnis des Urovesicaltractus unter Umständen eine tetanische Genese der Koliken in Frage kommt. Läßt sich eine solche Entstehungsweise der Symptomatologie sicherstellen, so ergeben sich daraus neue und anders geartete therapeutische Konsequenzen, und dem Kranken können unter Umständen Eingriffe erspart werden. Die Abhandlung des Kapitels Tetanie im Handbuch für Urologie soll dazu dienen, dem Urologen Hinweise auf ein Krankheitsbild zu geben, das — bei oft negativem urologischen Befund — gegebenenfalls den Koliken zugrunde liegen könnte. Einmal auf die tetanische Symptomatologie aufmerksam gemacht, wird der Urologe dem einen oder anderen Patienten helfen können, wo dies sonst vielleicht nicht möglich gewesen wäre. Die Abhandlung des Kapitels Tetanie führt uns somit in ein krankhaftes Geschehen, das sich nicht primär von den Harnwegen herleitet, das vielmehr genetisch den ganzen Organismus befällt, sich aber im Bereich des Urovesicaltractus in schweren Schmerzanfällen entladen kann.

## B. Einführung in den Krankheitsbegriff Tetanie

Als Tetanie bezeichnet man den „Zustand einer allgemeinen zentralen nervösen Übererregbarkeit, die zur Erniedrigung der neuromuskulären und sensiblen

Reizschwelle führt und mit der Entstehung neurovegetativer und motorischer Reaktionszentren einhergeht" (KRÜCK). Die Tetanie mit ihren verschiedenen Entäußerungen ist keine Krankheit an sich, sondern ein Symptomenkomplex bzw. ein Syndrom, das sich aus verschiedenen Anlässen entwickeln kann. Offenbar ist in jedem Menschen die tetanische Reaktionsweise in mehr oder weniger starker Ausprägung vorgebildet, beim Kind in der Regel noch wesentlich stärker als beim Erwachsenen. Das tetanische Syndrom ist (nach QUANDT und PONSOLD) eine vorwiegend subcorticale Reaktionsform des zentralen Nervensystems, wobei im tetanischen Krampfanfall selbst extrapyramidale Bewegungsabläufe auftreten. Diese Reaktionsform tritt nach völliger Ausreifung der Hirnrinde nicht mehr spontan in Erscheinung, es sei denn, daß die corticale Dämpfung nachläßt oder eine isolierte Steigerung der subcorticalen Erregungsabläufe zu verzeichnen ist.

Die Möglichkeit des Ausbruchs tetanischer Erscheinungen ist individuell durchaus verschieden; es müssen eine Anzahl von Vorbedingungen gegeben sein, welche das Manifestwerden deutlicher Tetaniesymptome ermöglichen. Die Diagnose Tetanie (S. 176, 194) kann man nur dann mit völliger Sicherheit festlegen, wenn im Verlauf des Krankheitsgeschehens ein klassischer tetanischer Anfall (S. 178) beobachtet worden ist. Wenn ein solcher Anfall niemals auftritt, so ist es oft außerordentlich schwierig, wenn nicht unmöglich, aus der häufig sehr vielgestaltigen Begleitsymptomatik der Tetanie die sichere Diagnose des Vorliegens dieser Erkrankung zu stellen.

Unter den Symptomen, welche bei der Tetanie außerhalb des echten tetanischen Anfalls beobachtet werden, befinden sich auch solche, die durch tetanische Sensationen in der nicht vom Willen abhängigen Muskulatur hervorgerufen werden; d. h. also, daß bei der Tetanie auch Krampfzustände der glatten Muskulatur vorkommen und beobachtet werden können. Diese Tatsache ist unter anderem der Grund, weshalb dem Krankheitsbild der Tetanie im „Handbuch für Urologie" ein besonderer Platz eingeräumt wurde.

Noch vor einigen Jahren herrschte vielfach die Anschauung, daß das Bestehen einer Tetanie in jedem Fall mit Störungen des Kalkstoffwechsels, und zwar mit einer Herabsetzung des Blutkalkspiegels unter die Norm, verbunden sei. Diese Auffassung hat sich als irrig erwiesen. So bedeutungsvoll auch der Blutcalciumgehalt für die neuromuskuläre und sensible Erregbarkeit ist, so ist doch das Auftreten tetanischer Entäußerungen, insbesondere auch des großen tetanischen Anfalls, nicht unbedingt von einer pathologischen Erniedrigung des Blutkalkgehalts abhängig. Es kommt hinzu, daß das Verhalten des Calciums im Blut nicht allein die neuromuskuläre Erregbarkeit bestimmt, sondern daß auch andere Ionen für diese von Bedeutung sind.

Entscheidend wichtig ist nämlich auch der Zustand des neuromuskulären Apparates als solcher für die Frage der Ausprägung tetanischer Symptome.

In Anbetracht dieser heute feststehenden Tatsachen ergibt es sich, die Tetanien in zwei verschiedene Formen aufzugliedern:

1. Tetanie, bei welcher der Blutkalkgehalt erniedrigt ist: hypocalcämische Tetanie,

2. Tetanie, bei welcher der Blutkalkgehalt der Norm entspricht: normocalcämische Tetanie.

Wir werden sehen, daß auch jede dieser 2 Formen an sich kein einheitliches Geschehen darstellt. Insbesondere ist die normocalcämische Tetanie die Ausdrucksform verschiedener pathophysiologischer Zustände.

# C. Die hypocalcämische Tetanie

Das Hauptkriterium der Diagnostik dieser Tetanieform ist die Erniedrigung des Blutkalkspiegels unter die Norm. Wir rechnen mit einem Normalwert des Blutkalkspiegels von 9 bis etwa 11 mg-%. Wird der Wert von 9 mg-% deutlich unterschritten, so steht bei entsprechendem klinischem Krankheitsbild die Diagnose einer hypocalcämischen Tetanie fest.

## I. Zusammensetzung des Blutcalciums

Der *Blutkalkgehalt* setzt sich aus 2 bzw. 3 Komponenten zusammen (Abb. 1). Das Blutcalcium ist zu etwa 50% an das Albumin des Blutes, als sog. Calciumproteinat, gebunden; bei den restlichen etwa 50% handelt es sich um ionisiertes Calcium, dem die entscheidende Bedeutung bei der Aufrechterhaltung der optimalen Schwelle der neuromuskulären und sensiblen Erregbarkeit zukommt. Schließlich existiert noch eine dritte, sehr kleine Calciumfraktion, ein Calciumkomplexsalz, dessen besondere Bedeutung noch wenig bekannt ist. Es gibt heute keine zuverlässige Methode, welche es erlaubt, die zwei großen Fraktionen des Blutes voneinander gesondert zu bestimmen; man kann sie allerdings anhand der gleichzeitigen elektrophoretischen Messung der Bluteiweißkörper mit Hilfe einer von MCLEAN und HASTINGS angegebenen Tabelle schätzen, ohne daß man in jedem Fall mit Sicherheit annehmen kann, daß diese Auswertung den wirklichen Verhältnissen genau entspricht.

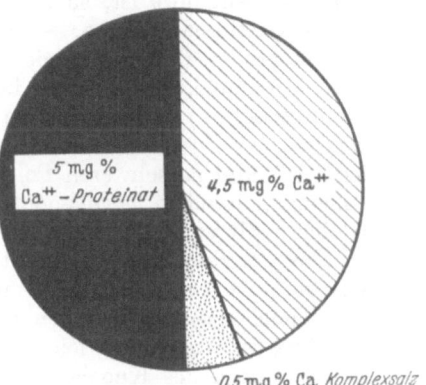

Abb. 1. Die Verteilung der Ca-Fraktionen im Blutplasma. (Nach MCLEAN und HASTINGS, HARNAPP)

## II. Bestimmung des Blutcalciumgehalts

Die Bestimmung des Gesamtcalciums im Serum erfolgt entweder chemisch mit Hilfe der Methode von CLARK bzw. von STÜRMER-SCHWARZENBACH; am elegantesten und sichersten aber heutzutage mit Hilfe der Flammenphotometrie. Äußerst wichtig ist die exakte Blutentnahme zur *Calciumbestimmung*. Die zum Auffangen des Sanguis bestimmten Gläser müssen vorher völlig calciumfrei gemacht werden. Praktisch bedient man sich bei der Blutentnahme am besten der sog. Venülen, deren Calciumfreiheit garantiert ist. Will man für genauere Bestimmungen absolut sicher verwertbare Calciumwerte erhalten, so muß der Proband 5 Tage vor der Blutabnahme möglichst kalkfrei ernährt werden, d. h. er darf an diesen Tagen weder Milch noch Milchprodukte, insbesondere Käse, zu sich nehmen; selbstverständlich auch keine Kalkpräparate. Bei der Routinebestimmung genügt aber ohne weiteres die Untersuchung des nüchtern entnommenen Blutes ohne vorangehende Diäteinhaltung.

## III. Calciumaufnahme, -abgabe und Deponierung

Der Calciumgehalt des Blutes stellt keine autonome Größe dar; seine Höhe hängt verständlicherweise von dem Zustand jener Organe ab, welche etwas mit der Calciumaufnahme und -abgabe und der Calciumdeponierung im Organismus zu tun haben. Die *Calciumaufnahme* durch den *Magen-Darmkanal* hängt von der Menge des Calciumangebotes der Nahrung ab, deren Optimum bei der heutigen Ernährung (etwa 1 g pro Tag) in der Regel garantiert sein dürfte, wobei hervorzuheben ist, daß die beste Calciumresorption aus der Milch und den natürlichen Milchprodukten erfolgt. Von entscheidender Bedeutung ist der Zustand des Magen-Darmkanals; das Vorliegen einer schweren Gastroenteritis mit etwaiger Bildung von unlöslichen Kalkseifen erschwert die Resorption des Nahrungskalks unter Umständen erheblich. Auch das Fehlen der Magensalzsäure ist der Calciumresorption nicht förderlich. Besonders wichtig ist die Anwesenheit von *Vitamin D* im Organismus, dessen Aufgabe in bezug auf den Magen-Darmkanal vor allem darin besteht, die langsame Resorption des Calciums aus dem Darm in den Organismus zu fördern. Da bei schweren Störungen des Magen-Darmkanals oftmals auch die Resorption der Fette und der fettlöslichen Vitamine, z. B. das Vitamin D, behindert ist, so erhellt daraus die große Bedeutung des Vitamin D für die Calciumaufnahme. — Als Ausscheidungsorgane für das in den Organismus aufgenommene Calcium fungieren in erster Linie die Nieren. (Auch im Dünndarm wird Calcium ausgeschieden, insbesondere mit den täglich abgesonderten Verdauungssäften.) Störungen der *Calciumausscheidung der Nieren* im Sinne des Zuviel oder Zuwenig können den Kalkspiegel des Blutes in erheblichem Maße irritieren und zu schweren Folgeerscheinungen führen: soweit es sich um Hypocalcämien handelt, gegebenenfalls zur Ausprägung tetanischer Entäußerungen. Gleiches gilt von Störungen der Calcium-Resorption aus dem Magen-Darmkanal.

Das *Calciumdepotorgan* stellt das *Skelet* dar, in welchem der über den Blutweg aufgenommene Kalk als unlösliche Calciumphosphatverbindung in Form des Knochenapatits ziemlich fest verankert wird. An der riesigen Oberfläche der Apatitkristalle sind leichter abspaltbare Calciumionen chemisch angelagert. Die Funktion des Knochens besteht im Hinblick auf den Kalkhaushalt unter anderem darin, daß das Calciumdepot des Knochens als Nachschuborgan für den Blutcalciumgehalt dienen kann. (Von dem Phosphathaushalt soll hier nicht die Rede sein.) Das Skelet ist aber kein totes Kalk-Phosphat-Depot; es herrscht vielmehr ein dauerndes Kommen und Gehen, wie an Hand von Untersuchungen mit markiertem Phosphor nachgewiesen wurde (v. Hevesy). Soweit ein Zuviel des Blutkalks nicht durch die Nieren ausgeschieden wird, kann es gegebenenfalls im Knochen deponiert werden; soweit der Blutkalkgehalt durch Bremsung der Calciumabgabe und Steigerung der Calciumaufnahme (bzw. vice versa durch Erhöhung der Calciumabgabe und Herabsetzung der Calciumresorption) nicht auf die Norm einreguliert werden kann, steht das Depot des Knochens als Aufnahme- bzw. Abgabeorgan für die Aufrechterhaltung des optimalen Blutkalkgehalts zur Verfügung. Für die Knochenverkalkung spielt das Vitamin D eine entscheidend wichtige Rolle. Außerdem sind für die Skeletverkalkung, aber auch für die Calciumaufnahme aus dem Magen-Darmkanal und die Calciumabgabe durch die Nieren verschiedene Hormone von mehr oder weniger großer Bedeutung. Unter ihnen ist in erster Linie das Inkret der Nebenschilddrüsen zu nennen.

## IV. Einige Daten über die Bedeutung der Nebenschilddrüsen

Die Tatsache, daß nach der Entfernung der Nebenschilddrüsen bei Schilddrüsenresektion eine Tetanie zur Entwicklung kommt, hat zur Aufdeckung der *Funktion der Nebenschilddrüsen* und ihrer zentralen Stellung im Kalkstoffwechsel den entscheidenden Anstoß gegeben. Die Verknüpfung der hormonalen Funktion der Nebenschilddrüsen (bzw. Epithelkörperchen) mit dem Kalkhaushalt wurde durch die Entdeckung des Parathormons durch KENDALL und HANSON weitgehend geklärt. Zur weiteren Aufhellung der Bedeutung der Nebenschilddrüsen im Kalkstoffwechsel trug fernerhin die Erkennung des Krankheitsbildes der Osteodystrophia fibrosa generalisata durch v. RECKLINGHAUSEN (vor ihm durch ENGEL) bei, insbesondere die Beseitigung dieser schweren Knochenerkrankung durch Entfernung eines Nebenschilddrüsenadenoms, welche zum erstenmal von MANDL ausgeführt wurde. Die Urologie wird durch die Klärung der bedeutsamen Rolle der Epithelkörperchen im Calciumstoffwechsel und die Tatsache, daß langdauernde Hypercalcämien sehr häufig zum Auftreten massiver Kalkablagerungen im Nierengewebe (Nephrocalcinosis) und zur Entwicklung von kalkhaltigen Nierenbecken- und Uretersteinen führen, in erheblichem Maße berührt.

## V. Funktion der Nebenschilddrüsen im Calciumhaushalt

Die Nebenschilddrüsen sind — neben anderen Faktoren, die demgegenüber weit in den Hintergrund treten — die *Hauptregulatoren des Calciumstoffwechsels*. Alles, was zu einer Herabsetzung des Blutkalkspiegels führt, wirkt auf die Nebenschilddrüsen im Sinne einer Steigerung ihrer Tätigkeit; alles, was mit einer Steigerung des Blutkalkspiegels einhergeht, veranlaßt die Nebenschilddrüsen zu einer Reduktion ihrer hormonellen Aktivität. Wenn die Nebenschilddrüsenfunktion gestört ist, so kann sie der von ihr verlangten Funktionsänderung unter Umständen nicht nachkommen, so daß eine Störung des Kalkstoffwechsels eintritt, die krankmachend wirkt. Das Nebenschilddrüsenhormon hält den Kalkspiegel des Blutes auf seiner normalen Höhe, indem es die Ablagerung bzw. Abgabe von Calcium im Knochensystem überwacht. Stärkere Überschwemmung des Blutes mit Nebenschilddrüsenhormon steigert den Blutkalkgehalt, wie z. B. bei der Ostitis fibrosa generalisata Recklinghausen oder etwa im Experiment, indem das Hormon die Herauslösung von Calcium aus dem Knochensystem fördert (und wahrscheinlich auch die Rückresorption von Calcium, das primär durch die Nierenglomeruli ausgeschieden wurde, begünstigt — CRAWFORD). Eine Unterproduktion von Nebenschilddrüsenhormon, wie z. B. bei dem Krankheitsbild der parathyreogenen Tetanie, führt zum Absinken des Blutkalkspiegels und zur Kalkablagerung in bestimmten Organen, wie z. B. der Augenlinsen (Tetaniestar), des Gehirns (Verkalkungen im Bereich der Stammganglien), sowie zu einer Schädigung bestimmter Anhangsgebilde der Haut, solange diese wachsen, wie z. B. der Zähne, der Nägel und der Haare (s. S. 178). Auch im Knochensystem kommt es bei Nebenschilddrüsenunterfunktion zu einer verstärkten Kalkanlagerung.

## VI. Funktion der Nebenschilddrüsen im Phosphathaushalt

Die Funktion der Nebenschilddrüsen beschränkt sich nicht allein auf die Regulation des Calciumstoffwechsels, sie wirkt auch auf den *Phosphathaushalt* des Organismus. Bei der verstärkten Abgabe von Nebenschilddrüsenhormon werden die Phosphate, deren Spiegel beim Erwachsenen etwa zwischen 3 und 4 mg-% im Serum liegt, herabgesetzt; bei der Unterproduktion von Nebenschilddrüsenhormon sind sie in der Regel gesteigert. Das Nebenschilddrüsenhormon beeinflußt somit das Blutcalcium und die Blutphosphate gegensinnig antagonistisch. Die Ausscheidung der Phosphate durch die Niere wird durch Nebenschilddrüsenhormon gefördert, indem die tubuläre Rückresorption abgebremst wird.

# VII. Hypo- und Hypercalcämie

Im folgenden interessieren (entsprechend unserem Thema) nur diejenigen Regulationsstörungen des Kalkstoffwechsels, welche mit einer Hypocalcämie einhergehen; denn nur die Hypocalcämie führt zur Tetanie. Bei der Hypercalcämie tritt das Gegenteil ein: die neuromuskuläre Erregbarkeit wird herabgesetzt, und die meisten Folgeerscheinungen der chronischen Hypercalcämie verhalten sich praktisch entgegengesetzt den Folgeerscheinungen der Hypocalcämie.

Aus dem EKG kann man Rückschlüsse auf die Blutkalkverhältnisse ziehen. Bei Hypocalcämie ist die sog. Q-T-Strecke deutlich verlängert, während das Q-T-Intervall über eine lange Distanz in der isoelektrischen Linie verläuft. Bei der Hypercalcämie ist die Q-T-Strecke im Gegensatz dazu verkürzt.

# VIII. Symptomatik der hypocalcämischen Tetanie

Die *Diagnostik der hypocalcämischen Tetanie* beruht, wie bereits betont, auf dem Vorliegen der *Erniedrigung* des nüchtern entnommenen *Blutkalkspiegels* unter der Norm von 9 mg-%. Zu diesem Symptom, mit welchem die Diagnose der hypocalcämischen Tetanie steht und fällt, gehören einige weitere charakteristische Krankheitszeichen, die zur Diagnose der hypocalcämischen Tetanie hinzugehören. Als wichtigstes ist *der tetanische Totalkrampf* zu nennen. Will man die Diagnose hypocalcämische Tetanie mit absoluter Sicherheit stellen, so ist das Auftreten eines derartigen Krampfes in seiner charakteristischen Weise ein sicheres Diagnosticum. Kann der tetanische Totalkrampf vom Arzt beobachtet werden, so sind weitere diagnostische Untersuchungen zur Sicherung der Diagnose — mit Ausnahme der Bestimmung des Blutcalciums — bei Vorliegen sonstiger charakteristischer Symptome kaum noch notwendig. Weitere Krankheitszeichen, welche die Diagnose hypocalcämische Tetanie gegebenenfalls sichern helfen, können in seltenen Fällen auch ohne Auftreten eines klassischen Totalkrampfes vorliegen. In einem solchen Fall ist man zunächst nur berechtigt, von „latenter Tetanie" zu sprechen; das weist aber darauf hin, daß der Eintritt des totalen Krampfanfalls erwartet werden kann. Wenn gesagt wurde, daß mit der Feststellung der Hypocalcämie die Diagnose einer parathyreogenen Tetanie steht und fällt, so muß hinzugefügt werden, daß beim symptomatisch geheilten Tetaniefall, z. B. nach optimaler Behandlung mit Dihydrotachysterin, ein normaler Kalkspiegel bestehen kann. Das Krankheitsbild der Tetanie kann in einem solchen Fall aber wieder zum Ausbruch kommen, wenn der Abbruch der gezielten antitetanischen Behandlung zum erneuten Absinken des Kalkspiegels führt. Ein wichtiges Leitsymptom der manifesten und latenten hypocalcämischen Tetanie ist die *Herabsetzung der neuromuskulären Erregbarkeit*, welche sich sowohl durch die *elektrische* als auch durch die *mechanische Untersuchung* der Nerven nachweisen läßt. Bekannt ist vor allem das *Erbsche Phänomen*, das darin besteht, daß die galvanische Reizung eines peripheren Nerven, z. B. des N. ulnaris, bereits bei Stromstärken zur Zuckung der zugehörigen Muskeln führt, die unter der normalen Reizschwelle liegen, d. h. weit unter 5 mA, bei Einwirkung der Kathodenöffnungszuckung. Man prüft die elektrische Erregbarkeit durch Anlegen der differenten Elektrode an den N. ulnaris im Sulcus nervi ulnaris am Ellenbogen. Die mechanische Erregbarkeitssteigerung weist man am besten an dem gut zugänglichen N. facialis im Bereich des Pes anserinus im Gebiet der Parotisdrüse vor dem Ohr nach. Die lege artis vorgenommene Beklopfung dieses Nerven führt beim Tetaniker zu einer blitzartigen Zuckung im Bereich der entsprechenden Mundmuskulatur. Nach unserer Nomenklatur bezeichnet man die Zuckung nur im Mundast als positiven *Chvostek I*, die Zuckung im Mund- und Nasenast als positiven Chvostek II, und diejenige in diesen 2 Ästen und dem Augen- bzw. Stirnast als positiven Chvostek III. Es gibt noch andere, z. B. an den unteren Extremitäten prüfbare Zeichen der Übererregbarkeit, die aber praktisch von gleicher Bedeutung sind. Man sollte es sich angewöhnen, bei jedem Fall mit Tetanieverdacht und mit Symptomen, über die noch im folgenden zu sprechen sein wird, die leicht ausführbare Überprüfung des Facialisphänomens vorzunehmen. Mit Recht wird davor gewarnt, die Bedeutung des Facialisphänomens (CHVOSTEK) zu überwerten. Man findet seinen positiven Ausfall mitunter nämlich auch bei Menschen ausgeprägt, bei denen keine Tetanie besteht, besonders häufig bei Kindern. Aber der positive Ausfall des Chvostekschen Phänomens sollte in jedem Fall veranlassen, nach dem Vorhandensein weiterer tetanischer Symptome zu fahnden, um damit das Spielen eines tetanischen Geschehens, und sei es auch nur latent, anzunehmen oder auszuschließen. Man kann das Chvostek-Symptom auch bei Gesunden, ebenso wie andere positive Übererregbarkeitszeichen der neuromuskulären Apparatur, durch den Kunstgriff der Hyperventilation manifest machen. Eine größere Bedeutung als das Chvosteksche Phänomen hat das *Phänomen von* TROUSSEAU, wenn es positiv ausfällt, im Hinblick auf die Diagnostik einer hypocalcämischen Tetanie. Das vorübergehende Abbinden des Oberarms, z. B. beim Messen des Blutdrucks, führt innerhalb weniger Minuten durch mechanischen Druck auf den N. brachialis zum Auftreten eines tetanischen Krampfes (Carpalspasmus) an der entsprechenden Hand (Geburtshelferstellung, eventuell Pfötchenstellung), womit das Vorliegen eines tetanischen Mechanismus aufgedeckt wird.

## IX. Der Hyperventilationsversuch

Für die Diagnose der Tetanie spielt der Hyperventilationsversuch eine wichtige Rolle, sofern diese nicht bereits durch den Ablauf eines klassischen tetanischen Krampfes sichergestellt ist. In der größten Mehrzahl der Fälle von echter Tetanie gelingt es, einen tetanischen Anfall durch eine etwa 5 min dauernde forcierte Hyperventilation, bei welcher besonders auf ausgiebige Ausatmung zu achten ist, zu provozieren. Bekanntlich führt die Hyperventilation durch starke Abrauchung der Kohlensäure des Blutes zu einer vorübergehenden Verschiebung der aktuellen Blutreaktion nach der alkalischen Seite hin. Dabei wird der Gehalt des Blutes an $Na_2CO_3$ erhöht. Diese „hypocarbische Alkalose" (LENGGENHAGER) hemmt das Freiwerden von Calciumionen im Blut und steigert vorübergehend die neuromuskuläre Erregbarkeit. Entsprechend der Györgyschen Formel basiert letztere nicht allein auf der absoluten Höhe des Blutkalkspiegels; sie ist vielmehr noch von verschiedenen anderen ionalen Faktoren abhängig, so daß die neuromuskuläre Erregbarkeit auch durch Veränderung der Blutphosphate, der Carbonate und des Kaliums auf der einen Seite, des Magnesiums und der H-Ionen auf der anderen irritiert werden kann. Ionisiertes Calcium und H-Ionenwerte des Blutes laufen agonistisch: durch H-Ionenherabsetzung wird die neuromuskuläre Erregbarkeit in gleicher Weise gesteigert wie durch Calciummangel im Blut; durch H-Ionensteigerung wird sie ebenso herabgesetzt wie durch Erhöhung des Blutkalkspiegels. Neuere Untersuchungen von QUANDT und PONSOLD lassen darüber hinaus daran denken, daß die Hyperventilation auf dem Wege über eine Veränderung der Hirndurchblutung zu einer Enthemmung subcorticaler Krampfzentralen führt, so daß die Entfesselung eines tetanischen Krampfes durch die Hyperventilation auch auf diese Weise

entstanden gedacht werden kann. Tatsache ist, daß es mit Hilfe der Hyper-
ventilationsprobe bei einem auf Tetanie verdächtigen Fall gelingt, einen mehr
oder weniger massiven tetanischen Totalkrampf auszulösen, falls eine latente
Tetanie besteht. Die Beseitigung eines durch Hyperventilation provozierten
Anfalls gelingt manchmal dadurch, daß man den Patienten auffordert, den
Atem so lange wie möglich anzuhalten bzw. daß man ihm ziemlich brüsk für
längere Zeit Mund und Nase zuhält, so daß eine Kohlensäurestauung im Blut
stattfindet. Das gleiche erreicht man verständlicherweise auch durch vorübergehende Inhalation eines Luftgemisches, das 5% Kohlensäure enthält bzw. durch
Rückatmung der eigenen Ausatmungsluft; natürlich auch durch die intravenöse
Injektion eines Calciumpräparates. Die Hyperventilation ist somit bei unklarer
Diagnose zur Aufdeckung der Tetanie (und zwar aller Formen der Tetanie)
wichtig; es handelt sich aber um eine ziemlich robuste Methode, die nur dann
ausgeführt werden soll, wenn sie zur Klärung des bestehenden Krankheitsbildes
unumgänglich ist. Die Beobachtung oder eindeutige Beschreibung eines tetanischen Anfalls bei der zu untersuchenden Person enthebt, wenn nicht außer-
gewöhnliche Situationen vorliegen, den Arzt der Anstellung des Hyperventilationsversuchs.

## X. Symptome an ektodermalen Organen

Wir haben bereits kurz auf eine Anzahl von Veränderungen aufmerksam
gemacht, die sich bei Menschen mit lange bestehender Hypocalcämie im Laufe
der Zeit entwickeln können. Sie spielen sich an Organen ektodermaler Herkunft
ab. So müssen bei jedem Kranken mit Hypocalcämie die Augen gründlich auf
das Vorhandensein eines *Tetaniestars* untersucht werden. Es handelt sich um
schalenförmige Kalkeinlagerungen in der Peripherie der Linse, die in den Anfangs-
stadien nur mit Hilfe der Spaltlampe entdeckt werden können. Des weiteren
untersuche man bei Menschen mit Hypocalcämie die Zähne, da diese mehr oder
weniger erhebliche *Schmelzdefekte* aufweisen können, falls die Tetanie bereits
in einer Zeit bestanden hat, wo die 2. Dentition noch nicht beendet war. Bei
Erwachsenen findet man nach FANKONI unter Umständen geringfügige Defekte
an den Wurzelspitzen der Zähne, fernerhin nicht ganz selten Zahnausfall. Gelegentlich bestehen auch auffällige Rillenbildungen an den Nägeln. Langjährige
Tetanien führen zuweilen zu verteilten Kalkeinlagerungen im Bereich der Stammganglien des Gehirns, die sich unter Umständen röntgenologisch durch die
Schädelübersichtsaufnahme nachweisen lassen.

## XI. Ablauf des tetanischen Anfalls

Der *tetanische Krampfanfall* zeigt in der Regel einen charakteristischen und
dramatischen Ablauf. Nicht immer kommt er völlig zur Ausprägung, insbesondere
dann, wenn er rechtzeitig coupiert werden kann. Er beginnt mitunter mit einer
Art Aura, in der sich der Patient nicht wohlfühlt. Dann kommt es zu Parästhesien
(Kribbeln, Ameisenlaufen, Gefühllosigkeit), die von den Finger- und Fußspitzen
zentral heraufkriechen, auch das Gesicht und den Mund befallen und schließlich
im Steifwerden der Extremitäten- und Gesichtsmuskeln enden. Die Hände
geraten in die sog. Geburtshelferstellung, indem der gestreckte Daumen gegen
die gestreckten Finger gezogen wird. Dabei ist der Arm oft im Ellenbogengelenk
angewinkelt: sog. Pfötchenstellung. Der mitunter eintretende Krampf des
Musculus orbicularis oris führt zum sog. „Karpfenmaul"; oft kann der Kranke
dann nicht sprechen. Im vollausgeprägten Totalkrampf liegt der Patient steif
wie ein Brett da. Im Gegensatz zum epileptischen Anfall ist der Muskelkrampf
(mit sehr seltenen Ausnahmen) tonisch, nicht klonisch. Die krampfenden

Muskeln schmerzen zuweilen erheblich. Das Bewußtsein ist im Gegensatz zur Epilepsie in der Regel nicht erloschen. Gleichzeitig kommt es nicht selten zu einem erhöhten Spannungszustand der Atemmuskulatur, die sich in dem Gefühl des Nichtdurchatmenkönnens („Atemsperre") äußert. Häufig entwickelt sich, besonders bei Kindern, ein Larynxkrampf (Laryngospasmus), der mit schwerer Atembehinderung einhergehen kann. Auch die glattmuskeligen Organe können an dem Krampf teilhaben. So kommt es mitunter zum Blepharospasmus, zu Schielstellungen der Augen (VELHAGEN), zu Krampfzuständen im Bereich des Herzens bzw. der Kranzgefäße (?) (Pseudo-Angina-pectoris tetanica), zu Krampfungen der großen, abführenden Gallenwege, zu Darmspasmen, zum Ureterenspasmus, zu Krampfzuständen im Bereich des Sphincter vesicae und damit eventuell zu vorübergehender Harnsperre. Bei spontanem Aufhören oder nach Beseitigung des Anfalls etwa durch eine intravenöse Calciuminjektion, lösen sich dann sämtliche Krampferscheinungen ebenso wie die Parästhesien. Für den Sphincterkrampf der Blase bedeutet dies, daß es nach dem Anfall in manchen Fällen zu Harndrang und zur Absonderung größerer Harnmengen kommt, wenn die Blase während des Krampfes gefüllt war (Fall 8).

## XII. Prätetanische Symptomatik

Wir werden bei der genaueren Beschäftigung mit der normocalcämischen Tetanie sehen, daß gewisse Krampfsymptome oder tetanische Äquivalente gerade bei dieser Form der Tetanie besonders häufig in den Vordergrund treten, und daß gerade sie mitunter weitgehend das Feld beherrschen. Sie können Wochen und Monate bestehen und lange Zeit die einzigen Zeichen des zugrunde liegenden Leidens darstellen. Da ein totaler Krampfanfall vorerst nicht zum Ausbruch kommt, sind sie nicht selten imstande, den Arzt in Anbetracht ihrer schillernden Symptomatik irrezuführen und ihn von dem Gedanken an die Diagnose Tetanie abzulenken. BERNHARDT sagt, daß die Tetanie sozusagen jede bekannte Krankheit nachäffen (imitieren) kann. Die im folgenden zu nennenden Symptome treten also zuweilen larviert auf; es ist aber notwendig, sie in ihrer Vielfalt und Buntheit zu kennen, um sie gegebenenfalls in das tetanische Syndrom einzuordnen oder nicht. Bei der hypocalcämischen Tetanie überwiegen die charakteristischen Totalkrampfanfälle weit mehr als die sog. larvierten Symptome. Sie kommen aber auch bei der hypocalcämischen Form vor, viel häufiger allerdings bei der normocalcämischen. Sie äußern sich außerhalb der Anfälle in Atemstörungen nach Art der „Atemsperre", in Druck- und Kloßgefühl in der Halsgegend, durch laryngospastische Phänomene bedingt, in ziehenden „rheumatischen" Schmerzen in den Muskeln auf Grund von spastischen Vorgängen, in anginösen Beschwerden am Herzen nach Art der genannten Pseudo-Angina pectoris tetanica, oder auch in Symptomen, die mit mehr oder weniger isolierten Krampfzuständen glattmuskeliger Organe im Zusammenhang stehen, wie z. B. Verkrampfungen im Bereich der Ureteren und des Blasenschließmuskels, des Magens, der Därme, des Pylorus, des Oesophagus oder der abführenden Gallenwege. Wir begegnen diesen larvierten Symptomen aber, wie nochmals betont sei, bei der normocalcämischen (neurogenen) Tetanie viel häufiger und bunter als bei der hypocalcämischen Form.

## XIII. Ätiologie der hypocalcämischen Tetanie
### 1. Parathyreogene Tetanie

Es gibt verschiedene Ursachen für die Entstehung der Hypocalcämie und damit der Entwicklung dieser Form der Tetanie. Die wichtigste und mit weitem

Abstand allerhäufigste ist die *parathyreogene Genese*, die sich nach Schilddrüsenresektion entwickelt, bei denen die Nebenschilddrüsen mehr oder weniger vollständig mit entfernt, oder wo diese durch Gefäßunterbindungen oder Anwendung
gewebsfeinlicher Stoffe intra operationem schwer geschädigt wurden. In über-
aus seltenen Fällen kann auch einmal eine Thyreoiditis auf die Nebenschilddrüsen
übergreifen oder eine zu intensive Röntgenbestrahlung der Glandula thyreoidea
die Nebenschilddrüsen schwer irritieren, so daß Hypocalcämie als Folge auftritt. Jede Beobachtung einer Tetanie muß daher den Arzt veranlassen,
anamnestisch nach einer etwaigen Schilddrüsenoperation zu fahnden und nach
der Kragennarbe am Hals zu suchen.

Es gibt noch weitere Ursachen der Hypocalcämie, die nicht in einer Schädigung der Parathyreoidea zu suchen sind.

## 2. Recalcifizierungstetanie

Bei der Recalcifizierungstetanie handelt es sich um die Folgen des massiven
Kalksturzes, der nach der chirurgischen Entfernung eines Nebenschilddrüsen-
tumors bei der Osteodystrophia fibrosa generalisata (RECKLINGHAUSEN) auf-
zutreten pflegt. Infolge Wegfalls der Parathormonproduktion kommt es zu
massivem Abströmen des Blutcalciums in das Skeletsystem und damit zum
Kalksturz im Blut.

## 3. Tetanie bei Osteomalacie und Rachitis

Ähnliches kann eintreten, wenn eine massive Vitamin D-Behandlung bei der
Rachitis oder Osteomalacie (unter Umständen auch eine intensive Ultraviolett-
bestrahlung) vorübergehend den Abstrom großer Kalkmengen aus dem Blut in
das Knochensystem hervorruft. Unter weiterer, konsequenter Verabfolgung von
Vitamin D kommt es dann zur Wiederherstellung der Normocalcämie, bei gleichzeitiger Besserung der gestörten Blutphosphatverhältnisse. Im Verlauf der
Osteomalacie kann es infolge Absinkens des Blutkalkgehaltes, neben dem Tief-
stand der Blutphosphate, in seltenen Fällen zum Auftreten schwerer tetanischer
Anfälle kommen, die durch Vitamin D-Verabfolgung günstig beeinflußt werden
können.

## 4. Enterogene Tetanie

Diese Form der Tetanie entsteht, wenn es bei bestehender schwerer, in der
Regel chronischer Gastroenteritis zu Resorptionsstörungen des Calciums, der
Phosphate, vor allem aber, in Anbetracht der vorliegenden Fettaufnahme-
behinderung, zu Vitamin D-Mangel kommt. Bekanntlich sind die Calciumresorption ebenso wie der Kalkanbau im Skelet bei Vitamin D-Mangel herabgesetzt. Dieses meist schwere Krankheitsbild ist in der Regel durch gleichzeitig
bestehende Resorptionsstörungen für andere Vitamine, für verschiedene Minerale,
für Eisen u. a. gekennzeichnet. Die Hypocalcämie führt zur Aktivierung der
Nebenschilddrüsen, so daß es durch Mobilisierung der Knochensubstanz zu
schweren Entkalkungen nach Art der Osteomalacie kommen kann. Es ist verständlich, daß die Hypocalcämie und ihre Folgen nicht durch perorale Zufuhr
von Calcium bzw. von Vitamin D behoben werden können; man muß diese
Stoffe (neben anderen) in solchen Fällen parenteral geben.

## 5. Toxische Tetanie

Die toxische Tetanie entsteht durch Fällung des Blutcalciums nach Ein-
nahme von Oxalsäure, z. B. Kleesalz, oder durch Aufnahme von Fluorpräparaten,

so daß der Blutkalk als Calciumfluorid ausfällt, zuweilen auch nach unkontrollierter Verabfolgung von Ionenaustauschern, die zum Abstrom von Calcium aus dem Organismus führen. Die durch die zuerst genannten Gifte hervorgerufene Tetanie ist absolut lebensgefährdend.

## 6. Tetanie bei schweren Nierenerkrankungen

Bei Niereninsuffizienz, insbesondere bei der sog. interstitiellen Nephritis und bei manchen schweren Glomerulus- und Tubulusschädigungen der Niere, kann es im Laufe der Zeit zu einem Absinken des Blutcalciums und unter Umständen zum Auftreten tetanischer Anfälle kommen. Die gleichzeitig bei der Niereninsuffizienz sich häufig entwickelnde Acidose des Blutes, verhindert wahrscheinlich — nach der Angabe verschiedener Autoren — in der Regel das Auftreten tetanischer Entäußerungen.

# D. Die normocalcämische Tetanie

## I. Allgemeines

Wie bereits betont, kommen Tetanien auch bei völlig normalem Calciumspiegel des Blutes vor. Wir bezeichnen diese Formen als normocalcämische oder neurogene Tetanie. Die neuromuskuläre Erregbarkeit ist nicht allein vom Calciummilieu des Blutes bzw. des Gewebes abhängig, sondern auch vom absoluten Erregungszustand des neuromuskulären Apparates. Ebenso wie bei der Epilepsie ist es wahrscheinlich, daß es im Gehirn nervale Aggregate gibt, von deren Funktionszustand die neuromuskuläre Erregbarkeit beeinflußt wird. Diese Gebiete werden im Pallidum und im Nucleus dentatus vermutet (ESSEN). So ist es zu verstehen, daß tetanische Anfälle bei bestimmten Gehirnschädigungen vorkommen können: cerebrale Tetanie (nach ZONDECK). Bei Hirntumoren, bei Durchblutungsstörungen des Gehirns, bei oder nach Entzündungsprozessen und bei pathologischen Vorgängen, die uns in ihrer Natur noch unbekannt sind, kann es, ähnlich wie unter gewissen Voraussetzungen zu epileptischen, so auch zum Auftreten tetanischer Krämpfe kommen. QUANDT und PONSOLD nehmen an, daß es in Fällen abnormer psychischer Erlebnisverarbeitung zu einer Enthemmung der genannten zentralen Aggregate kommen kann, offenbar dann, wenn die corticale Steuerung dieser Hirngebiete herabgesetzt ist. Bei diesen „Aggregaten" handelt es sich um „schlummernde" Mechanismen, die wahrscheinlich bei jedem Menschen präformiert vorhanden sind und die sich z. B. durch intensive Hyperventilation mehr oder weniger „erwecken" lassen. Ihre Erregbarkeit ist bei Patienten mit neurogener Tetanie offenbar gesteigert bzw. die Erregungsschwelle herabgesetzt. Bei der Entstehung mancher Fälle von normocalcämischer neurogener Tetanie spielen häufig psychische Faktoren eine wichtige Rolle, welche die Entwicklung von Verkrampfungen in die Wege leiten. Es ist auffällig (wie später noch mehr hervorgehoben werden wird), daß die neurogene, normocalcämische Tetanie besonders gehäuft bei Frauen auftritt, bei denen, wahrscheinlich im Zusammenhang mit den Schwankungen ihrer vegetativen und endokrinen Steuerung, das Auftreten neurogener tetanischer Entäußerungen leichter gegeben ist als beim Manne. Bei der Frau spielen die rhythmischen Schwankungen des Cyclus eine wichtige Rolle bei der Steuerung der neuromuskulären Erregbarkeit, was sich insbesondere darin zeigt, daß neurogene tetanische Entladungen sich besonders in der Zeit des Prämenstruums häufen. Ob bei den neurogen-tetanischen Entladungen auch der Calciumhaushalt als solcher mit berührt wird — etwa in Richtung einer Herabsetzung des schwer bestimmbaren ionisierten Calciums — ist zwar nicht sicher, aber auch nicht wahrscheinlich; es ist aber bemerkenswert, daß in Zeiten ansteigender Follikulinproduktion, wie in den Tagen vor der Periode, auch eine stärkere Inanspruchnahme des Calciumstoffwechsels besteht (HOLTZ und ROSSMANN). Über die Calciumverhältnisse im Gewebe, außerhalb des Blutes, sind wir nicht orientiert. Auch die Hypoglykämie ist unter Umständen von tetanischen Verkrampfungen begleitet, und nicht ganz selten sieht man bei der normocalcämischen Tetanie Zeichen einer Nebennierenrinden-Unterfunktion. Möglich, daß die bei letzterer Störung oft vorhandene Herabsetzung des Blutzuckers die Tetaniebereitschaft steigert (Tabelle 2).

## II. Formen der normocalcämischen Tetanie

Der Name „neurogene Tetanie" bei Normocalcämie besteht für einen sehr großen Anteil dieser Formen der Tetanie durchaus zu Recht, ist aber nicht für alle Formen ganz zutreffend. Es gibt normocalcämische Tetanien, bei denen die Veränderung blutchemischer Faktoren eine Rolle spielt. Hier ist besonders die Hyperventilationstetanie zu nennen, die, wie ausgeführt, bei jeder Tetanie hinsichtlich Auslösung bzw. Provokation eine wichtige Rolle spielt. Eine Hyperventilationstetanie tritt auch bei vorher völlig normalem Blutkalkgehalt auf, wenn Menschen bestimmter Prägung längere Zeit hyperventilieren. Daß bei dieser Form der Atmungstetanie Faktoren des Säure-Basengleichgewichts eine Rolle spielen, wird unter anderem auch dadurch wahrscheinlich gemacht, daß die Inhalation eines kohlensäurereichen Atmungsgemisches oder der länger erzwungene Atemstillstand diese Form der Tetanie, wie übrigens auch andere Formen der normocalcämischen Tetanie, günstig zu beeinflussen bzw. zu coupieren vermag. Bei vielen normocalcämischen Tetanien ist der Anfall mit dem Zwang zu verstärkter Ein- und Ausatmung verbunden. Die Hyperventilation ist in solchen Fällen vielfach nicht Ursache, sondern bereits Symptom der Tetanie. Der Patient hat eine tetanische Zwangsatmung, die ihn infolge der $CO_2$-Abrauchung freilich immer tiefer in das Krampfgeschehen hineinführt. Auch bei Patienten, die viel erbrechen (Magentetanie) und offenbar reichlich Säure verlieren, ferner bei Patienten mit starken Durchfällen bzw. mit erheblichen Mineralverlusten, auch aus anderen Gründen (z. B. Salyrgan-Entwässerung und Entmineralisierung), können tetanische Entladungen auftreten. Man muß aber bei allen derartigen Formen der Tetanie in jedem Fall durch subtile Untersuchungen, besonders des Blutes, die Entscheidung treffen, ob wirklich eine normocalcämische Tetanie vorliegt. Ob allein durch eine Steigerung des Blutkaliums, als einem der Antagonisten des Calciums, Tetanien entstehen können, ist nicht absolut sicher. Der Magnesiumgehalt des Blutes spielt aber für die Auslösung der Tetanie eine Rolle. So ist die *Grastetanie* der Rinder wahrscheinlich eine Krampfkrankheit infolge Magnesiummangels bei Alkalose im Blut. Beim Menschen ist die infolge vermehrter Produktion des Nebennierenrindenhormons Aldosteron auftretende Erkrankung, die als *Connsyndrom* bezeichnet wird, und bei der eine Tetanie auftreten kann, vermutlich durch Alkalose bedingt. Es gibt Menschen, bei denen durch alle möglichen Irritationen ein tetanisches Krampfsyndrom ausgelöst werden kann, so z. B. bei ärztlichen Eingriffen verschiedener Art, nach Operationen, nach Aufregungen, bei akuten und anhaltenden seelischen Erschütterungen. Zweifellos spielt eine besondere individuelle Konstellation bzw. Konstitution als Basis für die Entwicklung derartiger tetanischer Anfälle eine wichtige Rolle. Die Bereitschaft zur Auslösung tetanischer

Entäußerungen dürfte auf einer Herabsetzung der Erregbarkeitsschwelle cerebraler Areale und vielleicht auch ihrer peripheren Außenstationen beruhen; darauf weist unter anderem die Tatsache hin, daß die Krampfentladungen unter Umständen streng halbseitig lokalisiert sein können. Wie diese Alteration zentraler Areale zustande kommt, ob durch Durchblutungsveränderungen, durch entzündliche Irritationen oder deren Folgen, oder durch erbmäßig verankerte Faktoren, ist nur in seltenen Fällen mit Sicherheit zu entscheiden. Die Beobachtung einer Tetaniefamilie (RISAK, DENNIG, eigene Beobachtung) macht es wahrscheinlich, daß auch der Erbfaktor eine Rolle spielen kann. Anfälle, die durch Gelegenheitsirritationen ausgelöst werden, bezeichnen wir als *Situationstetanie* bzw. (nach JESSERER) als „tetanische Gelegenheitsanfälle". Bei diesen handelt es sich stets um die normocalcämische Form (Fall 1, 2, 3, 4).

Fall 1. H. Hermine, ♀, 34 Jahre. *Situationstetanie nach Tonsillektomie.* Die 34jährige Patientin hatte seit ihrer Kindheit schon über geringes Herzklopfen zu klagen, besonders bei Anstrengung, auch über Atemnot. Seit 8 Jahren jedes Jahr mehrfach Angina tonsillaris. Durchführung der Tonsillektomie am 6. 2. 57. Vier Tage nach der Operation plötzlich Druckgefühl in der Herzgegend, starkes Herzklopfen, Kribbeln in den Armen und Beinen, Steifigkeitsgefühl in den Händen und Füßen sowie um den Mund herum. Sofortige Coupierung der Beschwerden nach einer intravenösen Calciuminjektion. Wiederauftreten der gleichen Beschwerden in geringerem Ausmaß einen Tag später. Patientin gibt nachträglich an, daß sie seit 3 Jahren öfters ein Steifigkeitsgefühl im Hals und in der ganzen Schulter hat. Bei der Untersuchung der pyknischen Frau findet sich ein positiver Dermographismus, feinschlägiger Hand- und Fingertremor, kaltschweißige Handinnenflächen und Fußsohlen, Chvostek positiv, Calcium im Serum 10,4 mg-%. Kalium im Serum 24,5 mg-%. Im übrigen kein wesentlicher krankhafter Befund. Bei der Hyperventilation ließ sich nach 5 min der gleiche Zustand wie bei dem oben beschriebenen Anfall reproduzieren.

Es handelt sich im vorliegenden Fall um eine normocalcämische neurogene Tetanie, die im Anschluß an einen operativen Eingriff (Tonsillektomie) zum Ausbruch kam. Offenbar bestand eine Tetaniebereitschaft. Wir nennen diese Form der Tetanie Situationstetanie. Durch intravenöse Calciuminjektion gelang es, den Anfall schlagartig zu coupieren.

Fall 2. Z. Lissy, ♀, 26 Jahre. *Situationstetanie nach retrograder Urographie.* Bei einer 26jährigen jungverheirateten Frau kam es nach Durchführung einer Cystopyelographie, die ohne Schwierigkeiten überstanden wurde, nach Rückführung der Patientin in ihr Krankenzimmer zum Auftreten von Kribbeln in den Händen, Angstgefühl, Beklemmung im Bereich der Brust, Atemsperre; im Anschluß daran entwickelte sich ein universeller Steifigkeitszustand der oberen und unteren Extremitäten mit Geburtshelfer- und Pfötchenstellung, Schnauzkrampf sowie Würgegefühl im Hals (Laryngospasmus). Durch eine sofortige intravenöse Calciuminjektion gelang es, den Anfall zu coupieren. Bei der Patientin sind später, wie genaueste Nachforschungen ergaben, tetanische Anfälle niemals mehr in Erscheinung getreten.

Es handelt sich um eine neurogene, normocalcämische Tetanie, die im Anschluß an einen, die Patientin stark beeindruckenden ärztlichen Eingriff (Cystopyelographie) zum Ausbruch kam. Diese Form der neurogenen Tetanie wird als Situationstetanie bezeichnet. Die Tetanie blieb, soweit die Erkundigungen ergaben, im Leben der Patientin ein einmaliges Ereignis und kamen später nicht mehr zum Ausbruch.

Fall 3. S. Willi, ♂, 29 Jahre. *Auslösung einer Situationstetanie während der intravenösen Injektion zur Urographie.* Der 29jährige Küfer war uns seit 3 Jahren wegen abdomineller Beschwerden bekannt, die durch ein Ulcus duodeni bedingt waren. Diesem entsprach eine entsprechende Deformation des Bulbus bei der Röntgenuntersuchung. Er hatte Spätschmerz, Nüchternschmerz und Sodbrennen. Die Nabelgegend erwies sich als druckschmerzhaft. Der Magensaftbefund zeigte deutlich gesteigerte Säurewerte. Während des stationären Behandlung bekam der Patient mehrfach kolikartige Beschwerden im rechten und linken Unterbauch. Diese strahlten bei einer starken linksseitigen Schmerzkolik in den Hoden aus. Nach dieser Kolik waren vereinzelt Erythrocyten im Harn nachweisbar. Bei der Ausführung des ersten intravenösen Pyelogramms bekam der Patient während der intravenösen Injektion einen tetaniformen Anfall. Er hyperventilierte stark, klagte über Kribbeln und schließlich über Steifigkeitsgefühl in den Händen und Füßen. Die Untersuchung mußte daher abgebrochen werden. Bei der Wiederholung einige Tage später fand sich ein doppeltes Nierenbecken rechts, ein Konkrement konnte nicht gefunden werden. Calcium im Blut 10,1 mg-%.

Es handelte sich bei dem 29jährigen Mann um ein Ulcus duodeni, während dessen Behandlung kolikartige Schmerzen auftraten, die das Vorliegen einer Nierenkolik annehmen ließen. Bei der Injektion zur intravenösen Pyelographie kam es zum Auftreten eines neurogenen tetanischen Anfalls im Sinne einer Situationstetanie. Möglicherweise spielte bei der Entstehung der Kolikbeschwerden eine rechtsseitige Nierenmißbildung eine Rolle.

Fall 4. F. Werner, ♂, 27 Jahre. *Nierenkolik bei Tetanie.* Ein 27jähriger Mann wurde mit typischen linksseitigen Uretersteinkoliken eingeliefert. Die starken linksseitigen Flankenschmerzen, die nach vorn zu in den Leib, in Blase und Glied ausstrahlten, führten zur Krankenhausaufnahme. In den ersten Tagen des Krankenhausaufenthaltes war laufend mikroskopisch eine spärliche Hämaturie nachweisbar. Während des Transportes zur cystoskopischen Untersuchung trat erneut eine Nierenkolik auf. Im Verlaufe dieser kam es zu einem typischen tetanischen Anfall, der mit Parästhesien an Händen und Füßen, mit Atemsperre und Druckgefühl im Halse begann und zu ausgesprochenen Carpopedalspasmen bei später positivem Chvostekschem Phänomen führte. Die Verabfolgung eines intravenös gegebenen Kalkpräparates (Calcistin) führte sofort zur Beseitigung des tetanischen Anfalls und der Kolikbeschwerden. In den nächsten Tagen war der Harn frei von roten Blutkörperchen. Bei einer Cystoskopie, die 14 Tage später durchgeführt wurde, ließ sich, auch röntgenologisch, kein Anhalt für einen Stein finden. Die Untersuchung des Blutes ergab einen normalen Kalkspiegel von 9,9 mg-%.

Es handelt sich um eine Nierenkolik bei normocalcämischer Tetanie.

## III. Unterschiede der Symptomatik der Tetanieformen

Die Symptomatik der neurogenen, normocalcämischen Tetanie gleicht in den Kardinalsymptomen weitgehend derjenigen der hypocalcämischen Tetanie, weist aber andererseits, wie schon angedeutet, gewisse Abweichungen und besondere Züge auf, welche ihr gegenüber der hypocalcämischen Form ein besonderes Gesicht geben. Verständlicherweise fehlen der neurogenen, normocalcämischen Tetanie alle jene Symptome, welche sich im Laufe der Zeit als Folge lang dauernden Calciummangels im Blut bei der hypocalcämischen Tetanie entwickeln. Hierzu gehören vor allem die Veränderungen an den ektodermalen Organen, welche bei der hypocalcämischen Tetanie beschrieben wurden. Der normocalcämischen Tetanie drohen deshalb auch nicht jene, unter Umständen gefährlich werdenden Kalkeinlagerungen in den Augenlinsen und im Gehirn, sowie gegebenenfalls die Verkalkungsstörungen an den Zähnen. Was die meisten Formen der normocalcämischen Tetanie, entsprechend der neurogenen Verankerung, besonders auszeichnet, sind die vegetativen und psychischen Störungen, die bei der neurogenen Tetanie oft besonders kraß in den Vordergrund treten. Mitunter gleitet die Symptomatik der neurogenen Tetanie in das Symptomenbild der sog. vegetativen Dystonie über.

## IV. Besonderheiten der normocalcämischen Tetanie

Der totale Krampfanfall des neurogenen Tetanikers unterscheidet sich praktisch nicht von dem Anfallsgeschehen beim hypocalcämischen Tetaniekranken. Auch bei der neurogenen, hypocalcämischen Tetanie beginnt der Anfall mit Parästhesien, führt zur totalen muskulären Verkrampfung und geht mit den bei der hypocalcämischen Tetanie genannten charakteristischen Symptomen, wie Geburtshelferstellung der Hände, Pfötchenstellung, Mundkrampf usw. einher.

Wir brauchen die Symptomatik hier nicht zu wiederholen (vgl. S. 176). Man findet aber, wie bereits betont, bei der neurogenen Tetanie viel ausgeprägter und häufiger die vegetative „Begleitmusik", die unter Umständen sogar stärker in den Vordergrund tritt. Zu Beginn und mitunter auch während der Anfälle, vor allem aber in den Anfallsintervallen, sind die verschiedensten larvierten Tetanie-Symptome und Äquivalente ausgeprägt, welche die *absolut sichere* Diagnose einer neurogenen Tetanie erst dann erlauben, wenn ein richtiger Krampfanfall beobachtet worden ist. Es gibt aber gerade bei der neurogenen Tetanie Zustandsbilder, wo der Anfall nicht oder *noch nicht* aufgetreten ist, wo man aber auf Grund der charakteristischen Symptomatik das Spielen tetanischer Entladungen verschiedener Valenz annehmen muß. Dabei braucht das tetanische Geschehen nicht die Grundkrankheit zu sein, sondern die tetanischen Symptome können am Krankheitsgeschehen teilhaben — im Sinne der bereits genannten Begleitmusik.

## V. Die larvierten Symptome der neurogenen, normocalcämischen Tetanie unter besonderer Berücksichtigung der urovesicalen Entäußerungen

Welche larvierten Symptome sind bei der neurogenen Tetanie besonders häufig? Es handelt sich hier vor allem um Entladungen von Krämpfen im Bereich von Organen und Organsystemen, die weitgehend autonom arbeiten, so der Atmung und des Herzens, des Magen-Darmkanals, des Urovesicaltrakts, der Gallenwege und des Larynx (vgl. Tabelle 1). Diese Patienten klagen nicht selten über anginöse Beschwerden im Sinne der *Pseudoangina pectoris tetanica*. Diese anginösen Entladungen entsprechen nicht einer organischen Erkrankung der Coronararterien und gehen deshalb in der Mehrzahl der Fälle auch nicht mit Veränderungen im EKG einher, wie man sie bei der echten Coronarinsuffizienz antrifft. Hier sei sogleich bemerkt, daß diese anginösen Sensationen des Herzens auf intravenöse Calciumverabfolgung, nicht aber auf Nitrite reagieren, wie es bei der Coronarinsuffizienz der Fall ist. Besonders häufig findet man das Symptom der *Atemsperre* bei der neurogenen Tetanie; dieser Beschwerdekomplex besteht darin, daß die Kranken mitunter stundenlang nicht durchatmen können. Diese oft sehr quälenden Zustände entsprechen (wie betont) wahrscheinlich tetanischen Spannungen von Muskeln, welche an der Atmung beteiligt sind, etwa dem Zwerchfell oder den Intercostalmuskeln — vielleicht auch der Bronchialmuskulatur, ähnlich wie beim Asthma bronchiale, zu dem es übrigens gewisse Übergänge gibt. Nicht ganz selten sieht man intestinale Krisen, z. B. hypermotorische Zustände der Speiseröhre (Abb. 3) oder des Magen-Darms (Abb. 2, Fall 5), die zuweilen bei nicht sorgfältiger Untersuchung unter der Flagge eines Magengeschwürs, einer Gallenkolik (Fall 6), einer Appendicitis oder anderer Magen-Darmstörungen segeln können. Mitunter ist eine spastische Krise im Bereich des Sphincter vesicae Symptom der neurogenen Tetanie. Auch Ureterenkrämpfe kommen vor, meistens unilateral. Diese Einseitigkeit des Auftretens tetanischer Entladungen ist bei der neurogenen Tetanie an sich nichts Ungewöhnliches; so gibt es z. B. anfallsweise auftretende Halbseitentetanien, die nur eine Seite des Körpers befallen. Selbstverständlich muß man bei der Diagnose einer Ureterentetanie die etwa in Frage kommenden organisch ausgelösten Krampfzustände des Ureters, insbesondere den Ureterstein, mit aller Sorgfalt differentialdiagnostisch ausschließen. Dies hat klinisch, cystopyelographisch und röntgenologisch zu geschehen. HENI und RIETHMÜLLER beschrieben 1948 Fälle mit einseitiger abnormer Krampfbereitschaft des Nierenbeckens,

Tabelle 1

| Intestinale Krisenzustände bei Tetanie | Pectorale Krisenzustände bei Tetanie |
|---|---|
| Oesophagusspasmen, | Bronchospasmen, |
| Magenkrämpfe, | Atemsperre |
| Darmspasmen (Pseudo-Ileus) | Angina pectoris tetanica, |
| Dyskinesie der Gallenwege, | Gefäßkrämpfe usw. |
| Ureterenspasmen | |
| Sphincterspasmen, | |
| Metropathia spastica, | |
| Habitueller Abort usw. | |

Tabelle 2

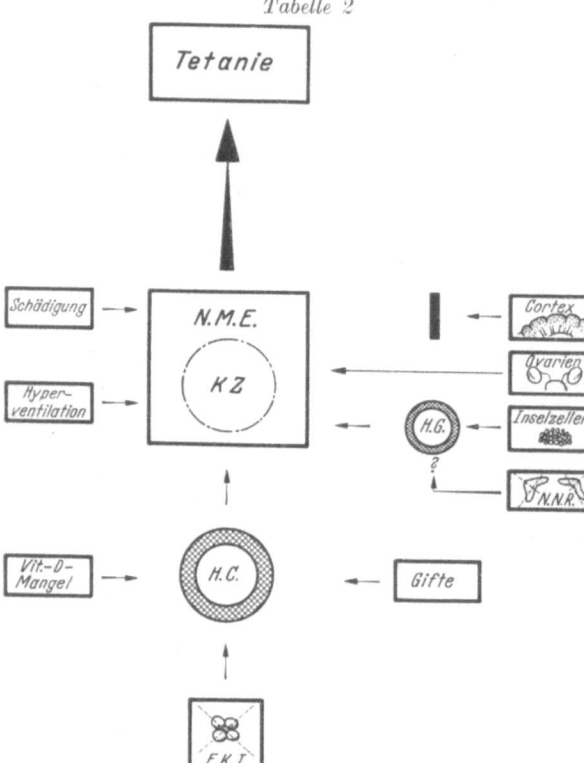

*Erklärung.* Die nebenstehende Abbildung versucht, verschiedene Möglichkeiten der Entstehung der Tetanie zu verdeutlichen. Im Zentrum des Bildes steht die neuro-muskuläre Erregbarkeit (N.M.E.) und die encephale Krampf-Zentrale (K.Z.). Die neuro-muskuläre Erregbarkeit wird durch den Calciumgehalt des Blutes gesteuert. Bei der Hypocalcämie (H.C.) kommt es zu einer Erregbarkeitssteigerung der Krampfzentrale bzw. des neuro-muskulären Apparates (bzw. zu einer Herabsetzung der Erregungsschwelle dieser Appatur). Bei Epithelkörperchen-Insuffizienz (E.K.I.) entsteht auf dem Wege über die Hypocalcämie die Tetanie. Auch verschiedene Gifte (Citrate, Guanidin, Kationenaustauscher) können Hypocalcämie erzeugen; ebenso der Vitamin D-Mangel.

Die Hemmung der Erregbarkeit der Hirnrinde (Cortex) führt zu herabgesetzter Bremsung subcorticaler Zentren und damit zu einer Steigerung der Erregbarkeit der Krampfzentrale. Die Schwelle der Erregbarkeit der Krampfzentrale kann auch durch unmittelbare Schädigung herabgesetzt werden. Hyperventilation führt auf dem Wege über eine Änderung der aktuellen Blutreaktion und wahrscheinlich durch corticale Schädigung zur Steigerung der Erregbarkeit der Krampfzentrale. Verstärkte Funktion der Ovarien (Hyperfollikulinie) bzw. Hypoprogesteronämie ändert ebenfalls die neuro-muskuläre Erregbarkeit im Sinne einer Steigerung. Auch bei Hypoglykämie (H.G.), z. B. durch Überfunktion der Inselzellen, wird die neuro-muskuläre Erregbarkeit unter Umständen gesteigert, so daß sich Tetanie entwickeln kann. Bei Zuständen von Nebennierenrindenunterfunktion (N.N.R.) ist zuweilen die neuro-muskuläre Erregbarkeit gesteigert. Möglicherweise entsteht diese Steigerung auf dem Wege über eine Erniedrigung des Blutzuckers.

bei denen ein aberrierendes Gefäß vorlag, das bei der Auslösung der spastischen Zustände unterstützend mitwirkte. Unter ihren Kranken befanden sich 3, die nach der Durchtrennung des Gefäßes keine Besserung zeigten, bei denen aber klinisch und nach dem Ausfall der elektrischen Erregbarkeitsprüfung eine Tetanie vorlag. Diese wurden nach antitetanischer Behandlung beschwerdefrei. HENI und RIETHMÜLLER fanden wiederholt, daß der Symptomenkomplex des spastischen Nierenbeckens durch eine Tetanie bedingt sein kann. Wir selbst verfügen über eine Anzahl von Tetanie-Fällen, bei denen mit großer Wahrscheinlichkeit Ureterkrämpfe anzunehmen sind. Auch der Krampf des Blasensphincters während des tetanischen Anfalls ist nicht ganz ungewöhnlich. Manchmal gehen die durch diesen hervorgerufenen Beschwerden in dem dramatischen Beschwerdekomplex des totalen Krampfes unter. Nach der Lösung eines solchen Sphincterkrampfes — z. B. durch eine intravenöse Calciuminjektion — kommt es dann vielfach zur Entleerung großer Harnmengen, deren Abgang durch den Sphincterkrampf während des Anfalls offenbar verhindert wurde. PFLAUMER hat schon 1926 auf die günstige Beeinflußbarkeit mancher Blasenkrämpfe durch Verabfolgung von Calcium aufmerksam gemacht, und SCHWARZ nennt das Calcium an erster Stelle bei den Mitteln, die den Sphincter vesicae zur Erschlaffung bringen. Tatsächlich ist der therapeutische Test der Calciuminjektion bei der Vermutung tetanischer Nierenbecken-, Ureteren- oder Sphincterkrämpfe von praktischer Bedeutung, wenngleich er allein natürlich nicht genügt, um eine sichere Diagnose zu stellen. Bei den von uns beobachteten Fällen mit tetanischen Ureterenkrämpfen handelte es sich immer um solche, bei denen die Diagnose einer neurogenen Tetanie oder einer tetanischen Reaktionsweise auf Grund weiterer Symptome sichergestellt war und wo die tetanische Entladung im Bereich des Urogenitaltrakts ein Teilsymptom des gesamten tetanischen Geschehens darstellte.

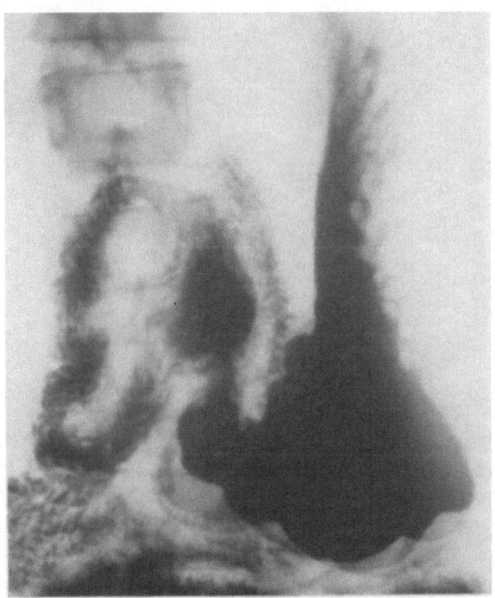

Abb. 2. M. F., 36jähriges Fräulein mit schwerer neurogener Tetanie. Man sieht die lebhafte Peristaltik, die in mehreren Wellen über den Magen abläuft. (Mehrere, hintereinander photographierte Aufnahmen auf derselben Platte: Riedertechnik)

In diesen Fällen lassen sich die Sensationen im Urovesicalbereich in der Regel beenden, wenn gleichzeitig die tetanische Gesamtstörung therapeutisch günstig beeinflußt wird (Fall 7, Fall 8).

Fall 5. F. Maria, ♀, 36 Jahre. *Tetanische Ureteren- und Magenkrämpfe.* Die 36jährige Patientin war uns schon seit vielen Jahren wegen ihrer schweren neurogenen, normocalcämischen Tetanie bekannt. Der Calciumspiegel schwankte zwischen 10 und 11 mg-%. Die bei ihr bestehenden hochgradigen tetanischen Anfälle, die in typischer Weise verliefen und in der Regel durch die hochgradige Atemsperre kompliziert wurden, traten in verstärktem Maße im Prämenstruum auf, hielten sich aber nicht ausschließlich an diese Zeit. Intravenöse Calciuminjektionen waren in den ersten Jahren regelmäßig erfolgreich und beseitigten die schweren tetanischen Entäußerungen. Die Tetanie erstreckte sich auch auf die Intestinalorgane, z. B. den Oberbauch. Hinzu kamen bei der Patientin außerhalb der Anfälle kolikartige Schmerzen in der rechten Nierengegend, die bis in die Scheide ausstrahlten. Auch diese Anfälle ließen sich durch Calciuminjektionen coupieren. Die gründliche Durchuntersuchung der Harnorgane ergab keinen pathologischen Befund; insbesondere ließ sich das Vorliegen eines Uretersteins ausschließen. Auch im Bereich des Magens zeichnete sich die Hypertonie deutlich ab (Abb. 2). Im Jahre 1955/56 wurden die Anfälle so schwer, daß eine künstliche Sistierung der Menses angezeigt erschien, zumal die Anfälle sich prämenstruell besonders stark häuften. Da die Patientin in Anbetracht ihres Alters eine Röntgenkastration ablehnte (wozu von uns auch nicht geraten wurde), wurde die Kastration vorübergehend hormonell durch große Testovirondosen durchgeführt. Während dieser Therapie hörten die tetanischen Anfälle völlig auf, aber bei der Patientin entwickelten sich ausgesprochen männliche Züge: tiefe Stimme, Steigerung der sexuellen Aktivität, Vergröberung des Gesichts, Bartwuchs, Acne. Im Laufe der nächsten Monate schlichen wir uns mit der Testovironverabfolgung wieder aus, und die vermännlichten Züge, einschließlich der Acne, gingen wieder völlig zurück. Die Patientin bekam wieder ihr weibliches Aussehen und ihre weibliche Wesensart. Während der Zeit der Virilisierung kamen auch die Nierenkoliken völlig zum Stillstand. Später entwickelte sich das tetanische Krankheitsbild wieder deutlicher, und auch die spastischen Zustände im Bereich der abführenden Harnwege kamen wieder zum Durchbruch.

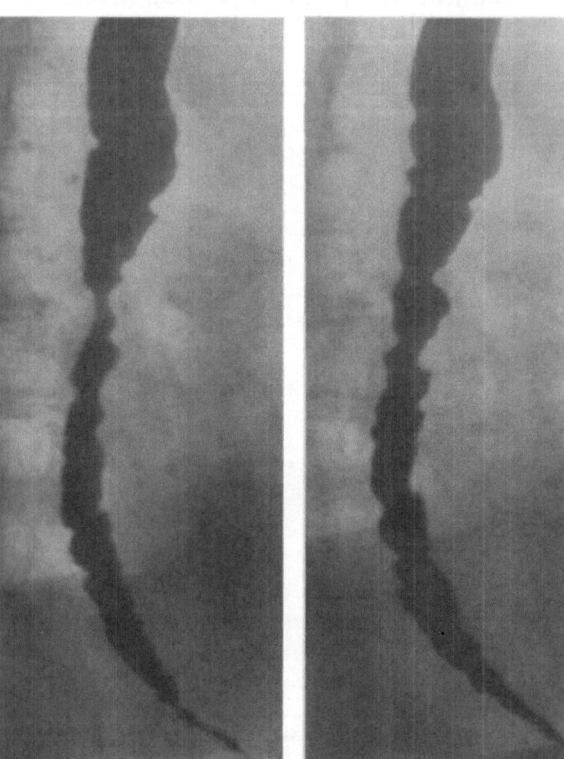

Abb. 3. A. R. (70 Jahre), mit hochgradigen Spasmen des Oesophagus bei normocalcämischer (neurogener) Tetanie. (Wesentliche Besserung der Beschwerden durch Verschiebung der aktuellen Blutreaktion mit Hilfe von Diamox)

Bei einer schweren neurogenen, normocalcämischen Tetanie bestanden außer typischen tetanischen Anfällen häufige Nierenkoliken, die in den ersten Jahren durch Calciuminjektion beseitigt werden konnten. Im Laufe der Jahre gelang es nicht mehr in gleicher Weise, die tetanischen Anfälle durch Calciuminjektion völlig zum Verschwinden zu bringen; dies unter anderem auch deshalb, weil die Venen der Patientin zu Injektionen nicht mehr geeignet waren. Eine vorübergehende hormonelle Kastrierung der Patientin ließ sowohl die tetanischen Anfälle als auch die Ureterkrämpfe aufhören.

Fall 6. B. Berta, ♀, 19 Jahre. *Dyskinesie der Gallenwege bei Tetaniebereitschaft.* Bei der 19jährigen Patientin bestanden Schmerzanfälle im rechten Oberbauch, die bei sonst negativen Untersuchungsbefunden an das Vorliegen von Gallenkoliken denken ließen. Bei der Röntgenuntersuchung der Gallenblase und der abführenden Gallenwege ließ sich kein krankhafter Befund nachweisen. Auch die Untersuchung auf Lamblien und Würmer verlief negativ. Die BSG war völlig normal. Die Schmerzanfälle in der rechten Oberbauchgegend kamen häufig nach Aufregungen und fielen regelmäßig in die Zeit vor der Periode. Der „Chvostek" war laufend positiv. Beim Hyperventilationsversuch ließ sich ein klassischer tetanischer Anfall provozieren. Auch bei der Magenaushebung kam es zu einem tetanischen Anfall. Während dieser Anfälle verstärkten sich die Schmerzsensationen im rechten Oberbauch. Der Calciumspiegel des Blutes war normal, desgleichen das EKG. Die tetanischen Anfälle ließen sich prompt durch intravenöse Calciuminjektionen beseitigen, desgleichen auch die anfallsartig auftretenden Schmerzsensationen im rechten Oberbauch.

Es handelte sich um eine latente Tetaniebereitschaft (neurogene, normocalcämische Tetanie). Die Auslösung der tetanischen Entäußerungen erfolgte durch Hyperventilation, aber auch durch Magenaushebung. Es ist anzunehmen, daß die Dyskinesie der Gallenwege durch die gesteigerte neuromuskuläre Erregbarkeit unterhalten bzw. provoziert wurde. Es ist wahrscheinlich, daß den Krampfbeschwerden im Bereich der Gallenwege eine (konstitutionelle?) Bereitschaft zugrunde lag.

Fall 7. F. Margot, ♀, 40 Jahre. *Nierenkoliken bei schwerster, normocalcämischer Tetanie.* Bei einer schwersten neurogenen, normocalcämischen Tetanie (Calciumwert zwischen 10,4 und 11 mg-% schwankend), die schon seit etwa 15 Jahren wegen dieses Leidens in ärztlicher Beobachtung stand und Anfang Februar 1957 mit dramatischen tetanischen Anfällen in unsere Klinik eingeliefert wurde, traten außerhalb der Anfälle immer wieder krampfartige Schmerzen im rechten Nierenlager, die in die rechte Flanke bis zur Scheide ausstrahlten, auf. Da es sich um eine außerordentlich schwere Tetanie handelte, gelang es nur selten, die Anfälle allein durch intravenöse Calciuminjektionen zu beseitigen. Außerhalb unserer Klinik war sie zur Linderung der schweren tetanischen Anfälle zeitweilig sogar mit Curare behandelt worden, während sie bei uns meist SEE-Injektionen erhalten mußte. Die Patientin, die im Laufe früherer Jahre und während des monatelangen Aufenthaltes in unserer Klinik genauestens durchuntersucht worden war, insbesondere auch im Hinblick auf eine etwaige organische Hirnerkrankung, verlor ihre Anfälle schlagartig nach Anwendung hoher Cortisondosen (Prednison), die auch die häufigen kolikartigen Schmerzen im Bereich der rechten Niere und des rechten Ureters völlig ausschalteten. Die eingehende Untersuchung der Harnwege, sowohl röntgenologisch, cystoskopisch als auch mikroskopisch (laufende Harnuntersuchungen) hatte ergeben, daß kein Anhalt für das Vorliegen einer Erkrankung der ableitenden Harnwege, insbesondere eines Steins bestand. Es sei hier hinzugefügt, daß Februar 1957 nach Einlieferung der Patientin in unser Krankenhaus wegen der schweren Anfälle eine Röntgenkastration vorgenommen worden war, deren Anteil an der Beseitigung der dramatischen tetanischen Anfälle und der Krämpfe im Bereich der abführenden Nierenwege hier nicht erörtert werden kann.

Bei einer schwersten normocalcämischen Tetanie bestanden neben den dramatischen Anfällen häufig Koliken und Schmerzen im Bereich der rechten Niere und des rechten Ureters. Mit dem Aufhören der tetanischen Anfälle verschwanden auch die Nierenkoliken vollständig. Bei der Beseitigung der Tetanie spielt (neben der Prednisontherapie) die Aufhebung des weiblichen Cyclus durch Kastration eine Rolle. Wie dargelegt, fördert der weibliche Cyclus, wahrscheinlich die Follikulinproduktion, die Ausprägung tetanischer Anfälle; das Aufhören des Cyclus, z. B. nach Einsetzen der Klimax oder infolge Kastration, hat auf die normocalcämische, neurogene Tetanie einen bremsenden bzw. beseitigenden Einfluß.

Fall 8. M. Luise, ♀, 18 Jahre. *Ureterkrampf, Sphincterspasmus tetanischer Genese.* Bei dem 18jährigen jungen Mädchen entwickelte sich die Tetanie in der Diphtherie-Rekonvaleszenz im Anschluß an eine Tonsillektomie. Das Mädchen wurde mit einem zunächst unerklärlichen schweren Krampfzustand in der linken Nierengegend eingeliefert, an den sich später ein Sphincterkrampf der Blase anschloß. Die eingehende Untersuchung der abführenden Harnwege und des Urins ließ mit Sicherheit das Vorliegen einer organischen Erkrankung der Harnwege, insbesondere einer Lithiasis, ablehnen. Die Patientin litt neben den linksseitigen Nierenkoliken, derentwegen sie zunächst eingeliefert worden war, unter schwersten tetanischen Anfällen, die sich bis zum Status tetanicus steigerten. Während dieses Zustandes bestand häufig eine Hyperthermie zwischen 40 und 41°, ohne Pulsbeschleunigung und Erhöhung der Blutsenkungsgeschwindigkeit. Der Kalkspiegel des Blutes war normal. Eingehende Untersuchungen, die sich mit der Frage des Vorliegens einer Encephalitis befaßten, blieben negativ. Insbesondere war die Occipitalpunktion ohne krankhaften Befund. Zeitweilig litt die Patientin unter starken anginösen Herzbeschwerden. Vorübergehend bestand eine 12 Std andauernde paroxysmale Lähmung beider Beine mit vorübergehender Areflexie, die wieder verschwand. Außerhalb der Anfälle bestanden typische Zeichen der Tetanie, wie positiver Chvostek und Trousseau. Die Durchführung des Hyperventilationsversuchs war unnötig. Calciuminjektionen waren in diesem außerordentlich schweren Fall meistens nicht imstande, die tetanischen Anfälle zu beseitigen, hatten aber einen mildernden Einfluß auf die Schmerzen im Bereich der linken Nierengegend. Nach Abklingen des tetanischen Anfalls kam es in der Regel zu einer starken Harnentleerung. Außer den geschilderten und anderen, hier nicht näher zu beschreibenden Symptomen fiel bei der Patientin der häufige bedrohliche Laryngospasmus auf. Zwei Jahre später wurde die Patientin nachuntersucht. Es ergab sich, daß sie seit 1 Jahr völlig gesund war und seit dieser Zeit überhaupt keine Krampfanfälle mehr gehabt hatte. Lediglich der positive Chvostek erinnerte noch an die latent bestehende neuromuskuläre Übererregbarkeit.

Bei dem 18jährigen jungen Mädchen war die Tonsillektomie der Anlaß (offenbar nicht die Ursache) zum Auftreten der ersten tetanischen Sensationen. Besonders bemerkenswert waren die linksseitigen Nierenkoliken, nach deren Lösung eine starke Urinentleerung erfolgte. Es wird angenommen, daß während der Krampfanfälle ein Sphincterspasmus bestand, nach dessen Lösung sich eine vorher gefüllte Blase entleerte. Bemerkenswert ist die Tatsache, daß die Tetanie nach Jahren wieder völlig verschwand.

Wir fügen hier an, daß wir (bisher) sichere tetanische Urovesicalverkrampfungen bei Fällen von hypocalcämischer Tetanie nicht gesehen haben, wollen damit aber nicht ohne weiteres ausschließen, daß sie auch bei der hypocalcämischen Tetanie vorkommen. Auch die anderen genannten Krampfzustände der glatten Muskulatur sind nach unseren Erfahrungen bei der normocalcämischen Tetanie weit häufiger als bei der hypocalcämischen; sie kommen hier aber vor.

## VI. Bedingende Faktoren des tetanischen Lokalkrampfes

Wir haben noch die Frage zu beantworten, wie es kommt, daß beim Krankheitsbild der Tetanie *lokalisierte* Krampfungen auftreten können. SÄKER hat gezeigt, daß es mit Hilfe des Hyperventilationsversuches oft gelingt, latent vorhandene, sozusagen präformierte pathologische Reaktionsweisen manifest zu machen. So ist es z. B. bei manchen Kranken möglich, Pyramidensymptome (wie etwa den Babinski-Reflex), die bei der üblichen Untersuchung negativ oder fraglich ausfallen, durch den Kunstgriff der Hyperventilation positiv werden zu lassen. Bei der Ausprägung der Halbseiten-Tetanie z. B. liegt offenbar eine nerval bedingte, möglicherweise auf einer Vorschädigung beruhende, einseitige Herabsetzung der Erregungsschwelle vor, die beim Einsetzen der Tetanie nur die eine Körperseite ansprechen läßt. Bei der Entscheidung der Frage, welches Organ sich bei einer allgemeinen Steigerung der Erregbarkeit als erstes oder überhaupt nur meldet, spielen mit großer Wahrscheinlichkeit besondere Prädispositionen dieser Organe bzw. Organsysteme eine Rolle. Diese Bereitschaft zu frühzeitiger tetanischer Entäußerung beruht nicht selten auf Vorerkrankungen oder Vorläsionen, die dieses Organ betroffen haben (vgl. SÄKERs Feststellungen). So äußert sich nach unseren Beobachtungen z. B. der einseitige Ureterkrampf nicht selten bei Fällen, deren Harnleiter bereits vorher durch eine organische Schädigung (z. B. Steindurchgang oder Anomalie) irritiert worden war (Abb. 4). In diesem Zusammenhang sei auf die einseitigen Nierenbeckenkrämpfe bei Vas aberrans hingewiesen (HENI und RIETHMÜLLER). Auf solche Kombinationen und die dadurch bedingten diagnostischen Schwierigkeiten hat z. B. ESSEN hingewiesen. Die tetanisch bedingte Auslösung oder ihre Beteiligung kann nur durch die exakte Feststellung eines tetanischen Grundleidens oder Begleitleidens sichergestellt werden. Dazu gehört gegebenenfalls unter anderem der therapeutische Test, d. h. das Schwinden des schmerzhaften Lokalkrampfes nach der intravenösen Injektion eines geeigneten Calciumpräparates (Fall 9).

Fall 9. B. Toni, ♂, 47 Jahre. *Auslösung von Ureterkoliken bei früheren Steinleiden auf der Basis einer tetanischen Übererregbarkeit.* Der 47jährige Mann hatte 1948 einen linksseitigen Ureterstein, der mit der Schlinge entfernt werden konnte. Vorher hatten gehäufte Koliken bestanden. Nach der Entfernung wurde der Patient bis zu seiner Aufnahme bei uns völlig beschwerdefrei. Seit einem Jahr klagt er über rechtsseitige, in den rechten Hoden ausstrahlende Oberbauchkoliken. Die von zwei namhaften Urologen durchgeführte, sehr sorgfältige Untersuchung ergab keinen pathologischen Befund; insbesondere keinen Anhaltspunkt für das Vorliegen eines Lithos im Bereich der abführenden Harnwege. Die weiteren Untersuchungen, insbesondere der Magen-Darmwege und ihrer Anhangsgebilde, ergaben keinen krankhaften Befund. Die erneute intravenöse Pyelographie lieferte ebenfalls keine neuen Gesichtspunkte. Während der stationären Beobachtungen wurden mehrere kolikartige Anfälle beobachtet. Bei diesen Anfällen war das Chvosteksche Phänomen positiv. Die Kalkbestimmung im Serum ergab 9 bzw. 9,1 mg-% bei normalem Phosphorspiegel. Es gelang regelmäßig, die „Ureterkoliken" durch intravenöse Injektion eines Calciumpräparates

zu beseitigen. Später bleibt der Patient frei von den beschriebenen Koliken. Einige Monate darauf kam es bei ihm erneut zu rechtsseitigen kolikartigen Beschwerden, die in den Hoden ausstrahlten. Die erneute Untersuchung der Harnwege ergab keinen krankhaften Befund. Beim Hyperventilationsversuch trat ein stark positiver Chvostek beiderseits auf, und es stellten sich Schmerzen im rechten Nierenlager ein, die nach unten ausstrahlten und durch intravenöse Calciumgaben coupiert werden konnten. Die später laufend durchgeführten Untersuchungen des Harns ergaben weder mikroskopisch noch makroskopisch eine Hämaturie.

Wir nehmen im vorliegenden Fall das Bestehen einer neuromuskulären Übererregbarkeit an, die im Bereich des „überempfindlichen" rechten Ureters zum Ureterkrampf führte. Es ist natürlich schwer, mit Sicherheit zu entscheiden, ob die späteren Koliken nicht doch hie und da mit dem Abgang von Konkrementen verbunden waren, deren Nachweis nicht ge

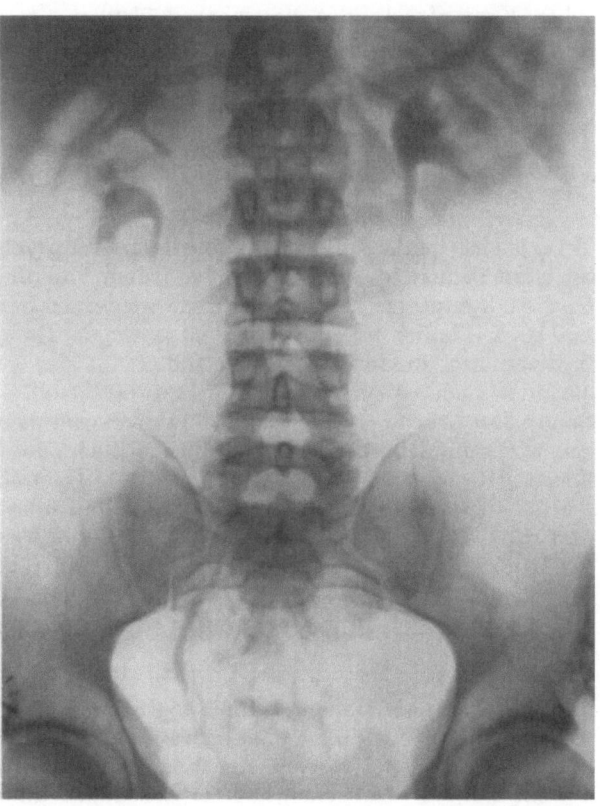

Abb. 4. W. St., Urogramm eines 29jährigen Mannes mit tetanischen Ureterkrämpfen bei gleichzeitiger Anomalie des rechten Nierenbeckens und rechten Ureters (doppeltes Nierenbecken)

lang. Die in dieser Beziehung durchgeführten sorgfältigen Untersuchungen sprachen dagegen. Die Feststellung einer Tetaniebereitschaft, die Auslösung der Schmerzen durch Hyperventilation und die prompte Aufhebung der Kolikanfälle durch die Calciuminjektion machen es wahrscheinlich, daß die neuromuskuläre Übererregbarkeit auf der Basis einer latenten neurogen-normocalcämischen Tetanie bei dem Auftreten der Anfälle eine mitwirkende Rolle spielte.

## VII. Weitere Krampfphänomene bei der neurogenen Tetanie

Der Laryngospasmus ist kein seltenes Symptom beider Tetanieformen. Oft äußert er sich in Mißempfindungen verschiedener Färbung im Halsbereich, mitunter nach Art des sog. Globusgefühls. Von weiteren, mehr isoliert auftretenden Krampfzuständen bei der Tetanie nennen wir den schon erwähnten Blepharospasmus, der besonders von VELHAGEN beschrieben wurde. Bei der an Tetanie leidenden Frau scheint es zu vermehrtem Auftreten von Aborten zu kommen, was wahrscheinlich mit vorzeitigen Verkrampfungen der Uterusmuskulatur in Zusammenhang zu bringen ist (RIML und TSCHERNE). Mitunter werden Zustände beobachtet, die denen der Bronchotetanie der Kinder ähnlich sind, mithin Anklänge an das Zustandsbild des Asthma bronchiale (s. auch S. 185 und Tabelle 1). Bei einer von uns beobachteten Tetaniekranken, die übrigens 8mal spontan abortiert hatte, kam es gleichzeitig mit den Vorstadien eines allgemeinen tetanischen Krampfzustandes zu einem quälenden „tetanischen" Husten, der durch intravenöse Calciumgaben coupiert werden konnte und der mit der Beseitigung des tetanischen Krankheitsbildes ebenfalls vollständig verschwand. Solche eigenartigen, „nervösen" Hustenanfälle sieht man hie und da bei der neurogenen Tetanie.

## VIII. Vegetative Dystonie

Es sei nochmals betont, daß die Fälle von neurogener normocalcämischer Tetanie eine bunte Fülle von vegetativen und psychischen Irritationen aufweisen, die chamäleonartig schillern und bei jedem Fall oft anders in Erscheinung treten. Gewisse Symptome kehren aber doch wieder, so Neigung zu Herzklopfen, manchmal sogar ähnlich wie die echte paroxysmale Tachykardie, Zustände von Atembeklemmung, in der Regel verbunden mit der genannten Atemsperre, Angstzustände und psychische „Verkrampfungen", stenokardische Sensationen, Schweißausbrüche u. a. Diese bunten vegetativ-nervösen Bilder der neurogenen Tetanie leiten mitunter kaum merklich zu dem oft so schwer definierbaren Krankheitsgeschehen der sog. vegetativen Dystonie über; dies insbesondere in jenen Fällen, wo der große tetanische Krampf überhaupt nicht beobachtet wurde und wo hie und da nur prätetanische Zustände wie Parästhesien in den Händen, Atemstörungen, Teilverkrampfungen usw. auftreten.

## IX. Verschiedene Formen der normocalcämischen Tetanie

Es ist oft schwierig, zu eruieren, wie man sich das gerade vorliegende Krankheitsbild der neurogenen Tetanie pathogenetisch zustande gekommen denken soll. Wir bringen im folgenden eine Zusammenstellung von neurogen-tetanischen Zuständen, die bei verschiedensten Grundstörungen vorkommen (vgl. auch Tabelle 2, 3). In Anbetracht der Tatsache, daß tetanische Anfälle bei organischen Hirnprozessen beobachtet werden, muß das Vorliegen eines derartigen Geschehens in jedem Fall nach Möglichkeit ausgeschlossen werden. Es ist aber zu betonen, daß die grob organisch bedingte cerebrale Tetanie keineswegs besonders häufig ist. In der Anamnese Tetanie-Kranker hört man nicht selten von Schädeltraumen, von Commotio cerebri u. ä. Wir besprachen die normocalcämische Tetanie nach Hyperventilation, mußten aber auch hier das Reservat machen, daß die Hyperventilation nur das letzten Endes auslösende Moment bei vorhandener Bereitschaft darstellt. Normocalcämische Tetanien kommen ferner gelegentlich nach starkem Erbrechen und nach schweren Durchfällen vor. Schließlich bei dem sehr seltenen Krankheitsbild des Connsyndroms (Hyperaldosteronismus), wo weniger ein erniedrigter Calciumgehalt des Blutes für das Auftreten der tetanischen Erscheinungen maßgebend ist, als vielmehr der Abfall des Magnesiums im Blut bei gleichzeitiger Alkalose. Bei diesen letzteren Formen sind somit Mineralverschiebungen im Blut für das Auftreten der Tetanie mit von Bedeutung. Bemerkenswerterweise finden sich bei tetanischen Frauen nicht ganz selten ähnliche Symptome wie bei Hypophysen-Nebennierenrindenunterfunktion.

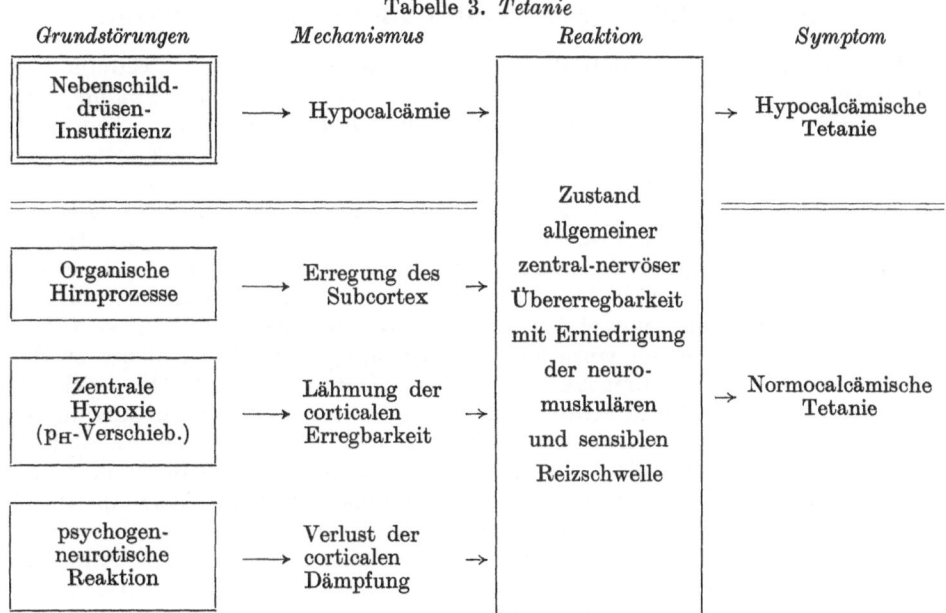

Tabelle 3. *Tetanie*

| *Grundstörungen* | *Mechanismus* | *Reaktion* | *Symptom* |
|---|---|---|---|
| Nebenschild-drüsen-Insuffizienz | → Hypocalcämie → | Zustand allgemeiner zentral-nervöser Übererregbarkeit mit Erniedrigung der neuro-muskulären und sensiblen Reizschwelle | → Hypocalcämische Tetanie |
| Organische Hirnprozesse | → Erregung des Subcortex → | | |
| Zentrale Hypoxie (pH-Verschieb.) | → Lähmung der corticalen Erregbarkeit → | | → Normocalcämische Tetanie |
| psychogen-neurotische Reaktion | → Verlust der corticalen Dämpfung → | | |

# X. Psychogene Tetanie

Wichtig sind diejenigen neurogenen Tetanien, bei denen offenbar die vegetativ-nervale Irritation als Hauptfaktor für die Entstehung der tetanischen Entladung maßgebend ist. In diesen Fällen spielen psychische Irritationen akuter und noch häufiger chronisch-schwelender Art eine entscheidende Rolle. Wie betont, nehmen QUANDT und PONSOLD an, daß die gestörte Erlebnisverarbeitung unter Umständen zu einer Herabsetzung der corticalen Steuerung vegetativer Zentren führt und damit zur Steigerung der Erregbarkeit jener Zentralen, zu denen auch die Krampfaggregate im Mittelhirn gehören. Langjährige eigene Beobachtungen haben uns gezeigt, daß schwere psychische Irritationen bei manchen Menschen (und zwar besonders beim weiblichen Geschlecht) im Laufe der Zeit zu einer Bereitschaft führen, die sich schließlich in tetanischen Entäußerungen verschiedener Art, unter Umständen im tetanischen Totalkrampf entlädt. Bei der Erhebung der Anamnese derartiger Kranker — es handelt sich fast immer um Frauen im geschlechtsreifen Alter — erschließt sich dem geübten Arzt oft eine Fülle von ungelösten Schwierigkeiten, mit denen die betroffene Patientin sich dauernd beschäftigt und mit denen sie zu kämpfen hat. Diese Fälle bedürfen einer außerordentlich intensiven Beschäftigung mit dem persönlichen Schicksal der Kranken, und die häufige Aussprache über die sie bewegenden Probleme, die immer wieder durchgeführt werden muß, ist nicht ganz selten imstande, die innere Verkrampfung bzw. die Verkrampfungsbereitschaft aufzuheben und damit die tetanischen Entladungen zurückzudrängen. Als besonders häufigen Anlaß zu dem Auftreten der neurogenen Tetanie, besonders der jungen Frauen, nennen wir das enge Zusammenlebenmüssen mit Familienangehörigen, besonders mit der Mutter des Ehemanns (Schwiegermutter), welche tetanieauslösend wirken können.

In der Tabelle 3 werden die Grundstörungen und der Mechanismus dargestellt, welche zu der Reaktion einer neuromuskulären Erregbarkeitssteigerung und damit zu Tetanie führen.

## XI. Normocalcämische Tetanie und weiblicher Cyclus

Wir betonten bereits, daß die neurogene normocalcämische Tetanie eine Krankheit ist, von der vorwiegend Frauen befallen werden. Sie kommt beim Manne seltener vor. Es ist bemerkenswert, daß sich die neurogene Tetanie in bestimmten Phasen des weiblichen Lebens gehäuft manifestiert; eine Steigerung der Tetanie-Bereitschaft findet sich besonders oft im Prämenstruum, wo an sich die vegetativ-nervöse Erregbarkeit bei vielen Frauen erhöht ist. Mitunter (keineswegs immer!) ist das Prämenstruum dieser Frauen mit Zeichen von Hyper-follikulinie bzw. Hypoprogesterinämie verbunden, die sich in zunehmender Spannung und Schmerzhaftigkeit der Brüste in dieser Cyclusspanne äußert. (Durch laufende Registrierung der rectal gemessenen Basaltemperatur lassen sich, falls nicht besondere Störungen vorliegen, die Beziehungen der Cyclusphase zu den Schwankungen der neuromuskulären Erregbarkeit verfolgen.) Oft, nicht in allen Fällen, hören die erhöhte Tetaniebereitschaft und die mannigfaltigen Tetanie-Masken mit dem Ausbruch der Menses auf. Hieraus wurden therapeutische Konsequenzen abgeleitet, die in charakteristischen Fällen darin bestehen, daß man die stärkere Einwirkung des Follikulins im Antemenstruum durch vorsichtige Gaben von Corpus luteum-Präparaten beeinflußt, wodurch es unter Umständen gelingt, der Manifestation der prämenstruellen Tetanie Einhalt zu gebieten. LACOUR beschrieb die Auslösung von Krämpfen am Urogenitalapparat durch Hyperfollikulinie, die therapeutisch durch Luteumhormon günstig beeinflußt werden konnten. Bei der größten Mehrzahl der Frauen verschwinden die neurogen tetanischen Sensationen während der Gravidität, um mit Wiederauftreten der Periode nicht selten wiederzukehren. Auch nach der Klimax pflegen die tetanischen Entäußerungen zu verschwinden. Völlig therapierefraktäre Tetaniefälle können unter Umständen durch Kastration geheilt werden (s. Fall 7, SANDOCK).

## XII. Die diagnostischen Kriterien der normocalcämischen Tetanie

Die Diagnose der neurogenen, normocalcämischen Tetanie basiert auf folgenden Symptomen:

1. Normocalcämie (Fehlen der Hypocalcämie): Abgrenzung gegenüber der hypocalcämischen Tetanie.

2. Fehlen der sekundären Veränderungen an den ektodermalen Organen, wie Augenlinse, Zähne, Haut, Haare, Gehirn usw.: im Gegensatz zur länger bestehenden hypocalcämischen Tetanie.

3. In der Regel Fehlen der Kragennarbe am Halse nach früherer Schilddrüsenresektion. (Diese Tatsache schließt nicht aus, daß auch bei früher Strum-ektomierten gelegentlich normocalcämische, neurogene Tetanien vorkommen können.)

4. Die bereits bei der hypocalcämischen Tetanie angegebenen Charakteristika, wie z.B. Parästhesien, tetanische Krämpfe. Dazu gehört auch der Hyperventilationseffekt, der bei der neurogenen Tetanie in der Regel in gleicher Weise auszulösen ist wie bei der hypocalcämischen. Bei der normocalcämischen Tetanie fehlt die Verlängerung der QT-Strecke im EKG; denn die Herabsetzung des Kalkspiegels ist die Ursache der QT-Streckenzunahme.

5. Therapeutischer Calciumtest. Hierzu ist folgendes zu sagen: Während bei der hypocalcämischen Tetanie in der Regel nach einer intravenösen Injektion von 10 cm$^3$ von 10—20%iger Calciumlösung der Totalanfall in wenigen Sekunden bis höchstens Minuten vollständig zu coupieren ist, gelingt dies bei der neuro-

genen, normocalcämischen Tetanie nicht immer. Dies ist verständlich, da, wie betont, im Anfall bereits Normocalcämie besteht. Man benötigt bei der normocalcämischen Tetanie zuweilen weit größere Calciummengen, bis der Anfall beseitigt ist. In ganz hartnäckigen Fällen gelingt die Anfallscoupierung zuweilen auch nicht mit Monstredosen. Die Tatsache aber, daß es mit Calciuminjektionen in der großen Mehrzahl der Fälle möglich ist, auch den neurogenen, normocalcämischen Anfall zu beseitigen, weist darauf hin, daß die bekannte, die Erregbarkeit dämpfende Wirkung des Calciums auch bei normocalcämischer Tetanie erfolgreich als Therapeuticum eingesetzt werden kann.

Es mag hier nochmals auf die bereits betonte Tatsache hingewiesen werden, daß besonders bei denjenigen Fällen von normocalcämischer Tetanie, wo die Hyperventilation für die Auslösung der Krämpfe eine wichtige Rolle spielt, die erzwungene Apnoe, die Rückatmung oder das Einatmen von Kohlensäuregasgemischen nicht ganz selten ausreichen, um den Anfall zu beseitigen.

6. Bei der normocalcämischen, neurogenen Tetanie sind die typischen tetanischen Entladungen in der Regel von den verschiedensten neurovegetativen Störungen begleitet, so daß das Bild der neurogenen Tetanie hinsichtlich der Symptomatik wesentlich bunter erscheint als die gewisse Einförmigkeit der hypocalcämischen Tetanie. Wie schon betont, bieten die neurogenen, hypocalcämischen Tetanieformen häufig viele Symptome dar, die bei der sog. vegetativen Dystonie vorkommen; z. B. vegetativ-nervöse Herzstörungen bis zu tachykardischen Anfällen, Störungen der Wasserausscheidung mit Polyurie nach dem Anfall, Schwitzen, anginöse Herzbeschwerden, Atemsperre, Angstzustände, seeische „Verkrampfungen" u. v. a. m.

# E. Die Therapie der Tetanie

## I. Die Behandlung der akuten Tetanie

Wie aus den vorangehenden Darstellungen bereits ersichtlich geworden ist, muß man grundsätzlich zwischen den therapeutischen Maßnahmen bei der hypocalcämischen und denen bei der normocalcämischen Tetanie unterscheiden. Immerhin haben beide Tetanieformen in bezug auf die Behandlung mancherlei gemeinsam. Insbesondere sind es der akute schwere tetanische Totalanfall und häufig auch die Äquivalente, bei denen die schlagartige *intravenöse Zufuhr von Kalkpräparaten* günstig wirkt. Wie schon betont, können wir bei der hypocalcämischen Tetanie in der Regel immer erwarten, daß der Anfall (bzw. seine Äquivalente) durch die intravenöse Calciumzufuhr in kurzer Zeit beseitigt werden; bei der normocalcämischen Tetanie hilft die intravenöse Calciuminjektion manchmal nur bei Anwendung hoher Dosen, dies aber auch nicht immer. Bei den tetanischen Entäußerungen an der glatten Muskulatur, z. B. bei intestinalen Krisen verschiedener Art, ist der Versuch mit einer intravenösen Calciuminjektion immer am Platze. Handelt es sich um einen durch tetanische neuromuskuläre Übererregbarkeit bedingten Krampf, etwa im Bereich der Ureteren oder des Sphincter vesicae, so können diese Beschwerden in der Regel durch Calciuminjektion beseitigt werden, gegebenenfalls allerdings nur für Stunden (PFLAUMER). In den ersten Stunden nach der intravenösen Calciuminjektion kommt es zu einem anhaltenden Anstieg des Blutcalciumspiegels, dem dann, zeitlich individuell verschieden, der Rückgang auf die Ausgangshöhe folgt. Die *perorale Verabfolgung von Calcium* ist sowohl beim tetanischen Krampfanfall als auch als Dauertherapie in der Regel erfolglos. Man kann also weder beim hypocalcämischen noch beim normocalcämischen Tetaniker durch enterale Calciumtherapie eine entscheidende Beeinflussung der Tetanie erwarten. Dies sei im Hinblick auf die heute noch vielfach geübte perorale Calciumtherapie bei derartigen Zuständen besonders unterstrichen.

Die intravenöse oder intramuskuläre Verabfolgung von Parathyreoideaextrakten, z. B. Parathormon, kommt praktisch nur bei der parathyreogenen, hypocalcämischen Tetanie in Frage. Sie wird heutzutage nur noch selten angewendet, zumal es beim tetanischen Krampfanfall zu lange dauert, bis durch die Einwirkung des Parathormons auf das Skelet genügend Calciumionen mobilisiert sind, welche den Blutkalkspiegel anheben.

## II. Dauerbehandlung der hypocalcämischen Tetanie

Hinsichtlich der *Dauertherapie der Tetanie* unterscheiden sich die hypocalcämische und die normocalcämische Form grundsätzlich voneinander. Die hypocalcämische parathyreogene Tetanie, in ihrer häufigsten Form nach Schilddrüsenresektion, kann heute praktisch in jedem Fall durch die moderne Behandlung mit Vitamin D bzw. Vitamin D-Abkömmlingen (= Dihydrotachysterin) therapeutisch so weit beherrscht werden, daß der Kalkspiegel des Blutes bei einer lege artis vorgenommenen Einstellung auf die eben genannten Mittel völlig auf die Norm zurückgebracht und bei Weitergabe der Erhaltungsdosis auf dieser Höhe für immer gehalten werden kann. Das von HOLTZ entdeckte Dihydrotachysterin, das unter den Namen AT 10 bzw. Antitetanin im Handel ist, kann über Jahre und Jahrzehnte verabfolgt werden, ohne, soweit bekannt, bei richtiger Einstellung irgendeinen Schaden zu verursachen. Auch das Vitamin D in Form von Vitamin $D_2$ bzw. $D_3$, etwa als Vigantolstoß oder in Form des ViDé (WANDER), ist nach JESSERERs Untersuchungen imstande, den Blutkalkspiegel völlig zu normalisieren. Die Behandlung der hypocalcämischen Tetanie sollte allerdings auf Grund einer längeren Beobachtung im Krankenhaus bzw. der Klinik eingeleitet werden, um die für jeden Kranken passende morbostatische Dosis von Dihydrotachysterin, z. B. AT 10 bzw. von Vitamin D in Form von Vigantol oder ViDé, herauszufinden, bei welcher der Tetaniekranke sich wohlfühlt und der Blutkalkgehalt auf der Norm verbleibt. Es muß beachtet werden, daß das Weglassen der Dauerbehandlung unter Umständen in ziemlich kurzer Zeit zum Abfall des Blutcalciums und damit zum Wiederausbruch tetanischer Entäußerungen führen kann. Für die hypocalcämische Tetanie ist deshalb die strikte Einhaltung der antitetanischen Therapie insbesondere auch deshalb von großer Bedeutung, weil die gefährlichen Kalkablagerungen in der Augenlinse (Katarakta tetanica) bzw. im Gehirn (Calcinosis cerebralis localisata) wieder zunehmen, wenn der Blutkalkgehalt für längere Zeit tief liegt. Man muß auch wissen, daß besondere Belastungen des Organismus mit einer erhöhten Beanspruchung des Kalkhaushalts bzw. der Parathyreoideafunktion einhergehen; das bedeutet, daß der Bedarf an antitetanischen Mitteln in bestimmten Belastungssituationen des Lebens steigen kann, so z. B. bei fieberhaften Krankheiten, bei schweren körperlichen Anstrengungen, bei lang andauerndem Sonnenmangel (Defizit an UV-Strahlen), in bestimmten Jahreszeiten, während der Schwangerschaft und in der Lactationsperiode, bei kalkarmer Nahrung, wahrscheinlich auch im Prämenstruum usw. Die Dosierung des Dihydrotachysterins kann verschieden gehandhabt werden. HOLTZ, QUANDT u. PONSOLD empfehlen z. B. beim Blutkalkgehalt unter 6,5 mg-% den großen AT 10-Stoß von 100 cm³ 0,5%iges AT 10 bzw. 10 cm³ 5%iges AT 10; bei einem Kalkgehalt unter 8 mg-% 50 cm³ 0,5%iges AT 10 bzw. 5 cm³ 5%iges AT 10 in 12 Std. Danach steigt der Blutkalkspiegel in der Regel wieder auf die Norm. Man fährt dann am besten

mit kleineren Erhaltungsdosen fort. Man kann nach JESSERER beim Erwachsenen auch mit 90 mg Vigantol bzw. ViDé (WANDER) intramuskulär, eventuell
auf 3 Tage verteilt, beginnen und diese Mengen je nach Verhalten des Blutcalciums wiederholt injizieren. Wir selbst pflegen bei der hypocalcämischen
Tetanie mit 3 mal 30 Tropfen AT 10 (=6 cm³; 15 Tropfen = 1 cm³ 0,5%iges AT 10
bzw. 1 Perle 5%iges AT 10) per os zu beginnen und diese Behandlung unter
gleichzeitiger laufender Kontrolle des Blutkalkspiegels so lange fortzusetzen,
bis der normale Blutkalkgehalt wiederhergestellt ist. Die perorale Therapie
kann natürlich nur dann wirksam sein, wenn die enterale Resorption garantiert
ist; bei erheblicher Gastroenteritis wird man immer Vitamin D parenteral an-
wenden. Im Laufe der Behandlung ermittelt man schrittweise jene tägliche
AT 10-Dosis, bei welcher der Blutkalkgehalt bei normaler Beanspruchung durch
das tägliche Leben und den Beruf auf der Norm bleibt. Daß solche eingestellten
Fälle auch später in großen Abständen ambulant nachkontrolliert werden müssen,
ist selbstverständlich. Die Symptome einer länger bestehenden und damit
schädlichen Hypercalcämie müssen dem Kranken eingeprägt werden, damit er
rechtzeitig zum Arzt geht, um den Blutkalkgehalt kontrollieren zu lassen und
die antitetanische Dosis gegebenenfalls herabzusetzen bzw. neu einzustellen.
Die Zeichen der pathologischen Hypercalcämie entsprechen etwa denjenigen
der Vitamin D-Vergiftung, die bekanntlich zur pathologischen Erhöhung des
Blutcalciumspiegels führt. .Es kommt zu starkem Durst, zu Polyurie, Übelkeit
und großer allgemeiner Schwäche; schließlich zu den Zeichen der Nierenschädigung mit Steigerung des Reststickstoffs, Blutdruckerhöhung, Urämie. — Mitunter reicht die Dosis AT 10 (bzw. Vitamin D) aber nicht aus und muß erneut
auf ein Optimum eingestellt werden. Für die Praxis hat sich die Ausführung
der Probe nach SULCOWITSCH (Sulkowitsch-Test) zur Beurteilung des Calcium-
gehalts im Urin als brauchbar erwiesen (Tabelle 4). Jeder Mensch scheidet

Tabelle 4. *Sulkowitsch-Probe*
Zu 5 cm³ Harn 2 cm³ Sulkowitsch-Reagens tropfenweise hinzugeben.
*Sulkowitsch-Reagens:* Oxalsäure 2,5; Ammoniumoxalat 2,5; Eisessig 5,0;
Aqua dest. ad 150,0 cm³.

| | Grad | Calciurie |
|---|---|---|
| Fällung sofort und kompakt . | \| \| \| \| | Hyper |
| Fällung sofort und wolkig . . | \| \| \| | Hyper |
| Fällung nach 2 min deutlich . | \| \| | Normo |
| Fällung nach 2 min schwach . | \| | Normo |
| Keine Fällung . . . . . . . | Ø | Hypo |

täglich im Harn bei normaler Ernährung, die in unseren Breiten wohl immer
ausreichend Calcium enthält, entsprechende Mengen Calcium aus, die durch die
positive Sulkowitsch-Probe nachgewiesen werden können. Bei stark ausgeprägter
Hypocalcämie wird die Sulkowitsch-Probe negativ, d. h. es wird kein Kalk mehr
im Harn ausgeschieden. Der Arzt hat auf diese Weise mit der Sulkowitsch-
Probe ein Verfahren in der Hand, mit dem er sich schnell orientieren kann,
ob eine deutliche Hypocalcämie vorliegt oder nicht. Andererseits kann bei
Feststellung eines positiven Sulkowitsch-Testes mit größter Wahrscheinlichkeit
angenommen werden, daß der Blutkalkgehalt nicht unter der Norm liegt. Man
rechnet bei möglichst kalkfreier Ernährung (keine Milchprodukte) mit einer
täglichen Gesamtausscheidung von maximal 250 mg. Bei krankhaften Hypercalcämien (z. B. bei der Osteodystrophia fibrosa generalisata) liegt der 24 Std-
Wert weit darüber. Man kann, von gewissen Ausnahmen abgesehen, festlegen:

ein negativer Sulkowitsch-Test im Urin bedeutet Hypocalcämie, ein positiver Normocalcämie, ein stark positiver unter Umständen Hypercalcämie.

Für den Urologen sind die Folgeerscheinungen der Hypercalcämie bekanntlich insofern von Bedeutung, als die länger dauernde renale Kalküberflutung zu einer diffusen Einlagerung von Kalksalzen im Nierenparenchym führt, die als Nephrocalcinosis bezeichnet wird. Diese ist bei pathologisch-anatomischen Untersuchungen durch chemische Analyse des Nierengewebes unter Umständen schon festzustellen, bevor sie röntgenologisch sichtbar wird. Wenn es bei überdosierter Behandlung mit AT 10 oder Vitamin D schließlich zur Nierenschädigung kommt, so dokumentiert sich diese in der Nephrocalcinosis. Im ausgeprägten Zustand kann man sie röntgenologisch an Hand der diffusen Einlagerung feinkörniger Kalkpartikelchen in beiden Nieren erkennen. Gegebenenfalls kommt es zur Bildung von Calciumphosphatkonkrementen in den Nierenbecken mit ihren etwaigen Folgen.

## III. Dauerbehandlung der normocalcämischen Tetanie

Die Dauertherapie der normocalcämischen, neurogenen Tetanie gestaltet sich außerordentlich viel schwieriger als die der hypocalcämischen Tetanie. Liegt eine Grundstörung vor, bei der eine Veränderung des Mineralstoffwechsels bzw. des Säure-Basengleichgewichts anzunehmen ist, so ist die Grunderkrankung therapeutisch anzugehen, z. B. das Erbrechen, die Durchfälle bzw. die Gastroenteritis, gegebenenfalls auch die Neigung zu Hyperventilation, fernerhin eine etwaige krankhafte Überproduktion von Aldosteron im Sinne des Aldosteronismus (Conn-Syndrom). Daß bei einem organischen cerebralen Prozeß das Grundleiden nach Möglichkeit zu behandeln ist, versteht sich von selbst. In der Regel sind es aber (wie betont) nicht diese Krankheitsbilder, bei denen die normocalcämische Tetanie besonders gehäuft vorkommt. Zu den häufigsten gehören vor allem die psychogenen Formen, bei denen eine Störung der Erlebnisverarbeitung, und zwar in der Regel mehr oder weniger schwere, oft nagende psychische Irritationen vorliegen. Dabei handelt es sich, wie ausgeführt, in der großen Mehrzahl um Frauen. Man achte auf die Steigerung der Anfallsbereitschaft im Prämenstruum und versuche gegebenenfalls, durch vorsichtige Zufuhr von Corpus luteum-Präparaten, am besten in Zusammenwirkung mit einem erfahrenen Gynäkologen, die Anfallsbereitschaft in dieser Zeit herabzusetzen. Die Behandlung mit Dihydrotachysterin versagt nach unseren Beobachtungen bei den Fällen von neurogener, normocalcämischer Tetanie praktisch immer. Die psychische Exploration und die psychogene Einwirkung auf dem Wege über häufig geübte Aussprachen zwischen Arzt und Kranken spielen die Hauptrolle bei der Herabsetzung der Neigung zu derartigen psychogen verankerten Anfällen. Im Zuge dieser Therapie muß versucht werden, die den befallenen Patienten bedrohenden menschlich-persönlichen Irritationen nach Möglichkeit abzustellen.

Die Herabsetzung der gesteigerten neuromuskulären Erregbarkeit kann durch Medikamente unterstützt werden, welche beruhigend und dämpfend wirken. Hierzu eignen sich unter anderem die Meprobamate, die heute unter verschiedenen Namen als sog. Ataraktica im Handel sind. Auch die bekannten Barbiturat-Präparate in möglichst niedriger Dosierung, über Tag und Nacht verteilt, können gegebenenfalls mit Vorteil eingesetzt werden. Diese Mittel müssen hinsichtlich ihrer individuellen Dosierung optimal auf jeden einzelnen Fall abgestimmt werden. Zu den eben genannten Maßnahmen kommt bei der neurogenen normocalcämischen Tetanie die Beseitigung der verschiedensten auslösenden Faktoren, welche mit dazu beitragen, die Erregbarkeit des zur Tetanie neigenden Patienten zu steigern.

Alle etwaigen organischen Irritationen, die neben der Tetanie ungünstig auf die neuromuskuläre Erregbarkeit einwirken können, müssen nach Möglichkeit behandelt, abgedämpft bzw. beseitigt werden. Das gilt unter anderem auch von Irritationen der Wirbelsäule, die gelegentlich die neuromuskuläre Übererregbarkeit mit unterstützen.

Wir hatten mehrfach darauf hingewiesen, daß man manchmal den tetanischen Anfall des Normocalcämischen durch lang dauerndes Atemanhalten bzw. Inhalieren von Kohlensäuregas beseitigen kann. Oft beginnen die Patienten nach Beseitigung des Anfalls (mittels Apnoe) allerdings erneut mit einer hyperventilierenden Zwangsatmung, so daß der Krampfanfall nach wenigen Atemzügen erneut einsetzt. Die Apnoe muß deshalb für längere Zeit erzwungen werden, und die Rückkehr zur Normalatmung darf bei erfolgreichem Effekt nur langsam und stufenweise vor sich gehen. Sehr geeignet ist für manche Fälle die sog. Rückatmung, d. h. der Patient atmet in einen entsprechend dimensionierten Beutel bzw. Tüte aus und aus demselben Behälter wieder ein. Diese Atemmethode muß natürlich sorgsam ärztlich überwacht werden. Aus diesem Versuch geht die Bedeutung der aktuellen Blutreaktion für die Aufrechterhaltung des Anfalls hervor, in dem Sinne, daß die Abrauchung der $CO_2$ des Blutes zu einer Verschiebung der Blutreaktionen nach der alkalischen Seite hin und damit zum Auftreten bzw. Bestehenbleiben des Anfalls führt. Aus diesem Grunde hat man versucht, durch Zufuhr von Stoffen, welche eine Verschiebung der aktuellen Blutreaktion nach der sauren Seite hin erzielen, das Auftreten tetanischer Entladungen zu verhindern. Nach den Arbeiten von BÜHLMANN, LABHART, HOLTMEIER und SPÜHLER, sowie von KRÜCK, gelingt es durch Hemmung des Gewebsferments Carboanhydrase, die Hydratisierung der Blutkohlensäure abzustoppen, so daß die aktuelle Blutreaktion mehr nach der sauren Seite hin tendiert. Im Diamox liegt ein Carboanhydrase-Inhibitor vor. Die Verabfolgung von Diamox vermag eine Verschiebung des Blutes nach der alkalischen Seite hin abzubremsen und im Sinne einer Acidose des Blutes zu wirken; es ist also unter Umständen geeignet, im gegebenen Fall die Tetaniebereitschaft herabzusetzen. In Fällen von neurogener Tetanie, wo die Hyperventilation als auslösendes oder verstärkendes Moment häufig eine wichtige Rolle spielt, eventuell auch in anderen Fällen von normocalcämischer Tetanie, ist der Versuch einer Behandlung mit Diamox durchaus zu empfehlen. Das Mittel ist auf eine optimale individuelle Dosis einzustellen, durchschnittlich auf 125—150 mg pro die (= 5 bis 6mal $^1/_2$ Tablette Diamox). Dabei ist die Alkalireserve des Blutes zu verfolgen und deren Senkung auf einen Wert von etwa 25 ($HCO_3$ mmol/C) anzustreben. Man verhindert so das Auftreten von tetanischen Entladungen. (Diese Therapie hat man übrigens auch mit Erfolg bei Epilepsie-Äquivalenten angewandt.) Es ist nach einigen Tagen, eventuell 2—3 Wochen notwendig, das Mittel langsam abzubauen. Wenn man etwa mit 6mal $^1/_2$ Tablette (=4stündlich $^1/_2$ Tablette) in 24 Std begonnen hat, geht man langsam auf 5mal $^1/_2$ Tablette auf 24 Std verteilt usw. herunter, um schließlich die optimale Dosis herauszufinden, bei welcher tetanische Entladungen nach Möglichkeit ausbleiben. Unter Umständen kann man sich völlig mit dem Mittel ausschleichen. Es ist notwendig, die Alkalireserve des Blutes in größeren Abständen immer wieder zu kontrollieren.

## IV. Prognose der neurogenen Tetanie

Die Prognose der neurogenen normocalcämischen Tetanie ist (nach unseren Erfahrungen) nicht schlecht. Wir verfügen über eine große Zahl von Kranken mit schwersten tetanischen Anfällen, die sich unter ärztlicher Führung wieder völlig zurückbildeten. Voraussetzung dafür ist, daß alle ungünstig einwirkenden Faktoren, unter denen die psychischen an erster Stelle zu nennen sind, nach Möglichkeit eingeschränkt, in den Hintergrund gedrängt oder ausgeschaltet werden. Mit dem Abklingen der Tetaniebereitschaft, d. h. der Heraufsetzung der neuromuskulären Erregbarkeitsschwelle, gehen auch die tetanischen Entäußerungen im Bereich der glatten Muskulatur, z. B. des Urovesical-Apparates, zurück. Sind sie nur Erscheinungen, die einem Grundleiden parallel laufen oder durch dieses geweckt wurden, so hören sie in der Regel in gleichem Maße auf, wie das Grundleiden zum Abklingen gebracht wird.

# F. Schluß

Aus der gegebenen Darstellung sollte hervorgehen, daß es spastische Krampfzustände der glattmuskeligen Organe gibt, denen kein organisches Leiden des betroffenen Systems zugrunde liegt, die vielmehr auf der Basis einer neuromuskulären Erregbarkeitssteigerung entstehen können. Die Tetanie stellt eine wichtige Ursache derartiger Krampfzustände dar, von denen im Bereich des Urovesicaltractus sowohl die Ureteren als auch die Blase befallen werden können. Bemerkenswerterweise ist es fast ausschließlich die normocalcämische Form der Tetanie, bei welcher sich derartige Krampfzustände im Bereich der abführenden Harnwege entwickeln. Fernerhin muß hervorgehoben werden, daß das weibliche Geschlecht häufiger von der normocalcämischen Tetanie und damit den tetanischen Entäußerungen im Bereich des Urovesicaltractus befallen wird als das männliche. Dies hängt, wie ausgeführt wurde, mit großer Wahrscheinlichkeit mit der gesteigerten Labilität der Frau zusammen, wobei die große Rolle endokriner Schwankungen beim weiblichen Geschlecht besonders hervorzuheben ist. Nach der Symptomatik der Tetanie muß man in der Anamnese und im Befund sorgfältig suchen. Man kann das Vorliegen tetanisch bedingter Entäußerungen erst dann mit Wahrscheinlichkeit postulieren, wenn organische Ursachen im Bereich der betroffenen glattmuskeligen Organsysteme ausgeschlossen werden können. Wichtig, aber nicht allein entscheidend, ist der therapeutische Test, d. h. die Feststellung, ob eine oder mehrere intravenöse Injektionen eines geeigneten Calcium-Präparates (z. B. Calciumgluconat) imstande sind, den Krampfanfall zu beseitigen. Es ist aber nicht gestattet, die Diagnose einer tetanischen Genese allein auf den therapeutischen Effekt einer intravenösen Calciuminjektion zu gründen. Man bedenke, daß eine derartige intravenöse Injektion mit dem oft bemerkenswerten und den Patienten beeindruckenden Eintreten des Wärmegefühls auch erhebliche psychische Effekte haben kann. Wenn aber weitere Symptome, wie sie dargestellt wurden, für eine tetanische Genese sprechen, so gewinnt die Diagnose „ex juvantibus", also der therapeutische Calciumtest, besondere Bedeutung. Es sei zum Schluß noch einmal besonders unterstrichen, von wie großer Bedeutung die sorgfältige Erhebung der Anamnese für die Diagnosestellung ist und wie wichtig es ist, nach weiteren tetanischen Phänomenen zu fahnden, um die Annahme einer tetanischen Bedingtheit der Krampfzustände abzurunden. Wie dargestellt, kommen mitunter auch Komplikationen organischer Störungen im Bereich des Urovesicaltractus bei gesteigerter neuromuskulärer Erregbarkeit mit tetanischen Entäußerungen vor; insbesondere kann die Lenkung tetanischer Krampfzustände in dieses oder jenes Organ bzw. in die eine oder andere Körperseite, mit einer Bereitschaft bzw. Vorschädigung des betroffenen Organs oder Körperteils zusammenhängen. Auch in solchen Fällen kann die Beachtung einer tetanischen Komponente

(,,tetanische Begleitmusik") für die Erkennung und Therapie des betreffenden Falles von Bedeutung sein.

Wie in der Einleitung betont, sollte die vorangehende Darstellung insbesondere dazu führen, den Urologen auf funktionelle und spastische Zustände im Bereich des Urovesicaltractus hinzuweisen, welche nicht durch die bisher bekannten organischen Störungen im Bereich dieses Systems zu erklären sind, sondern die durch andere Bedingungen von allgemeiner Bedeutung hervorgerufen werden können. Unter diesen Bedingungen spielt das tetanische Syndrom eine wichtige Rolle.

## Literatur

ALDENHOVEN, H.: Therapiewoche 6, 244 (1952). — ALTROCK, T.: Über die Behandlung von Dysmenorrhoen und Spasmen im Bereich des Urogenitalsystems. Medizinische 1955, 1418. — BERNHARDT, H.: Med. Klin. 1948, 428. — BÜHLMANN, A., A. LABHART, H. J. HOLTMEIER u. H. SPÜHLER: Helv. med. Acta 20, 323 (1953). — CRAWFORD, J. D.: In A. LABHART, Klinik der inneren Sekretion (M. WERNLY), S. 825. Berlin-Göttingen-Heidelberg: Springer 1957. — DECOURT, J., et C. TARDIEU: Presse méd. 1939 I, 469. — DENNIG, H.: Dringliche Krankheiten in der inneren Medizin. Stuttgart: Ferdinand Enke 1942. — EGER, W.: Mat. Med. Nordmark 7, 7—11 (1955). — ESSEN, K. W.: Therapiewoche 1953, H. 1/2. — Dtsch. med. Wschr. 1953, 402. — Med. Klin. 1955, Nr 2, 89. — Fortschr. Med. 73, H. 2 (1955). — FANCONI, G.: Dtsch. med. Wschr. 1953, 85. — Schweiz. med. Wschr. 1954. — Handbuch der inneren Medizin, Bd. 7, Teil I. 1957. — GLAUNER, W., u. P. SCHWARZ: Med. Klin. 1950, Nr 33, 1024. — HENI, F., u. H. U. RIETHMÜLLER: Z. Urol. 41, 236 (1948). — HOLTZ, F.: Z. physiol. Chem. 1, 1 (1930). — Klin. Wschr. 1934, 104; 1937, 1557. — HOLTZ, F., u. A. KRAMER: Naturwiss. 24, 177 (1936). — Münch. med. Wschr. 1936, 1332; 1939, 485. — HOLTZ, F., u. A. PONSOLD: Z. ärztl. Fortbild. 1951, 468. — HOLTZ, F., u. E. ROSSMANN: Z. Geburtsh. Gynäk. 116, 187 (1938). — JESSERER, H.: Praxis 37, 481 (1948). — Dtsch. med. Wschr. 76, 1552 (1951). — Ärztl. Wschr. 1951, 748. — Wien. klin. Wschr. 1953; 1954, 711. — Ärztl. Fortbild. 1955, H. 6. — JESSERER, H., u. W. HENNETZ: Enterogene Tetanie nach Ileo-Transverostomie. Dtsch. med. Wschr. 1957, 1369—1372. — KRÜCK, F.: Ärztl. Wschr. 1956, Nr 31, 673. — LACOUR, A.: Zit. nach F. HENI u. H. U. RIETHMÜLLER. — LENGGENHAGER, K.: Schweiz. med. Wschr. 1951, 548. — NISSEN, K.: Landarzt 1954, H. 10. — PARADE, G. W.: Med. Welt 1950, 39; 1951, 20, 1265, 1309. — Dtsch. med. Wschr. 1949, Nr 16, 495; 1950, 47; 1951, 10, 51; 1952, 1. — Therapie-Kongr. Karlsruhe 1949 u. 1950. — Dtsch. med. Rdsch. 1949, 12, 336. — Klinik der Gegenwart, Bd. VI, S. 303. München u. Berlin: Urban & Schwarzenberg 1958. — Med. Klin. 1955, 1988. — PFLAUMER, E.: Handbuch der Urologie von A. v. ZIRSTENBERG, F. VOELCKER u. H. WIDBOLZ, Bd. I, S. 361. Berlin: Springer 1926. — QUANDT, J.: Nervenarzt 23, 261 (1952). — Wiss. Z. Univ. Halle 2, 63 (1952). — Z. Psychother. med. Psychol. 1953, 133. — Samml. Abh. Psychiatr. u. Neurol. 1954, H. 11. — QUANDT, J., u. W. PONSOLD: Münch. med. Wschr. 1953, 977. — RIML, O., u. E. TSCHERNE: Dtsch. med. Wschr. 1953, Nr 42, 1429. — RISAK, E.: Wien. klin. Wschr. 1938, 1004. — Klin. Wschr. 1939, 257. — SÄKER, G.: Nervenarzt 1950, H. 8, 348. — SCHWARZ, P.: Handbuch der Urologie von A. v. ZIRSTENBERG, F. VOELKER u. H. WIDBOLZ, Bd. I, S. 432. Berlin: Springer 1926. — STÜRMER-SCHWARZENBACH, W.: Zit. nach G. W. PARADE. — VELHAGEN, H.: Zit. nach HOLTZ.

# Male Sterility

By

WALTER W. WILLIAMS

With 35 Figures

## Introduction

Since the time of Leewenhoek, over two hundred years ago, it has been recognized that spermatozoa are essential for reproduction, but it was not generally appreciated that differences in the health of the ejaculated spermatozoa dictated differences in potential fertility until 1925 when WILLIAMS and SAVAGE reported their observations on the relationship of spermatic structure to the reproductive fitness of bulls. Prior to this, CARY had pointed out that spermatic abnormalities, the reduction of sperm concentration and reduced sperm motility played an important role in male infertility, but his observations went essentially unnoticed because of his failure to record in precise terms his cytologic observations and to document his material so as to bring out the clinical correlations which were so obvious to him. About ten years elapsed before the more precise and better documented observations on animal breeding revealed the close correlation between spermatic pathology and the reproduction efficiency of various species of animals. It was then realized that fundamental spermatic disease played a very significant role in the etiology of infertility in various species. Such correlations of spermatic pathology to the fertility potential were reported with respect to the bull by WILLIAMS and SAVAGE 1925 and 1927, LAGERLÖF 1934, BROCHART in 1951, on the cock by CONKLIN in 1929, the stallion by SAVAGE, WILLIAMS and FOWLER in 1930, BIELANSKI in 1951, and the ram in 1937 by McKENSIE and BERLINER. Similar results were reported with relation to spermatic disease in man by MOENCH in 1931, WILLIAMS in 1937 and 1939, WILLIAMS and SIMMONS in 1942, and HAMMEN in 1944.

The observations by these and other investigators have clearly indicated that a very large segment of male infertility is associated with a fundamental, intrinsic fault of the germinal epithelium which prevents formation of adequate numbers of normal fertile spermatozoa. Thus barring intercurrent disease or sexual excesses, the ability to form normal numbers of spermatozoa, as well as the percentage and degree of motility and the structure of the spermatozoa produced, remains as more or less fixed attributes of the individual, and decides his potential fertility. Apparently, the greatest barrier to progress in the subject of male infertility during the past decade has been the reluctance to consider that faulty germ plasm is often incapable of forming other than faulty gametes and that the cytology of the ejaculated spermatozoa mirrors the fundamental health of the germ plasm from which it is derived.

Because of the relatively high incidence of incurable male infertility which can be recognized by means of a semen examination, it is generally considered desirable in the study of infertile matings that the examination of the male should precede that of the female partner and thus obviate much needless work on the latter.

During the past few years, there has been an increasingly greater integration of the studies of infertile marriages so that gynecologists, urologists and other specialists have complemented each other to bring about more thorough diagnostic studies. Unfortunately, much male infertility is, however, still being treated without any precise knowledge concerning the status of the male gametes and the general health factors which may influence their viability and fertility. Indeed, there still exists in many quarters a considerable reluctance or even antipathy to the inclusion of a comprehensive semen analysis for the evaluation of male fertility.

# A. Etiology

Male sterility or impaired fertility exists whenever any factor seriously interferes with the production of or availability of normal fertile spermatozoa. Such may be the result of an intrinsic weakness or abnormality of the spermatozoa, it may be due to an organic or functional disorder of the generative organs or to some somatic factor which either indirectly lowers the vitality of the spermatozoa or interferes with the normal function of the generative organs. A physiochemical alteration of the seminal fluid or of the spermatozoa may be associated with such disorders. Potential fertility varies according to differences in the health of different sperm populations. Consequently, the evaluation of male fertility requires more than some simple procedure such as a flighting glance at a cover-glass preparation of semen or perhaps an examination of the prostate, but rather a general consideration of various somatic factors, the health of generative organs, and the intrinsic health of the mature ejaculated spermatozoa.

The efficacy of resolving the male infertility problem depends to a considerable degree upon whether the concept of etiology is based upon secure scientific evidence, since this will govern the nature and scope of diagnostic procedures, the prognosis and the type of therapy.

## I. Somatic health

### 1. Age

The age of the male has much less influence on fertility than the age of the female. Although the male fertility does diminish with age, it is evident that this dimunition is very gradual so that fertility may be maintained in man until well after seventy years of age. In one instance, the fertility was authenticated at the age of ninety-four years (SEYMOUR). It is reported that the incidence of neonatal deaths increases with the age of the male parent as well as with the female (YERUSHALMY). However, where much spermatic pathology is present, the spermatic picture may deteriorate with age and one will observe an extensive spermatic disorder in a previously fertile individual, suggesting that there may occasionally be a change in the character of the ejaculated spermatozoa as age advances. Although age in itself does not exert an outstanding influence upon fertility during the ordinary reproductive life of the individual, the intercurrent disorders encountered with advancing years may exert a considerable influence.

## 2. General health

It is usually exceedingly difficult to correlate statistically various somatic or general health problems with a lowering of fertility of the male because of the lack of adequate control series. One does, however, frequently observe a transitory lowering of sperm motility and concentration in association with such factors as a common cold or high fevers. As a part of infertility studies and the subsequent fitness for parenthood, one should always consider the possible influence of the general health of both partners, and that good health is always an asset to normal reproduction even though this relationship may not be statistically proven. Unfortunately, the influence of many supposed etiologic items such as psychologic, are often based largely upon hearsay evidence, and their precise clinical significance is not proven.

## 3. Nutrition

In cases of malnutrition or debilitating diseases, there is apt to be an impairment in spermatogenesis, sperm motility and decreased interest in sex life, according to the severity of the disorder. Cases with severe dietary deficiencies are rarely concerned with the infertility problem, but dietary disorders of a minor nature such as a moderate vitamin or protein deficiency are commonly observed and may be significant.

Metabolic disturbances are frequently indicated by overweight or underweight. Clinically, it seems that patients do best if on a balanced diet, which includes meat, butter, eggs, milk, fresh fruits and fresh vegetables or their equivalent. Various vitamin deficiencies have been held responsible for infertility from time to time. Experimentally, it has been shown that vitamin deficiencies of various types can cause sterility and abortion in experimental animals. Comparable deficiencies are, however, not ordinarily encountered in the human subject. The effect of vitamins is best considered from the viewpoint of general health and not as providing some special fertility factor. Although various clinical avitaminoses such as scurvy, and beri-beri or a general vitamin deficiency may prevent reproduction, these diseases almost never occur amongst the group of patients studied because of infertility. Subclinical multi-avitaminosis may possibly, however, be a factor in some cases.

Metabolic diseases, such as diabetes, chronic liver disorders, or other factors which interfere with nutrition must all be considered as important when they exist. Since the liver plays an important role in steroid metabolism, it is frequently concerned with abnormal gonadal function. Blood dyscrasias, particularly a simple anemia, are so common that a complete blood examination is in order with all cases of both male and female infertility. A hyper or hypoglycemia may interfere with fertility, and should always be brought under control.

## 4. Exercise, overweight, underweight

An adequate amount of exercise contributes materially to good health. This does not need to be of a strenuous character, but should be rather regular from day to day, even if consisting of only a brisk out-of-doors walk. It is desirable that the weight of a person should not vary too widely from the normal averages as influenced by height, sex, age and family characteristics. Overwork and excessive exercise may be detrimental to general health and lessen sexual capacity. It will often be found that a balanced program of proper rest, recreation and exercise is desirable for good somatic health and may favorably influence the sperm picture and fertility. This applies to man and animals alike. For instance, breeders of various species of domestic animals recognize that a reasonable amount of exercise and good nutrition are very important in maintaining a high fertility of the male. Although in man the procreative ability cannot be measured as it is with domestic animals, clinical experience with man suggests that the same principles apply in the human race as with the breeding of domestic animals in respect to the relation of general health to fertility. In human, however, we encounter additional emotional or psychosomatic factors which, in some instances, affect reproduction because of the deterioration in general health. In other cases, the emotional stress provides a functional basis for impotency or prompts sexual overactivity and the consequent reduction in the number and quality of the ejaculated spermatozoa.

## 5. Environment, toxic factors and allergies

Under certain circumstances, environmental and occupational factors may exert considerable influence upon reproduction, although in general, man is a very versatile creature and adapts himself to great variations in environment. High altitudes such as encountered high in the Andes are reported to interfere with fertility. In experimental animals, it has been shown that low oxygen tension may depress spermiogenesis (WALTON). It is reported that the extreme heat of some regions in the tropics lowers fertility. On the other hand, the extreme heat encountered in connection with industrial occupations, such as stoking blast furnaces is not known to affect the fertility of individuals so exposed (CASTRO).

Very little factual information is available concerning the relation of toxic factors to male infertility. It seems to be well established that major intoxicants which influence the general health of the individual are detrimental to reproduction, and amongst these may be listed lead poisoning, chronic alcoholism, and narcotics when used especially to the point of addiction. Lowered fertility is often attributed to the excessive use of tobacco, but such is not a constant sequel, and it seems very likely that any deleterious effect of nicotine on reproduction must be attributed to its influence on general health and not because of any specific influence on the health of germinal cells. Indeed, with most persons, there is no evidence that nicotine is detrimental to generative function. In general, those who are suffering from severe toxins or allergies seek medical attention because of other complaints than their failure of reproduction and are therefore rarely infertility problems. Various industrial poisons are at times encountered, such as coal-tar products, paint and plastic solvents, but no specific effect on the character of the ejaculated spermatozoa has been attached to them. Although a vast array of etiologic factors, such as occupational, toxic, allergic, infectious, psychosomatic, etc., are constantly presented for consideration, much more information is needed concerning any specific effect which they may exert upon the character of the spermatozoa produced. In most instances, one should consider that adverse influences are often not specific but come about indirectly by altering the general health of the individual.

## 6. Infections

Various types of infection may either depress spermiogenesis because of the hyperthermia or cause direct injury to the testes or some other portion of the generative tract. A transitory reduction of spermatogenesis, sperm concentration and motility is observed with a common cold and other minor ailments, but epidemic parotitis is apparently the only acute general infection which specifically involves the testes. Other infections such as the granulomas and syphilis may involve various portions of the generative tract, but with the exception of gonorrhea, are not encountered with sufficient frequency in most countries to constitute an infertility problem. This does not, however, discount their significance in some parts of the world where such infections are particularly prevalent.

### a) Mumps (Epidemic parotitis)

Orchitis parotidea occurs as a complication of epidemic parotitis in about eight per cent of the males affected after the age of puberty, but apparently does not occur prior to this age. One or both testes may be involved, resulting in a severe inflammation, swelling and acute pain of the involved organs. This often terminates in such a profound atrophy of the involved testes that they may be represented after a period of three to eight weeks merely by a firm, fibrous mass no larger than two centimeters in diameter. When the clinical orchitis is unilateral, spermatogenesis is usually impaired or at least temporarily inhibited in the normal-appearing testis. In other instances, it is reported that degenerative changes occur in the germinal epithelium of both testicles in spite of the absence of any clinically cognizable orchitis (NORLANDER, BAYLE). This may result in the complete destruction of the germinal epithelium and thus permanent azoospermia. Coincident with the orchitis, there is a transitory epididymitis which does not, however, lead to occlusion. Clinically, it seems that the intense swelling under an unyielding tunica albuginea is partly responsible for the profound degeneration, since the testicles that are treated promptly with ice packs exhibit a better conservation of spermiogenesis. Recently, it has been reported that the use of cortisone (RISMAN) and diethylstilbesterol may greatly reduce the damage to the testes (HOYNE, SAVIN).

The first stage in the histopathology of mumps orchitis consists of a leukocytic infiltration of the stroma and small stromal hemorrhages. The seminiferous tubules are pushed apart with exudate, and this is usually associated with a swelling and extreme pain of the testis. Due to the heat, toxins and pressure, spermatogenesis ceases. The basal membrane of the seminiferous tubules is destroyed, and there is a leukocytic invasion of the seminiferous tubules which spreads rapidly throughout the testis so that within a few days, there may be a total destruction of the seminal epithelium. In some instances, a few of the tubules survive, but apparently due to some toxin, there is commonly a considerable damage to the seminal epithelium of the testis which is not clinically inflamed, so that spermatogenesis ceases. This aspermatogenesis is, however, apt to be transitory. Thus if the clinical orchitis is unilateral, the fertility of the individual may not be permanently destroyed. NORLANDER reports, however, that the rate of sperm production remains permanently lower even with a unilateral involvement, and also that destruction of the seminal epithelium may occur without clinical evidence of orchitis.

### b) Gonorrhea

A gonococcal infection has been and continues to be of considerable importance from the viewpoint of infertility because of the frequency with which it causes an inflammation, induration and obstructive lesions of the fine coiled tubules of the epididymis or of the vas deferens, a complication which not infrequently follows a gonorrheal urethritis and causes a permanent obstruction to the passage of spermatozoa. The globus minor of the epididymis is the most frequently involved portion of the ductal system and its induration is commonly detected by palpation. If the globus minor alone is obstructed, live spermatozoa may be found in the globus major for a period of years after the obstruction occurs, and an epididymovasectomy which brings together and establishes a connection between the proximal portion of the vas deferens and the globus major, may restore patency and permit spermatozoa to again appear in the ejaculate. Fertility may thus be restored with some cases, but it should be realized that male sterility due to epididymal obstruction is encountered in less than one per cent of infertile matings (WILLIAMS 1956) and that only a small portion of these can be corrected by surgery. Neisserian infection is playing a gradually diminishing role in the etiology of sterility of both male and female. In some communities, it is claimed that as much as fifty per cent of female sterility is due to a Neisserian involvement of the fallopian tubes. In such instances, there may be a corresponding high incidence of male sterility due to gonorrheal epididymitis, but where an active venereal disease control has been established, the amount of sterility due to specific venereal disease is almost negligible.

### c) Tuberculosis

A tubercular infection may involve particularly the epididymis and this may be suspected in case of an epididymal induration, azoospermia and the lack of history of gonorrhea, together with evidence of tubercular infection elsewhere in the body, particularly in the lungs.

## II. Miscellaneous pathology of generative organs

A wide variety of factors involving either the testes or the ductal system may either prevent testicular function or the egress of spermatozoa from the testes. Direct trauma to the testes or the epididymis may be of sufficient severity to injure the matrix of the testicle or the epididymis. Circulation of a testis or epididymis may be impaired as a complication of surgery, particularly with a herniorraphy, varicocelectomy or repair of a hydrocele, and lead to sterility. In the case of undescended testes, the circulation is restricted because of the inadequately developed testes, but here we are often concerned with a genetically unsound organ whose circulation is of little consequence. The testicle associated with a large varicocoele is commonly of smaller size than the testicle on the normal side, and presumably such testes are incapable of normal function. With bilateral varicoceles, an improved circulation and spermato-genesis may be favored by the excision or ligaturing of the varicoceles. With a unilateral varicocele, there is apparently a compensitory hyperfunction of the other testicle, with adequate spermatogenesis and the value of surgery for the unilateral varicocele is very questionable from the infertility viewpoint. Surgery is principally indicated to relieve the discomfort.

A spermatocele or cyst-like enlargement of the tubules of the epididymis is rarely encountered, but if present, will prevent egress of spermatozoa from the affected organ. Fertility is usually not impaired if the pathology involves only one testicle.

Tumors and newgrowths of the testes are not commonly encountered with those presenting themselves for infertility studies, but one must always suspect malignancy if a solid tumor mass is associated with the testicle, or if a testicle is of stone-like consistency, even though not significantly enlarged.

## III. Congenital or hereditary factors causing infertility
### 1. Abnormalities of the generative organs

A variety of congenital or hereditary factors may reduce or destroy fertility of the male. These may be recognized either by some gross abnormality in the development of the generative organs or by a developmental fault of the germ plasm. One observes rather infrequently such gross anomalies as infantile generative organs, epispadius, hypospadius, absence of the epididymis or vasa deferentia. The failure of testicular descent occurs much more frequently. It is commonly associated with a germinal hypoplasia or aplasia and consequently hypoplastic testicles. The injury to the germ plasm of a hypoplastic testicle is usually permanent even though the testis may later be brought into the scrotum either by means of surgery or by gonadotropic therapy. Thus such therapy is of very questionable value from the viewpoint of fertility, since a hypoplastic testis rarely if ever becomes capable of normal spermiogenesis.

A retarded descent of a normally developed testis may not interfere with its subsequent function. Also, unilateral cryptorchidism is usually of little or no significance from the viewpoint of infertility unless the scrotal testis is hypoplastic or that it represents a genetic defect which will be perpetuated. This hereditary aspect of cryptorchidism has been noted with various species of animals, such as equine, bovine, porcine and ovinae (W. L. WILLIAMS 1943, LAGERLÖF 1950).

### 2. Congenital disorders of the germ plasm

Of especial interest from the viewpoint of infertility is a congenital disorder of the germ plasm, whereby the germinal epithelium is inherently incapable of forming normal numbers of viable, fertile spermatozoa (WILLIAMS 1953). This may be associated with small flabby testes or testes of normal size and consistency. Such testes are commonly associated with a hypoplastic germinal epithelium, a condition which is usually not recognized until the reproductive phase of life when an explanation for infertility is sought.

The failure of normal development of the germinal epithelium may be secondary to some endocrine disorder, but such cases are very infrequently encountered in connection with the study of infertile marriages because men with pronounced endocrine disturbances, as well as those with marked anomalies of the generative organs, do not commonly acquire a mate. Male infertility or sterility is very frequently due to a congenital fault of the germ plasm whereby the seminal epithelium becomes permanently incapable of forming an adequate supply of normal, healthy spermatozoa. This damage may be evidenced by a fixed low sperm concentration in the seminal fluid, a constantly low viability of the ejaculated spermatozoa or the presence of a fixed high ratio of specific types of structurally abnormal spermatozoa, whereas under the influence of extrinsic factors, motility and sperm concentration may vary considerably with different specimens of semen from the same individual (WILLIAMS 1953).

The observations by KNUDSEN upon bovine spermio-cytogenesis is of considerable interest because of its analogy to observations in human. He has pointed out that the character of the cytologic changes in the spermatogonia and the spermiocytes decide the histologic picture of the germinal epithelium, the character of the ejaculated spermatozoa and the fertility of the individual. The anomalies which involve the chromosomes, the centrosomes and the spindles may furnish evidence as to whether the disturbance is of genetic or acquired origin.  Pathology of the ejaculated spermatozoa have their counterpart in the observed anomalies of the spermatogonia and primary spermatocytes to such an extent that the type of faulty spermiogenesis may often be identified by the nature of the anomalies observed in the ejaculated spermatozoa.

Acquired germinal cytopathology may result from such factors as febrile diseases and cause disturbances of the centrosomes and spindles.  This results in a faulty distribution of the chromosomes (Fig. 1, 2). During the metaphase in the primary spermiocytes, vacuoles may form in the cytoplasm and the centrioles. This is followed by a swelling and crumbling of the centrosomes, then a disintegration of the spindle fibers. The division and distribution of the chromosomes is thereby altered; and without the support of the fibers of the spindles, the nucleus becomes pyknotic. In some instances,

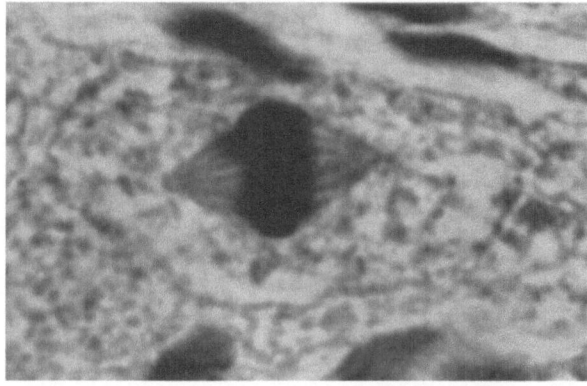

Fig. 1. *Normal primary spermiocyte in full metaphase.* Normal nuclear spindle. 3000×. (Courtesy of ODD KNUDSEN, Stockholm, Sweden)

without this support, the chromosomes proceed to divide but the nuclear membrane does not do so, thus resulting in a gamete with double the normal number of chromosomes. Since the centriolar bodies are intimately associated with motility, a disturbance in this area may lead to an immobilization of the affected spermatozoa (Fig. 3, 4).

In other instances, due to the formation of multiple centrosomes, multiple spindles will arise and this may result in the formation of giant cells, with multiple nuclei, which produce a characteristic seminal picture, with semen of a watery consistency and containing in the centrifuged sample multinucleated cells and cells with pyknotic nuclei. This particular type of anomaly was all observed in bulls belonging to the same family and is presumably the result of faulty recessive genes.

The primary disturbances of

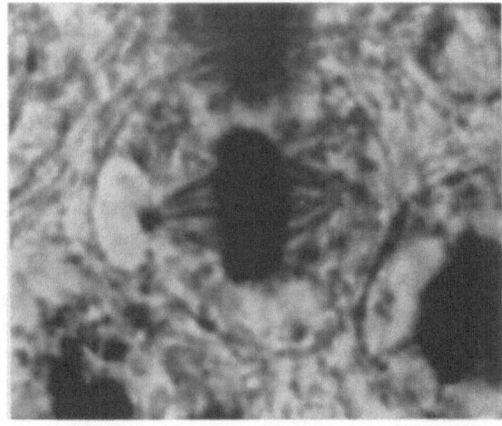

Fig. 2. *Pathologic primary spermiocyte in full metaphase.* With vacuolated cytoplasm and degeneration of the centrosomes. 3000×. (Courtesy of ODD KNUDSEN, Stockholm, Sweden)

the chromosomes were apparently the result of genetic or hereditary factors which were most frequently apparent in the primary spermiocytes. They did, however, involve the primary spermatogonia and led to a reduction in their numbers, and consequently to a hopeless type of sterility. In some cases, there occurred what KNUDSEN designates as "stickiness" of the chromosomes (Fig. 5, 6). The chromosomes of the spermatic epithelium become sticky and adhere together after the homologous chromosomes have paired together in the primary spermiocytes, and this prevents the bivalent chromosomes from migrating to the respective poles of the cell. With this disorder, there is generally a spermiogenic arrest in the primary spermiocyte stage, and if spermiogenesis progresses any further, the product consists of cells of the spermatid stage with pyknotic nuclei.

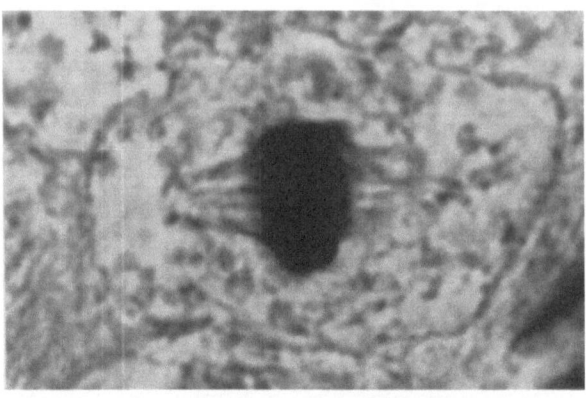

Fig. 3. *Primary spermatocyte with slightly destroyed spindle.* 3300×. (Courtesy of ODD KNUDSEN, Stockholm, Sweden)

In other instances, a segment of a chromosome would become paired with a non-homologous segment of another chromosome and although the number of chromosomes might not be altered, the disorder would prevent cell division or result in faulty, infertile mature gametes which if sufficiently extensive, would completely arrest further spermiocytogenesis. It is pointed out that such chromosomal anomalies are commonly associated with genetic infertility of cattle, and further that the disturbances which have been described in the spermatic epithelium, should occur to an equal degree in the germinal cells of the female. Various other types of genetic disorders of the gametes can be recognized.

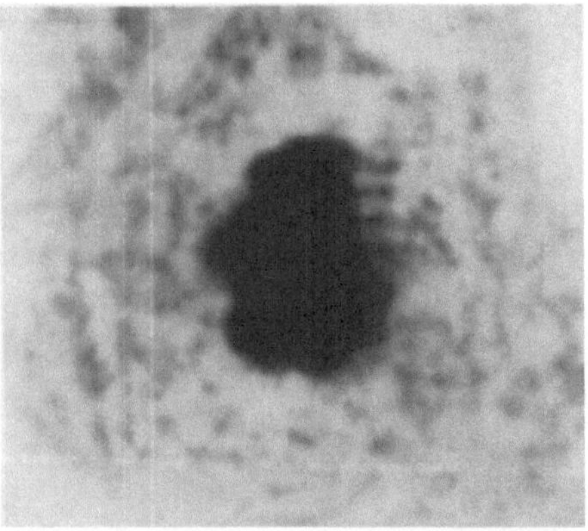

Fig. 4. *Primary spermatocyte with extensively disturbed spindle.* This type of anomalie may interfere seriously with the motility of the mature spermatozoön. 3000×. (Courtesy of ODD KNUDSEN, Stockholm, Sweden)

The observations by KNUDSEN and his co-workers are of particular interest in the field of human infertility, first because they tie together the cytologic picture as seen in the germinal epithelium with that observed in the ejaculated spermatozoa, and further they indicate strongly the genetic origin of much infertility. A little different light is cast upon the significance and the explanation of the histologic picture of testicular biopsies which in the past has been generally associated with hypothetical endocrine factors and studied largely by endocrinologists and not by cytologists or geneticists. Studies on human male infertility have largely been somewhat segmental in nature, with a dissociation of spermiocytogenesis, histology of the germinal epithelium, endocrinology, genetics and cytology of the ejaculated spermatozoa. Thus an integrated picture of the infertility problem becomes obscured. It is well to observe that there are certain fundamental laws which apply equally to man and the lower animals, and that this is particularly exemplified in respect to behavior of the germinal cells.

The various abnormalities of the mature sperm which arise from the different anatomical components of the immature cell, such as the nucleus, idiosome, and nebenkern, result in very distinctive abnormalities in the mature gamete. The constancy of ratio and types of these different spermatic abnormalities strongly suggest their derivation from a faulty primordal germinal cell which carries to each of the primary spermatogonia the same genetic potentialities and thus creates a constant supply of distinctive abnormalities which outcrop in given ratios in the mature gametes, irrespective of any extrinsic factors. It follows that such abnormalities must trace back to a faulty anlaga arising from the fusion of the antecedent ovum and sperm. Because the primitive germ plasm is involved, there is apt to be a lack of normal development of the seminal epithelium. This causes variable histologic pictures according to the extent of germinal involvement and the conditioning by various endocrine influences, such as may arise from a lack of development of Leydig cells, adrenals, pituitary or thyroid, whose dysfunction may likewise be of a genetic etiology. Sperm concentration and vitality may be altered by extrinsic factors which are of a transitory nature, whereas genetic factors cause a derangement which, if of sufficient magnitude, may involve permanently all of the gametes and result in total, irreversible sterility.

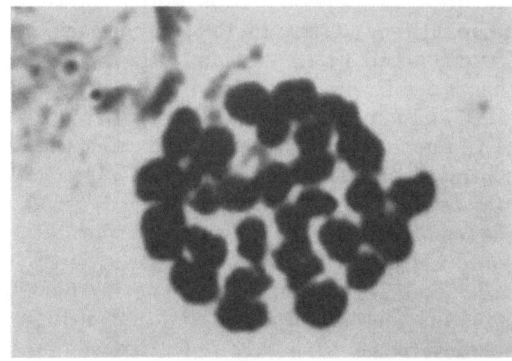

Fig. 5. *Normal primary spermiocyte.* Normal chromosomes in full metaphase. 3000 ×. (Courtesy of ODD KNUDSEN, Stockholm, Sweden)

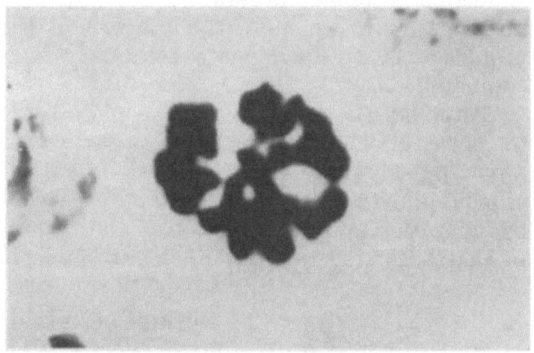

Fig. 6. *Pathologic primary spermiocyte with sticky chromosomes.* This type of disorder causes an arrest in spermiogenesis. 3000 ×. (Courtesy of ODD KNUDSEN, Stockholm, Sweden)

## 3. Histopathology of the testes

Histologic studies of testicular biopsies from individuals with low sperm concentrations in the ejaculated semen or with azoospermia commonly reveal various degrees of thinning and disorganization of the germinal epithelium and a corresponding arrest at various stages of spermatogenesis. With some, there is a lack in the development of the Leydig cells which cause various degrees of hypogonadism. Associated with this, there may be a peritubular fibrosis which may progress to a point of complete hyalinization of the seminiferous tubules and total destruction of the seminal epithelium (KLINEFELTER et al. 1942). This process may be reversible, and may be improved occasionally by androgen therapy. Such cases may be of endocrine etiology, but the paucity or absence of Leydig cells is probably of genetic etiology. In either case, whether genetic or endocrine, the sterility is almost always permanent if the derangement of the seminal epithelium is sufficient to cause azoospermia. Although many of the poorest prognoses of male infertility are associated with a spermatic dysplasia[1], very little attention has been given to the underlying cytologic abnormalities of the germinal cells which predicate the abnormalities of the mature spermatozoa. It is noted, however, that the types of spermatic abnormalities and the histologic changes in the testes observed in animals by FINCHER and FERGUSON and others are similar to those observed with man. In the case of hereditary infertility of Swedish cattle, KNUDSEN and LAGERLÖF (1957) have pointed out a disturbance of the chromosomes and a disarrangement of the genes which is associated with the formation of high ratios of pathologic spermia and a high incidence of abnormalities in the progeny of the bulls so affected. Thus, the observations on cytology reveal a close correlation between the condition of the ejaculated spermatozoa and the germinal epithelium, a condition which is commonly predicated by a genetic fault of the primitive germ cell. Then if this genetic damage involves too high a ratio of the sperm population, the fertility of the individual is impaired or lost.

Most cases of highly defective seminal epithelia are apparently of a congenital origin, associated either with a genetic fault which may or may not involve the Leydig cells or other cells supplying internal secretions. Frank endocrine disorders are rarely encountered in the male partner to infertile marriages, but are more the concern of the endocrinologists because of such problems as an inadequate secondary sexual development and inability to copulate.

Although the faulty histologic picture of the testicle seems to relate mostly to genetic etiology, such is not necessarily the case. Thus McENTEE and OLAFSON report a generalized hyperkeratosis of cattle and sheep due to the consumption of contaminated processed food and a part of the clinical picture is a peritubular hyalanization and degeneration of the germinal epithelium which is very similar to that occurring in the Klinefelter syndrome of man.

### a) Normal germinal epithelium

Histologic studies of biopsy specimens derived from normal functioning testes reveal a distinctive architecture of the stroma and seminiferous tubules, in which the various stages of spermiogenesis are represented. Spermatogonia with their dense nuclei may be observed adjacent to the basement membrane, then the primary and secondary spermatocytes with their abundant mitotic figures, spermatids and lastly the mature spermatozoa which are located more centrally. With normal active spermiogenesis, the tubules are lined with a thick layer of germinal cells, disposed in an orderly manner so that gametes in various stages of development may be identified. Many mature spermatozoa may be observed either lying free in the lumina of the tubules or with their heads still attached to the Sertoli cells (Figs. 7, 8).

### b) Germinal hypoplasia or aplasia

A germinal hypoplasia or aplasia commonly exists in association with azoospermia or with a marked reduction in sperm concentration in the semen. There may be an atrophy of the germinal epithelium of various grades, resulting in a thinning of the layers of the germinal cells and an arrest in spermiogenesis at any stage so as to prevent the formation of mature spermia. If the arrest occurs at the spermatogonia stage, only a few spermatogonia may line the

---

[1] Spermatic dysplasia signifies an abnormality in the development of the spermatozoa. In this respect, the term "teratospermia" has been very commonly and erroneously employed in the literature on sterility.

seminiferous tubules. The disorder may progress further so that all of the germinal epithelium disappears. A germinal hypoplasia usually arises prior

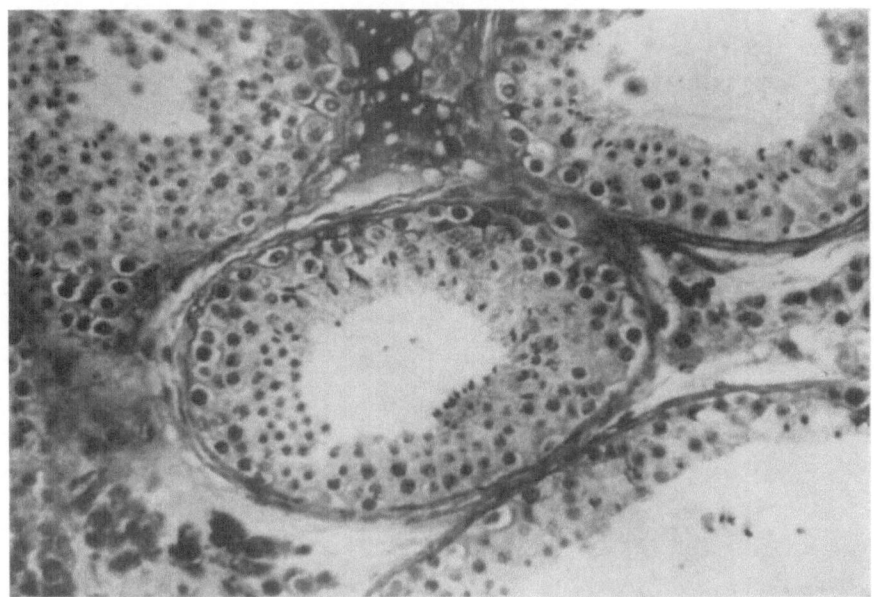

Fig. 7. *Normal germinal epithelium.* Note orderly arrangement of germinal cells, with the more immature cells, the spermatogonia at the periphery and the mature spermia in lumina of seminiferous tubes. One commonly observes collections of mature spermatozoa in the lumina of the seminiferous tubules, in addition to those still attached to the Sertoli cells, when spermiogenesis is normal. Low power magnification. (Courtesy of PAUL GETZOFF, M. D., New Orleans, Louisiana, USA)

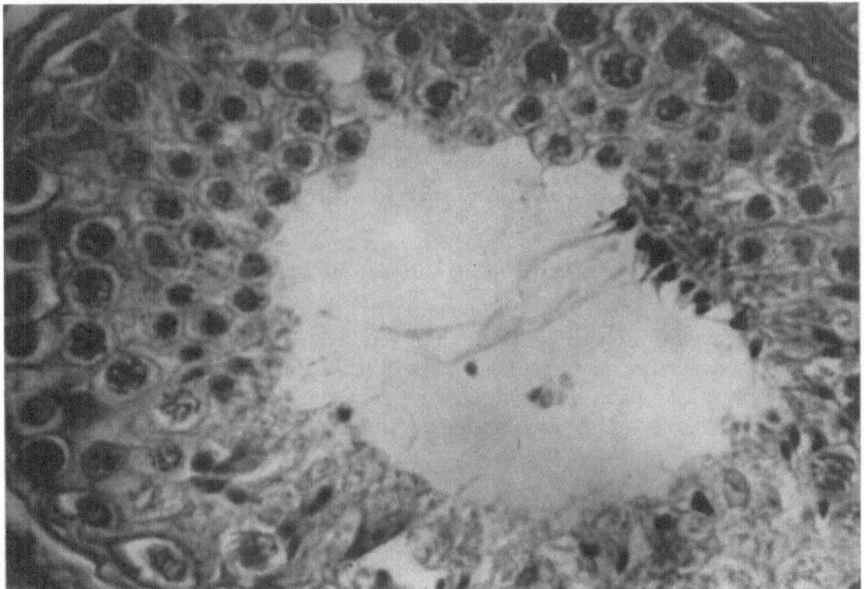

Fig. 8. Normal germinal epithelium. Same as Fig. 7. (High magnification)

to puberty. The consequent sperm concentration in the seminal fluid commonly tends to continue at a rather fixed level, irrespective as to whether this concentration is high or low, thus indicating that the disorder is not as a rule a progressive, degenerative process, but rather the result of a poor genetic endowment (Fig. 9).

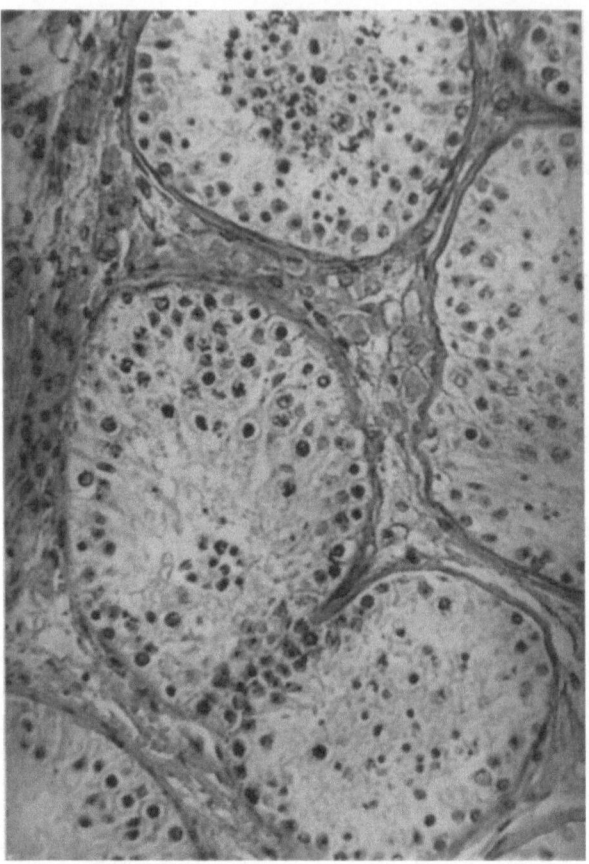

Fig. 9. *Germinal hypoplasia, with total arrest of spermiogenesis.* Spermiogenesis may become arrested at any stage. In many such instances, the lumina of the tubules are not developed and the arrest occurs in the first or second spermatocyte stage. Few or no mature spermatozoa are developed. (Courtesy of PAUL GETZOFF, M. D., New Orleans, Louisiana, USA)

### c) Peritubular fibrosis of testes

A low sperm concentration or azoospermia is occasionally associated with a peritubal fibrosis and hyalinization, followed by a hyalinization of the seminiferous tubules and the destruction of all of the germinal epithelium. This is commonly but not always associated with a reduced Leydig cell function and symptoms and signs of hypogonadism, the so-called Klinefelter syndrome (Fig. 10).

### d) Infantile germinal epithelium

According to the type and severity of the disorder, a spermatogenic arrest may occur at any phase of the spermatogenic process, and thus produce a wide variety of different histologic pictures. An arrest at the spermatogonia stage and the persistence of small infantile-type seminiferous tubules which are lined only by a few inactive spermatogonia occurs when the disorder occurs at the time of puberty (Fig. 11).

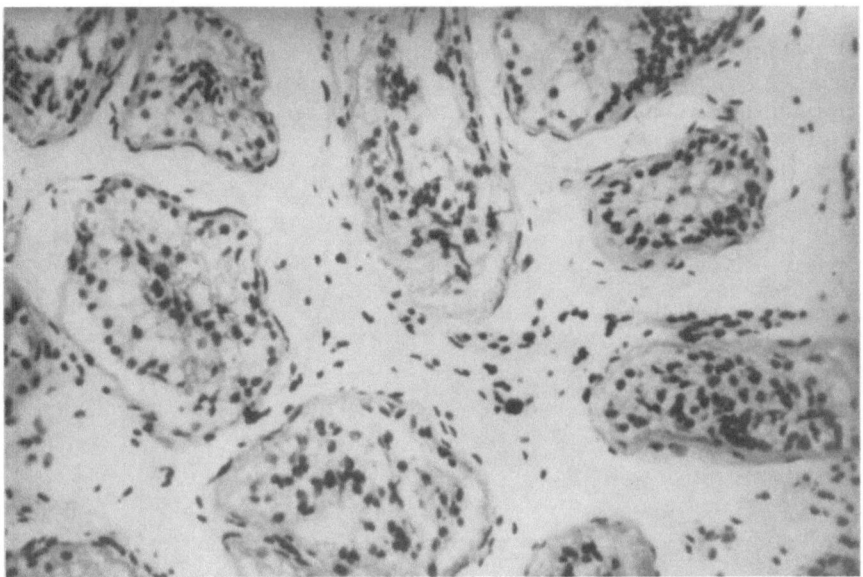

Fig. 10. *Peritubal fibrosis and hyalinization of the seminiferous tubules.* Kleinfelters syndrome.  Only Sertoli cell are to be observed if the tubules are not completely obliterated.  The Leydig cells are not affected. (Courtesy of PAUL GETZOFF, M. D., New Orleans, Louisiana, USA)

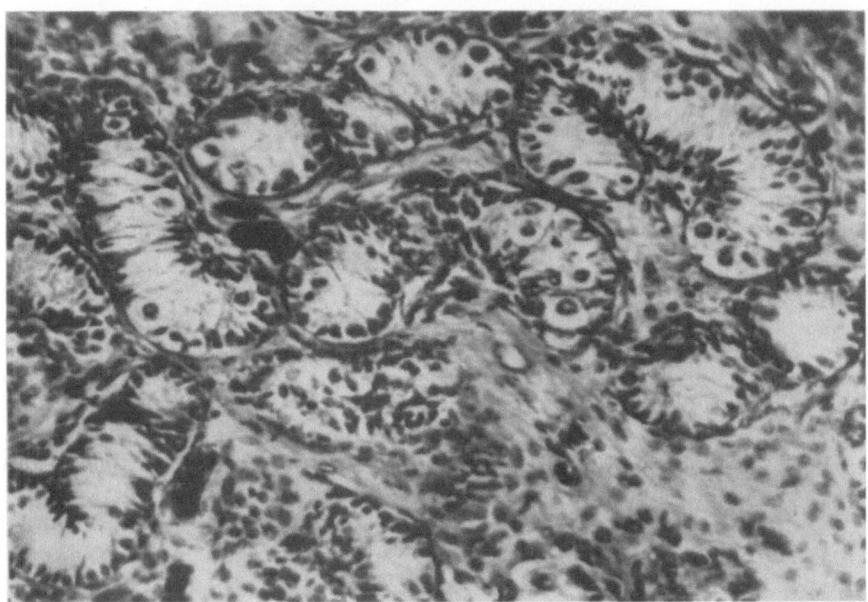

Fig. 11. *Infantile germinal epithelium.* With the typical prepubertal type of seminal epithelium, the tubules are lined with spermatogonia, with few or no spermatocytes. This type may be theoretically amenable to endocrine therapy because of the abundance of the spermatogonia which may possibly be enactivated. (Courtesy of PAUL GETZOFF, M. D., New Orleans, Louisiana, USA)

### e) Germinal aplasia

From aplastic germinal epithelia, no spermatogenesis is possible.  The histologic picture varies greatly, and one may observe in some instances a complete atrophy of the germinal epithelium except for the supporting Sertoli cells (Fig. 12).

## f) Dysspermatogenesis

A striking disorganization of the germinal epithelium is occasionally observed, so that the different layers or stages of spermiogenesis cannot be distinguished, — a condition which may be termed dysspermatogenesis. In some of these,

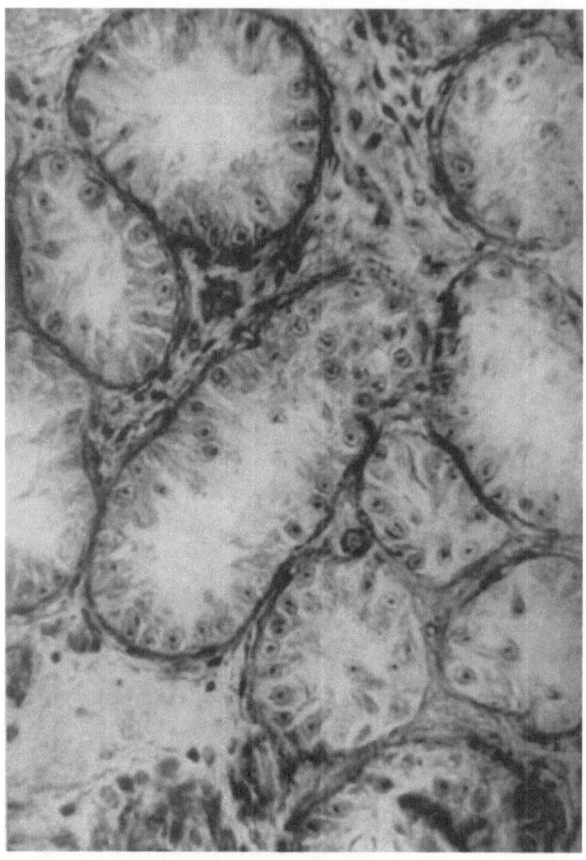

Fig. 12. *Aplasia of germinal epithelium.* No spermatogenic cells are present and the seminiferous tubules are lined only with Sertoli cells. (Courtesy of PAUL GETZOFF, M. D., New Orleans, Louisiana, USA)

there may exist a definite disturbance in karyokineisis which is due to faulty chromosomes and genes (KNUDSEN, LAGERLÖF 1957) (Fig. 13, 14).

When such a disturbance exists, the ability of spermiogenesis is inhibited or completely eliminated and the quality of any ejaculated spermia is greatly impaired.

A spermatogenic arrest in the spermatocyte stage is a very common feature, and may involve a part or all of the different tubules of the testicles. Some of the seminiferous tubules may have little or no lumina, and few or no adult type gametes are present. Other cases may be capable of producing a limited number of mature type spermatozoa, but insufficient to provide any spermatozoa in the ejaculate. A semen examination provides however a better means of measuring the quality of spermatozoa produced than can be accomplished by a testicular biopsy.

From the academic viewpoint, the histopathology and cytology of the testicle is of considerable interest. Clinically, however, the individuals whose testicles are incapable of providing a sufficient number of normal mature gametes in the ejaculate, present a hopeless prognosis, irrespective of the character of the histologic changes in the germinal epithelium.

## 4. Endocrine factors

Most cases of germinal hypoplasia present no clinical evidence of an endocrine etiology (NELSON, DEL CASTILLO). A lack of normal development of the genera-tive organs or of the germinal epithelium may result from various outstanding

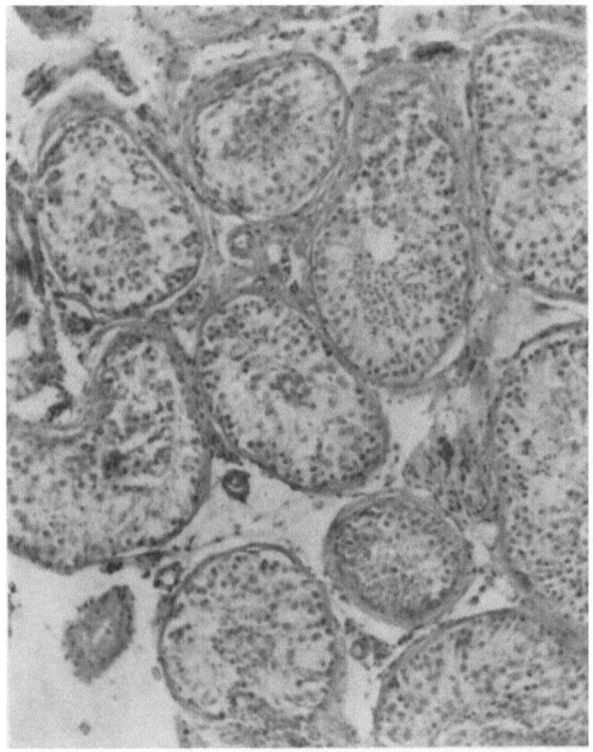

Fig. 13. *Dysspermatogenesis*. In some instances, there is a very marked disorganization of the different spermato-genic cells and a desquamation of the immature gametes, with no mature spermia being formed. In rare cases, these desquamated immature types of cells are observed in the ejaculated semen. (Low magnification.) (Courtesy of PAUL GETZOFF, M. D.,, New Orleans, Louisiana, USA)

glandular derangements, such as a decreased secretion from the Leydig cells of the testes, the thyroid, anterior pituitary and the adrenals, but such cases are not frequently encountered with infertile marriages, and when present, are so hopelessly infertile that they fall into the field of the endocrinologist rather than presenting an infertility problem. Most outstanding endocrinopathies cause an irreparable damage to the germinal epithelium of both testes which is already far beyond repair when first recognized, whether it be associated with Fröhlich's syndrome, insufficiency of the anterior pituitary, a disorder of the adrenal secretion or a deficiency of the Leydig cells.

Normal gametogenesis is dependent upon a very fine balance being maintained between the secretion of different glands of internal secretion. This balance is apparently maintained by means of a mechanism whereby an excessive secretion of one gland can exert an antagonistic effect on the action of another gland. The close relationship in the function of the adrenal, anterior pituitary and the

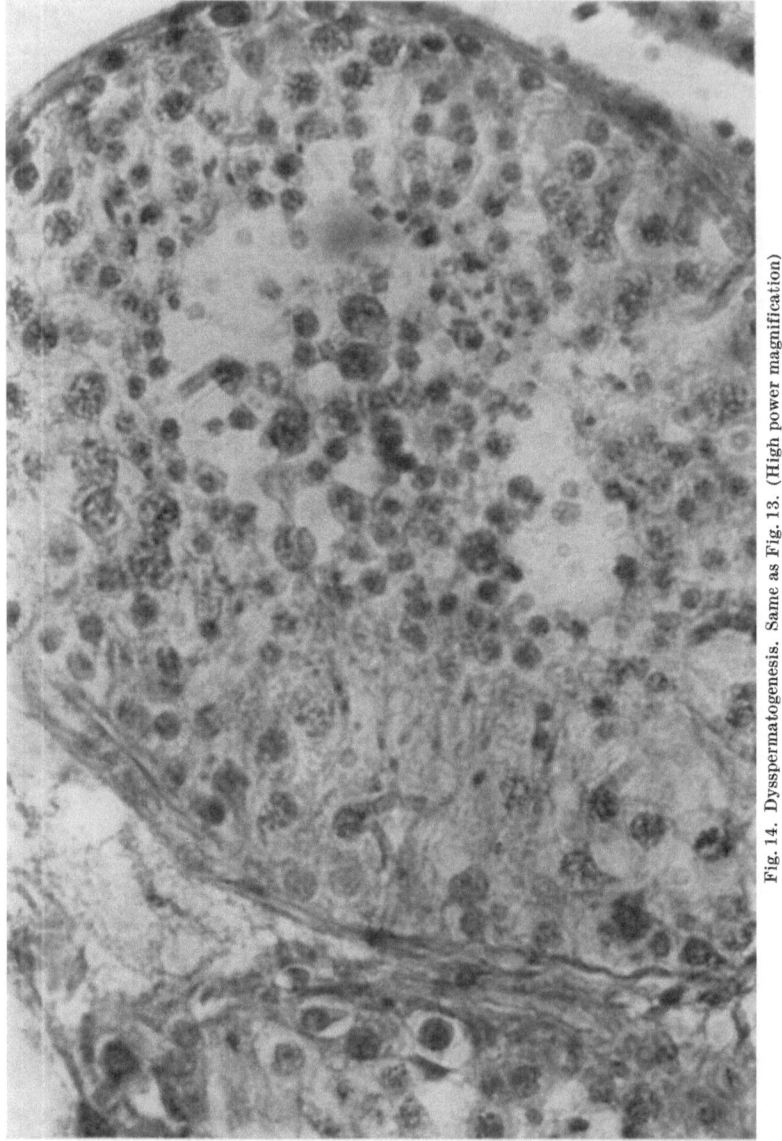

Fig. 14. Dysspermatogenesis. Same as Fig. 13. (High power magnification)

testicle and secretion of specific hormones produced by each of these glands is essential for gametogenesis. An excessive adrenal activity depresses the elaboration of pituitary gonadotropins. Such is also the case with androgen secretion. Thus, if the antagonistic action of the adrenal or of the androgen is withdrawn, there occurs in the urine an increase in F.S.H., or the anterior pituitary gonadotropins. On the other hand, if there is a failure of the anterior pituitary gland, as occurs in Fröhlich's syndrome, the urinary gonadotropins are reduced, and to a variable extent, there is a reduction in the 17-Ketosteroids which has resulted from a failure of Leydig cell stimulation by pituitary gonadotropins. Thus the germinal epithelium may be depressed either because of a primary defect of the Leydig cells or secondarily because a lack of stimulation by pituitary gonadotropins prevents an adequate androgen elaboration. Since a portion of the urinary 17-Ketosteroids is derived from the adrenals as well as from the Leydig cells, the urinary 17-Ketosteroid assay may not provide a true index to androgen elaboration. Excessive adrenal function exists in some instances and may be depressed by means of the administration of cortisone, which in turn would lessen the antagonistic action of the adrenal upon the pituitary. In a few instances, an increased spermatogenesis has been reported following the use of androgens in primary testicular failure; or the use of pituitary or anterior pituitary-like gonadotropins of placental origin has resulted in an increased spermiogenesis with cases which were not entirely devoid of germinal epithelium. However this may be, germinal disorders associated with infertility are so rarely of endocrine etiology, and endocrine damage to the germinal epithelium is so commonly irreparable that the endocrine approach to the problem of male infertility has essentially no value. Theoretically, it may seem possible to affect the character of spermiogenesis. This might occasionally be true were it not for the irreversible pathology of the germinal epithelium which exists so frequently in association with various types of clinically significant glandular disorders.

The effect of thyroid extract upon fertility has not been clearly evaluated, and many of the conceptions reported after its use are merely chance conceptions which are not related to therapy. Hyperthyroidism or Graves disease is seldom observed with infertility cases. Apparently an elevated basal metabolic rate is not detrimental to fertility, unless elevated sufficiently to produce symptoms of Graves disease. Thyroid extract does not exert any specific effect upon reproduction per se, and a lowered metabolic rate becomes important only when sufficiently depressed to affect the general health and well-being of the individual.

A basal metabolic rate which is not lower than minus twenty per cent seems to exert no perceptible influence upon the general health or upon fertility, and the empiric administration of thyroid to such cases does not as far as is known improve fertility or cause any significant alterations in the semen. If the basal metabolic rate is less than minus twenty per cent, thyroid therapy may improve the general state of health and vigor, and indirectly may favor a higher fertility. In general, the value of thyroid extract with infertility is limited to cases having a basal metabolic rate which is sufficiently lowered to affect the general health of the individual.

# IV. Functional, psychosomatic and emotional factors

## 1. Psychosomatic health

During the past few years, an increasing interest has been exhibited in psychosomatic factors as the cause of infertility. Psychosomatic aspects of fertility have been exceedingly difficult to evaluate because so frequently the accompanying general study of the infertility problem of one or both partners is inadequate. Thus, an improvement in the psyche may result from an improvement in somatic health, rather than the reverse. Most infertile couples desiring relief because of their infertility are emotionally very stable individuals and are not prone to psychosomatic episodes. They may be quite disturbed because of the failure of conception and the apparent hopelessness of their condition, but caution needs to be exercised that the cause and effect are not transposed. Those dealing with infertile marriages often observe that nervous tension promptly diminishes as soon as the patient commences to understand his condition and feels that the doctor is making a conscientious effort in his behalf.

Every doctor dealing with marital infertility must to a certain degree practice psychiatry. This does not mean that he should make a formal psychiatric examination, nor is it desirable that this be done. It will be found that some of the most valuable contributions to bringing emotional factors under control consist in their recognition and control during the course of other routine examinations, and in a manner that the patient is unaware that such an analysis is being made. Fears and anxieties are thus allayed.

The relatively high incidence of conception soon after the adoption of a baby is one of the most classical illustrations concerning the relation of the psyche or emotions to fertility. Some of these conceptions are apparently due merely to the lessening of the sexual load on the already overworked germinal epithelium of the male partner and the consequent increase in the fertilizing ability of the spermatozoa. With some, the same result might have been brought about by restricting the frequency of sexual relations, without adoption. On the other hand, anxiety and worry on the part of a woman subjected to rape does not seem to lessen the chances of conception. Various examples may be given where nervous or emotional influences affect ovulation, such as the mating of a rabbit which instigates ovulation, or when a woman under great emotional stress develops menstrual irregularities.

Psychic or emotional trauma affect the male in different ways. It may lead to excessive frequency of relations in a vain effort to compensate for the failure of conception. This serves to exhaust the germinal epithelium and lessen the viability of the spermatozoa. In other cases, the apparent futility of coitus seems to favor impotency, or the general health of the individual becomes impaired because the emotional upset has interfered with proper nutrition, sleep, rest and recreation. For this reason, it is important that the living habits, nutrition and sexual habits be explored. These various factors involving somatic health may arise from false ideas as to the means of overcoming infertility and this interferes with a normal healthy mode of living. Such emotional stresses and anxieties and their somatic manifestations commonly dissipate as a result of general health studies coupled with a free discussion of the factors involved. When the nervous system is so unstable that correction is not thereby accomplished, some question may arise as to the suitability of the individuals for parenthood and the desirability of a purely psychiatric approach.

## 2. Impotentia

Impotentia signifies the inability of the male to perform the sexual act and as commonly employed, it connotes the inability to attain or maintain an adequate erection of the penis. This is brought about principally by a psychic barrier or inhibition, but may also be due to some organic factor such as weakness of the ischiocavernosus muscle or to an interruption of the nerve pathways in the spinal cord, peripheral nerves or in the brain. In some instances, impotentia is associated with faulty nutrition, thyroid deficiency or other general health factors, but most commonly exists on a functional basis. Organic etiology of impotency includes such items as failure of adequate development of the generative organs, hernia, a large varicocele, large hydrocele, injury in perineal region, particularly involving the ischiocavernosus muscle in scar tissue, but these causes are indeed uncommon. An inflammation of the verumontanum may result in a premature ejaculation and impotentia.

Impotentia plays a role in the etiology of less than one-half per cent of the infertile marriages. Although it may occur at any age, it is more apt to develop as age advances. Occurring in individuals past the age of fifty, it is indeed rare that the ability to perform the sexual act will return under any type of therapy. Even with the younger age group, the chances for recovery after a few months of psychic impotentia is poor. Psychiatric therapy for this condition has not been highly satisfactory from the clinical viewpoint and many psychiatrists are loath to assume the responsibility for its therapy because of the poor results that they experience.

Psychic impotentia may be conditioned by various factors, such as

1. Lack of love of partner.

2. Fear or anxiety, such as fear of inadequacy either to satisfy his partner or properly demonstrate his male adequacy and satisfy his ego.

3. Homosexuality.

4. Masturbation, if employed as a substitute for sexual relations.

5. Fear of injury to himself or to his partner.

6. Feeling that sex act is unclean, improper or immoral.

7. Compulsion neurosis induced by inability to have coitus as frequently as desired. This may induce a vicious cycle in which the greater the effort, the less is the response.

8. Excessive frequency of coitus or masturbation.

Failure of erection may be partial or complete. In some instances, ejaculation results without erection, and with these, artificial insemination may overcome the infertility. Psychic impotentia is derived from diverse mental trauma which for its understanding may require the services of a physician experienced in psychoanalysis, thus bringing to the surface and into consciousness the inner repressions, tensions and inhibitions which have precipitated this difficulty. Occasionally, erection and ejaculation can be attained only by masturbation because a patient has conditioned himself in this manner and obtains no psychic response from the opposite sex. Impotentia following a long period of sexual overactivity is not uncommon, and with these especially, a laxness of the ischio-cavernosus muscle should be considered as the possible cause.

An anxiety or compulsion neurosis may play an important role with infertile marriages, especially if failure of conception prompts a frequency of relations in excess to normal tolerance. This excess then becomes to them an impelling necessity either to maintain their ego or unwisely compensate for the failure of the conception. Thus by exceeding their normal capacity, they condition themselves for impotentia, both mentally and physically.

Impotentia is not uncommon to unmarried men who are given to sexual excesses. These cases do not as a rule fall into the field of infertility and there is some question as to the ethical desirability of attempting to correct their impotency for the sole purpose of promiscuous sexual activity and bolstering their ego. The mental and emotional aspects of the subject seem to play a lesser role with the married men than with the unmarried. In either instance, but more particularly with the unmarried group, it is the oversexed individuals who develop the greatest difficulties and provide very refractory psychiatric problems. If their minds cannot be conditioned to the idea that it is possible for them to live more or less normal useful lives without the gratification of sexual desires as the principal purpose of living, nothing highly beneficial may be accomplished in their behalf.

# V. The character of seminal fluid

## 1. Volume

The volume of the ejaculated semen from most fertile men varies between 2 cc. and 7 cc., having a mean volume of 3.5 to 4.5 cc. Excepting for a small group of the infertile men with whom a testicular hypoplasia predicates a very small seminal volume, the volume range of the semen from the infertile and the fertile is similar. Because of this, the seminal volume furnishes no criterion whatever as to the quality of the sperm population and its potential fertility excepting when a volume of less than 1.5 cc. suggests a testicular and germinal hypoplasia. Such semen specimens with a small volume are commonly of a watery consistency. Likewise a volume of over 8 cc. is usually associated with permanent infertility in spite of the presence of apparently normal spermia (WILLIAMS 1953) (Fig. 15).

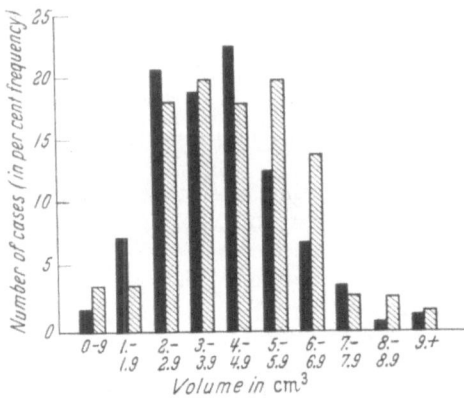

Fig. 15. *Relation of seminal volume to fertility.* Note that the incidence of conceptions is not materially different with the semen volumes ranging between two and seven cubic centimeters. When less than two cubic centimeters, a high incidence of pathologic spermatozoa is commonly present, which together with the low volume, may prevent cervical insemination with normal spermatozoa. A lowering of fertility associated with a semen volume of over seven cubic centimeters seems to be associated with two factors, an abnormality in the physiochemical properties of the substrat, or to an exhaustion of the seminal epithelium

357 Sterile cases ■■■ 150 Conceptions ▨

Ordinarily, there exists a regulating mechanism which provides that the volume of the ejaculate and the sperm concentration in it shall remain more or less constant for a given individual. Cases with a small seminal volume commonly exhibit a low sperm concentration and thus it becomes apparent that the function of the accessory glands may be influenced to a considerable extent by the same factor which is responsible for a germinal hypoplasia. Excessively long periods of abstinence fail to increase sperm concentration or seminal volume to any significant degree.

## 2. Physical properties

Seminal fluid is normally in a semi-gelatinous state when ejaculated. This is due to the presence of a fibrin-like substance which is soon acted upon by a fibrinolysin to cause its liquefaction so that within about fifteen minutes after ejaculation, the semen assumes a viscid or mucoid consistency. Because of this property, the semen is not so readily lost in its entirety from the vagina during the first few minutes after coitus, and sufficient time ordinarily elapses to permit the spermatozoa to find their way into the cervical mucus before the bulk of the seminal fluid is lost from the vaginal cavity.

Semen, as with estrual mucus, often presents considerable Spinnbarkeit, so that it may at times be pulled out into a string as long as twenty to thirty centimeters, although usually not more than four to five centimeters. The relation of its rheologic properties to fertility has not been evaluated, excepting that a thin, watery seminal fluid and a very thick viscid semen is frequently associated with a paucity of spermatozoa. The spermatozoa in these cases are often of poor quality and unsuitable for fertilization.

The color of seminal fluid is usually of a whitish or slightly yellowish hue, being colored by a pigment, and its varying opacity is largely determined by the concentration of spermatozoa. This opacity commonly increases after liquefaction if the sperm concentration is high. Specimens with a very low sperm concentration are more commonly translucent and of a watery consistency, and are a counterpart of faulty spermatogenesis; whereas the seminal fluid associated with azoospermia due to epididymal obstruction is usually of normal volume, consistency and color. Such semen without spermia may even present quite normal opacity because of a high leukocytic concentration. Semen ordinarily has a rather pungent odor which is apparently due to spermine.

## 3. Formed elements in the seminal fluid

One observes microscopically with the more normal semen, an abundance of normally shaped, highly motile spermatozoa migrating actively in a clear background which is essentially free of other formed elements. The presence of formed elements, such as cellular debris, cytoplasmic droplets, crystals, prostatic bodies, bacteria, white blood cells, immature spermatic cells or cells arising from different parts of the generative tract, generally indicate a disturbance of spermatogenesis or abnormal function of the accessory glands. Cytoplasmic masses and cellular debris are very commonly associated with faulty spermatogenesis. An abundance of spermine crystals assuming the shape of a truncated diamond are observed most frequently in association with low sperm concentrations. Leukocytes are frequently observed in the seminal fluid and are usually derived from the prostatic secretion. An acute urethritis as the source of leukocytes is not commonly encountered with infertility studies. The presence of leukocytes in the seminal or prostatic fluid seems to exert very little effect on the spermia and their potential fertility. Corollary to this, prostatic massage usually exerts very little effect upon the number of leukocytes in the prostatic secretion or on the fertility of the individual. The high leukocytic content of the prostatic secretion and of the semen in most infertility cases seems to occur because of a chronic passive congestion of the prostate, which is apparently not due to infection and does not respond to antibiotics.

One commonly observes in the seminal fluid large homogenous amyloid-like globules, known as prostatic bodies. They are several times the size of white blood corpuscles, may be mistaken for immature germinal cells at times, but in themselves are of no known clinical significance in so far as fertility is concerned.

## 4. Biochemistry of semen

The chemistry of semen is extremely complex and is altered by a large variety of factors. The fluid portion of semen is derived from a number of sources, such as the seminiferous tubules, the epididymides, the epithelium of the ejaculatory duct, the prostate, and the seminal vesicles. These structures contribute a variety of different chemical substances, so that the final product is a complex mixture of organic and inorganic substances, proteins, carbohydrates, the disintegration products of these anions and cations, enzymes, and other chemical substances such as those which are derived from the different anatomic components of the spermatozoa.

From the testes is derived hyaluronidase, an enzyme which was previously considered as possessing the property of breaking down the cells of the cumulus of the ovum and thus favoring the penetration of the ovum and its fertilization.

Both clinically and as the result of various laboratory observations, it seems that hyaluronidase possesses no such property and its clinical use fails to improve fertility (AUSTIN). It is claimed that the vasa deferentia and the ejaculatory ducts contribute fructose. The seminal vesicles produce fructose, cholin, carbonates, and a yellow pigment. From the prostate, such substances as acid phosphatase, spermin, and citric acid are derived, possibly some amino acids, fibrinogen, fibrokinase, a fibrolysin, and a proteolytic enzyme. Various other substances have been identified in the seminal fluid, including a bacterostatic substance, vitamin C, and vitamin B. Those desiring a more detailed survey of the chemical composition of the seminal fluid and its cellular components are referred to the work of MANN, HUGGINS and the general résumé of the biochemistry of the semen by GIAROLA.

Much of this work is merely of academic interest, and its clinical import at this time is not apparent. A few phases of the biochemical behavior of the seminal fluid and of the spermatozoa do, however, justify review, since they serve to furnish a better understanding of how alterations in the biochemistry of the sperm and the seminal fluid may influence the clinical evaluation of semen and the maintenance of fertility of the spermatozoa.

Various complex proteins which are present in the seminal fluid at the time of ejaculation, are soon acted upon by proteolytic enzymes and split into a variety of amino acids. Thus, the chemical composition of semen presents a changing picture owing to its original composition, the character of its cellular content, temperature, hydrogen ion concentration, the time elapsing since ejaculation, and many other factors. These changes serve to alter the motility and fertility of the spermatozoa.

Commencing within four or five hours after ejaculation, the degree of motility changes rapidly under the influence of the length of time that these seminal variables have operated and the intrinsic quality of the spermia. Accordingly, a motility examination may merely register the progress of a deteriorative process which is common to all semen and may not indicate the initial fertilizing ability. The chemical findings do, however, explain some of the marked changes occurring in the seminal fluid under different influences, and these should be taken into consideration when evaluating the significance of immotility of ejaculated spermatozoa. The knowledge that such changes do occur with all semen specimens unless the action of enzymes is depressed by freezing, suggests that most favorable conditions for a motility examination commence with the liquefaction of the semen, which usually occurs within fifteen minutes after ejaculation, and terminates within four to five hours. During this period there is very little loss of motility with specimens kept at 60° to 70° F., thus indicating a natural retardation of deteriorative processes over a brief period. Thereafter many changes occur which affect motility and sperm survival without necessarily giving any index of the fundamental vitality of the spermia. For instance, the normal vaginal acidity of about pH 4.5 is essential for the maintenance of vaginal bacteriostasis, but is not favorable for sperm survival within the vagina for more than two or three hours. If the vagina becomes alkaline, there will be an overgrowth of an unfavorable vaginal bacterial flora, which is much more detrimental to the spermia than normal acidity.

The mature sperm possesses highly specialized structures which are of a somewhat different chemical composition than those encountered with somatic cells or ova (GREEN, MARKUS). The different spermatic structures, such as the nucleus, acrosome, centriolar bodies, axillary filament, shell of the nucleus, sheath of the middle piece, and spiral filament, each make specific contributions to the chemistry of the spermatozoön (GIAROLA, WILLIAMS). Thus, one observes a chitinous-like covering of the nucleus which is quite distinctive of mammalian spermatozoa, and also the specialized structures of the caudal extremity, which present no analogues in form and chemistry to other types of cells.

The chemical composition of the ejaculated semen is affected by various intrinsic and extrinsic influences to which the seminal fluid and the spermatozoa are subjected, not only prior to ejaculation but also subsequently, either in vivo or in vitro. Thus after ejaculation the influences of proteolytic enzymes, bacterial growth, and sperm metabolism proceed rather rapidly, causing progressive changes in the chemical picture and motility according to the time elapsing since ejaculation. Such deteriorative influences advance much more rapidly at a temperature of 80⁰ to 90⁰ F. than between 60⁰ and 70⁰, since the higher temperature is more favorable to the destructive influence of enzymic action, bacterial multiplication, and the collection of sperm metabolites. The physiologic changes in the chemical composition of the seminal fluid are principally related to the metabolic processes associated with fructolysis and to enzymic activity.

Fructolysis is dependent upon the fundamental health of the spermatozoa, their concentration in the seminal fluid, their kinetic activity, the presence of an amylase, and the proper conditions as to temperature, hydrogen ion concentration, electrolyte balance, and osmotic pressure. The oxidation of glycogen and fructose furnishes the energy required for sperm motility (MANN, BIRNBERG) but there is no evidence that fertility is related to the rate of glycolysis (DAVIS). The metabolism of spermatozoa may be measured by means of the WARBURG technique (MACLEOD), which in effect measures the oxidation of glycogen associated with energy production.

If, following the technique of SORENSON, a given amount of methylene blue is added to semen, the methylene blue will be decolorized because of dehydrogenization of the spermia, liberating oxygen, which is accepted by the methylene blue and causes its decoloration. This reaction is dependent upon the concentration of motile spermatozoa and upon the degree of their motility. Since the life span of motile spermatozoa is very limited, the methylene blue decoloration test is dependent at any given time upon the age of the specimen on which the tests are conducted, unless there has been an artificial depression of metabolism by some factor such as low temperature or increased carbon dioxide tension. Corollary to this, live spermatozoa may be stained by various vital stains, or, on the contrary, devitalized spermatozoa can be identified by means of eosin staining, which stain is accepted only by the dead spermatozoa.

Thus the motility, glycolysis, vital staining, and the eosin live-dead staining method of BLOM run a parallel course in indicating diminished or absent metabolism. The ratio and degree of motility of the in vitro specimen generally represents a stage in the progressive deterioration and death of the sperm population, and is associated with a corresponding reduction in metabolism of the different spermia, according to differences in their fundamental health.

### Enzymic action, jelling of semen, and liquefaction

The temporary gelatinous state of the freshly ejaculated semen is due to the presence of fibrinogen and thromboplastin. Within a few minutes after ejaculation, the action of a fibrolytic enzyme which is apparently derived from the prostate causes liquefaction of the seminal fluid (HUGGINS).

There is a splitting of various protein substances present in the ejaculated semen by means of proteolytic enzymes, so that after two hours or so various free amino acids appear in the seminal fluid (LUNDQUIST). It seems likely that the presence of free amino acids exerts an important influence in the loss of fertility, since vitality endures longer if enzymic action is retarded by cold. The accumulation of lactic acid, hydrogen peroxide, and other products of enzymic action and metabolism serves to lessen the kinetic activity of the spermatozoa and their potential fertility, but the spermatozoa deposited at the external os, which migrate promptly into the cervical mucus, are liberated at once from various of these deleterious influences.

In the above respects, it is noted that the fundamental chemical processes which transpire in the semen and spermatozoa of different species of mammals are analogous, with the exception of minor specie differences. In general, if the circumstances required for optimum kinesis are provided, the above changes transpire more rapidly and the spermatozoa perish sooner because of exhaustion or the accumulation of products of enzymic activity, metabolism, or perhaps bacterial end products. This happens either in vitro or in vivo. In vitro, the lack of the buffer system and the lack of the bacteriostatic action of the cervical mucus favor earlier death of the spermatozoa than is the case with the more ideal environment of the normal cervical canal and the endometrium.

On the other hand, it has been shown with bovine spermatozoa that depressing the temperature of the semen by freezing with carbon dioxide ice to —79⁰ C. serves to prevent sperm metabolism and enzymic action, and thereby prolongs indefinitely the life and fertilizing ability of the spermatozoa. Under such circumstances, it has been found that skimmed milk is a satisfactory diluent to provide a desirable chemical balance for sperm survival and fertility. The addition of 5 to 10 per cent glycerol serves to prevent the crystallization incident to freezing and thereby lessens death from the shock of freezing. A buffered egg yolk extender is also used (DUNN). Although one would assume that human spermatozoa might survive freezing as well as bovine spermatozoa, the reports by BUNGE and SHERMAN of survival and fertility of human spermatozoa after deep freezing have not been confirmed. Employing the various techniques described for human semen and also that used in cattle breeding operations, the writer has observed that over 95 per cent of human spermatozoa usually perish during the freezing and thawing process and the remainder are only feebly motile. An improvement in the technical aspects of freezing and thawing of human spermatozoa will be necessary before frozen human semen can be successfully used for insemination.

## VI. The characteristics of sperm populations

For many years, it has been attempted to define a normal fertile sperm and what constitutes a normal sperm population. The great difficulty in accomplishing this is that spermatozoa follow the same rule of variability in viability, size, shape and general structure as pertains to every living thing in nature, and although there does exist a great predominance of very similar spermatozoa in the semen of the highly fertile, it is nevertheless true that a considerable variability exists even with the most fertile. Sperm populations composed mostly of definitely abnormal spermia may contain a few normal healthy spermatozoa which are perfectly capable of causing fertilization. Unfortunately, patient and physicians alike become discouraged when it is discovered that they cannot definitely differentiate the fertile and infertile and must deal with the law of probabilities with which there is no sharp line of distinction between the normal and abnormal, or the fertile and infertile.

A normal, highly fertile sperm population is composed of typically full oval-shaped spermatozoa which are surprisingly uniform in size and shape (Fig. 16). If the cells of such a population are measured and a curve plotted so as to show the variability in size, a normal monomodal curve results. On the other hand, many sterility cases show wide variations in size and shape of the cells. These exhibit wide variabilities in potential fertility, and if a group of cells are measured, either in respect to the longitudinal or transverse diameters of their heads, it is found that abnormal curves result, some of which are of a skew pattern because of the excessive frequency of either extremely small or large spermatozoa in the sperm population (SAVAGE, WILLIAMS and FOWLER; MOENCH).

Various portions of the sperm present abnormalities which may interfere with motility or with the fertilization of the ovum. These include the nucleus, acrosome, centriolar bodies and various portions of the caudal extremity. Aside from this, various apparently minor structures such as the thin outer covering of the acrosome, termed the galea capitis, and a thin covering of the nucleus, the nuclear shell, and the fibrillae of the tail likewise have an essential function to perform. Without these structures, fertilization does not occur.

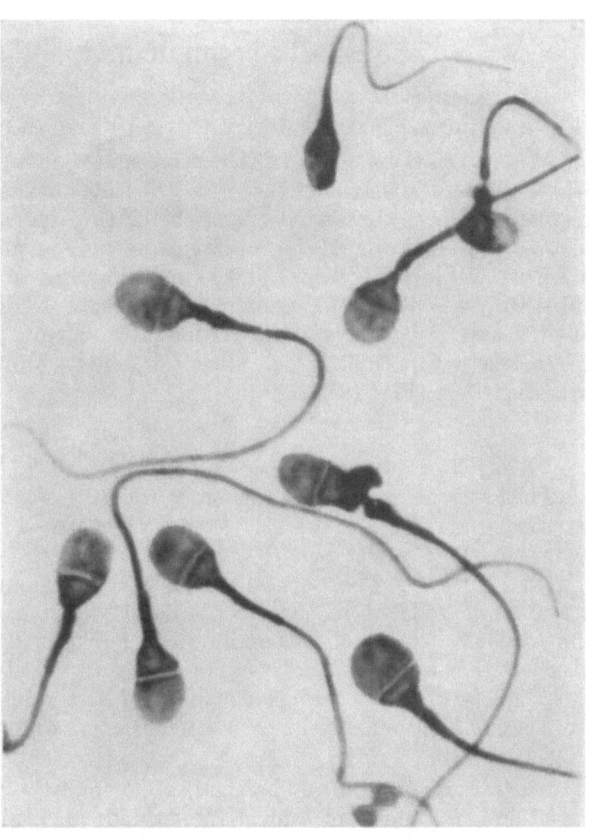

Fig. 16. *Normal sperm population.* Note the uniformity as to size and shape of the spermatozoa and the transverse line where the galea capitis contacts the shell of the nucleus

There is, however, a difference in the clinical significance of different types of spermatic abnormalities. Thus a given ratio of acrosomic abnormalities may have a somewhat greater significance from the viewpoint of infertility than the same ratio of nuclear abnormalities, and the presence of abnormalities of the mitochondrial sheath may be very highly significant even when less than five per cent of the sperm population is visibly involved. In rare instances, one observes a considerable number of immature gametes.

Accordingly, in the appraisal of fertility, it is desirable to know something of the nature of the abnormality as well as the extent to which the sperm population is involved. About fifty per cent of male infertility is associated with extremely high ratios of pathologic spermatozoa, and clinically it is very evident that the fertility of these individuals is permanently reduced or destroyed thereby. The clinical significance of these cases has been rather clouded by a somewhat prevalent teaching that the structure of the male gamete is unimportant and all that is needed is an abundant supply of motile, migratory spermatozoa, a viewpoint which seems to have been conditioned by the frequent omission of cytologic observations on spermatozoa of the suspected infertile, and disregarding the common clinical observation that a high incidence of acrosomic anomalies commonly provide a high ratio of actively migratory cells.

## 1. Spermatic morphology [1, 2]

For description, a spermatozoön may be divided into five principal parts, the head, neck-piece, middle-piece, tail-piece and end-piece (Fig. 17).

Wide variations occur in the different anatomic components of male gametes when spermiogenesis is pathologic, affecting one or more of its structures. This results in bizarre conformations of the mature spermatozoa, due to the variations in size and contour of its various anatomic components; and with different observers, this has prompted the manufacture of fantastic terminologies as a substitute for a knowledge of cytology and cytologic nomenclature. As a result of this and the failure to use adequate staining methods, a consideration of spermatic cytopathology is quite frequently omitted as a part of infertility investigations (Fig. 18).

### a) Head

The head of the spermatozoön is roughly of an oval contour when observed flatwise, but when viewed laterally, there is a marked narrowing anteriorly owing to the flatness of the acrosome which rests on the anterior pole of the rounded nucleus. The normal sperm head is about 4.6 microns long and about 2.6 microns wide at its largest diameter which usually lies slightly anterior to the nucleus. The nucleus commonly occupies a little less than one-half of the head at its caudal end and is capped over anteriorly by the acrosome into which the slightly rounded anterior aspect of the nucleus bulges. One observes a transverse line across the head where the acrosome and the nucleus meet (Fig. 16, 17, 19).

*Nuclear abnormalities.* Nuclear abnormalities are usually distinguished by variations in their size and shape. Such variations can be more readily distinguished if a staining process is used that will differentiate the nucleus from the acrosome and the caudal extremity. Commonly, the abnormal nuclei present various degrees of constriction of their transverse diameters and lengthening of their longitudinal diameters, although in some, the nucleus is of normal shape but either too large or small (Fig. 20).

*Acrosomic abnormalities.* Marked differences in both the size and shape of the acrosome are common to infertile patients, and if a sufficiently high ratio of the population is involved, this results in intractable sterility (Fig. 21). Usually this abnormality is tolerated up to a ratio of about fifteen to twenty per cent without any apparent effect upon fertility, but when this ratio is exceeded, the incidence of failures in conceptions rises. Vacuoles of various sizes are commonly observed in the acrosome of the normally fertile as well

---

[1] This description of the anatomy of the spermatozoön is from the volume "Sterility" by courtesy of the author, WALTER W. WILLIAMS.

[2] For the finer details of sperm structure as indicated by electron microscope studies, the reader is referred to the monograph by J. SCHULTZ-LARSEN, Published by VILLARS LUNN, Copenhagen, May 1958.

as the infertile individual, sometimes rupturing and leaving a nick in the surface of the acrosome. Occasionally, the acrosome is enlarged or markedly elongated, but the most common acrosomic anomaly consists of various degrees of deficient development. With a small acrosome, the head becomes more spherical in shape,

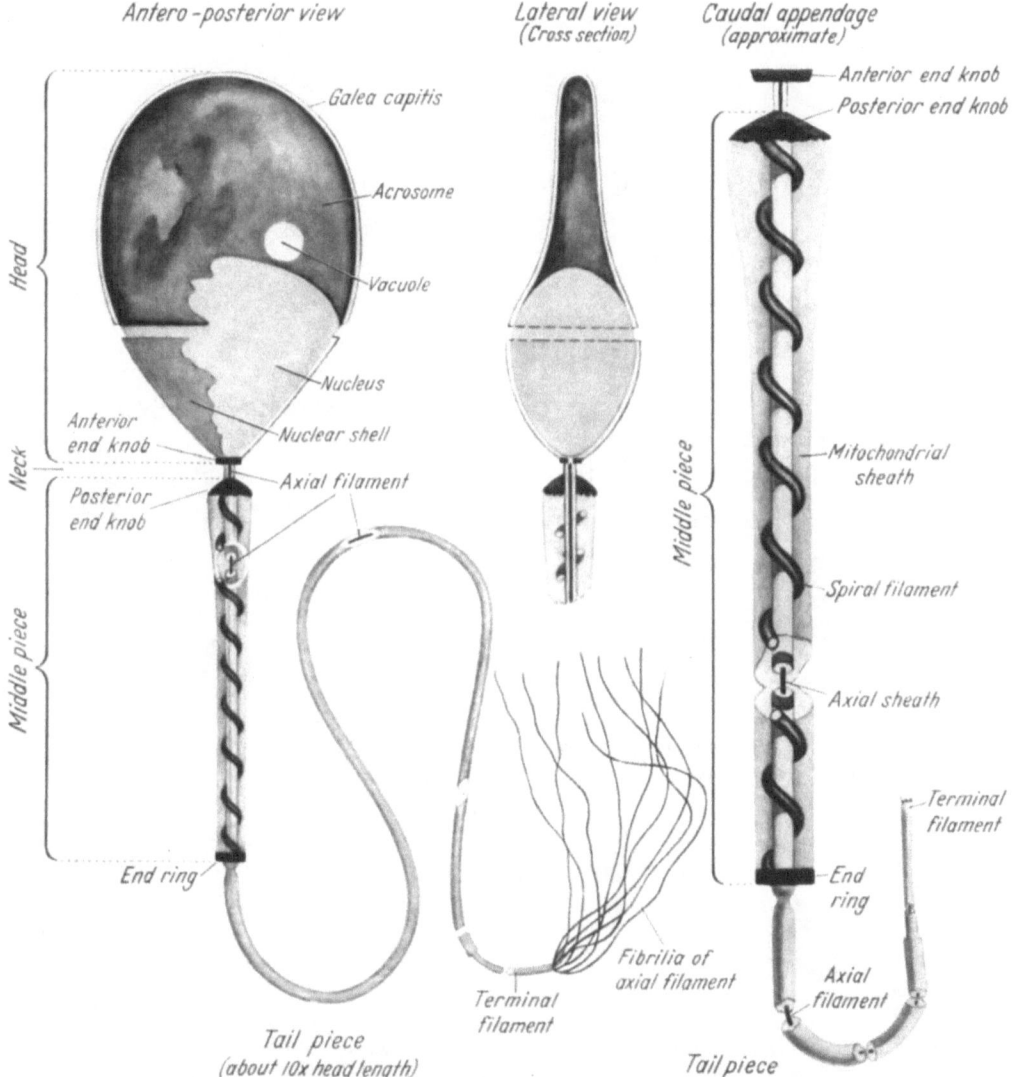

Fig. 17. *Structure of the spermatozoön.* A composite representation of structure based upon studies with the compound microscope, electron microscope and microchemical methods

and if absent, the sperm head stains only with a nuclear stain and appears as a globoid, homogeneous mass which is about one-half of the size of the normal sperm head. Such cells ordinarily possess normal caudal appendages and frequently exhibit high mobility.

*Galea capitis and nuclear shell.* Covering the acrosome and coinciding with its surface, is a very thin membrane termed the galea capitis. There is also an outer covering over the nucleus, termed the nuclear shell (MARKUS, WILLIAMS 1953), into which the nucleus fits as an acorn in its shell. Where the nuclear shell and the galea capitis meet, and corresponding to the line of contact between them, one observes a line transversely across the sperm head. The

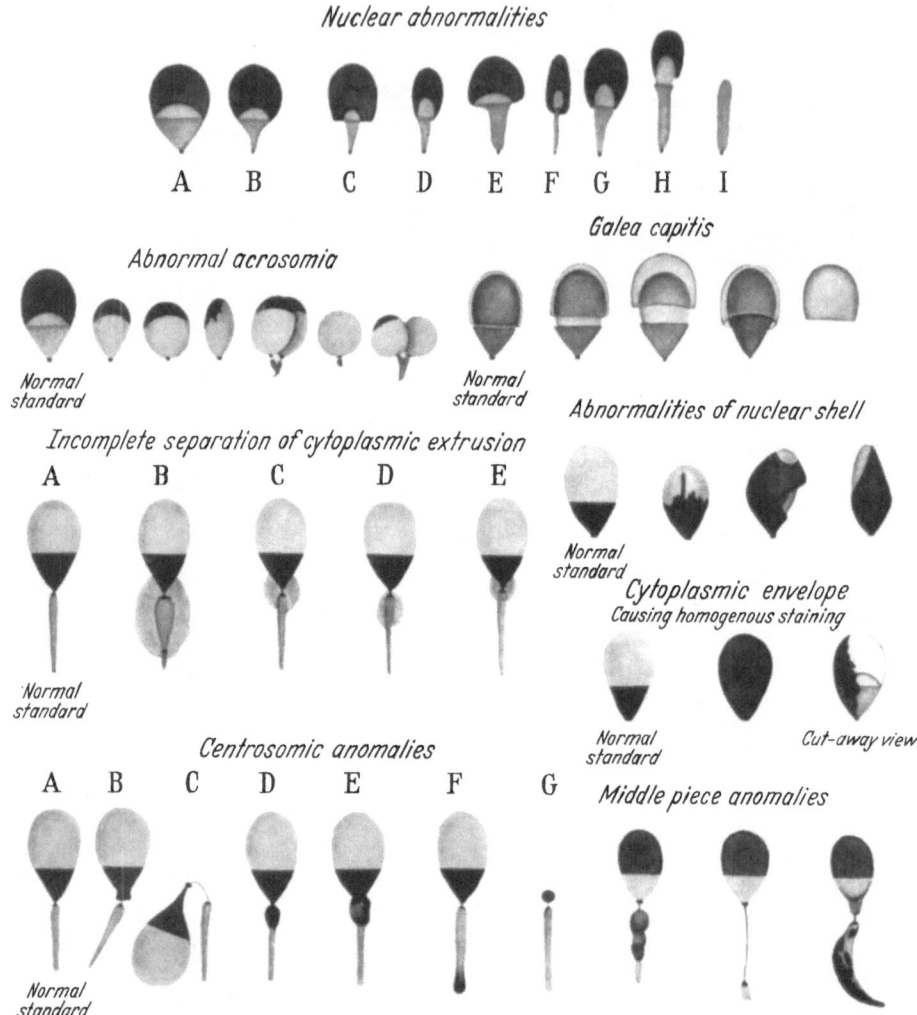

Fig. 18. *Miscellaneous spermatic abnormalities.* Each of the various anatomical components of spermatozoön are subject to pathologic changes. These cause a vast array of different types of spermatozoa according to the part or parts of the cell involved in the abnormality

galea capitis is readily identified with the spermia of some animals, particularly the bovine species (BLOM), where its loosening or separation from the acrosome is noted with the aging of the semen. With homo, however, the galea is an extremely delicate covering and is rarely observed, except in instances where its loosening and forward displacement may be recognized by the presence of a narrow band across the middle of the sperm head which results from the posterior margin of the galea pulling away from the nuclear shell (Fig. 16).

The nuclear shell is a thin membranous structure which overlies and usually coincides with the area occupied by the nucleus, excepting for the portion of the nucleus which arches upwards into the acrosome. It is very easily distinguished from the underlying nucleus by the difference in staining affinities. Its anterior margin meets the posterior margin of the galea capitis, where it ordinarily forms a single transverse line across the mid-portion of the nuclear head. Occasionally one observes a defect in this covering. In other instances, in association with a very marked elongation of the caudal end of the nucleus, the nuclear shell is pulled entirely off the nucleus and forms a bulbous mass at the caudal nuclear pole which may, without proper staining, be mistaken for the nucleus, an enlargement of the middle-piece or a cytoplasmic extrusion. The nuclear shell stains with crystal violet which is not removed with ninety five per cent alcohol, whereas this stain is not retained by the nucleus, cytoplasmic extrusions or any portion of the caudal extremity (Fig. 22).

*Anterior end knob or proximal centriolar body.* The centriolar body in the mature sperm is commonly observed as a small, discoid granule which is closely applied to the caudal end of the nucleus. It is best revealed by the use of a cytoplasmic stain. With the electron microscope, the centriolar body may be resolved as three distinct granules from which the fibrillae of the axillary filament of the caudal appendage arise. Abnormalities

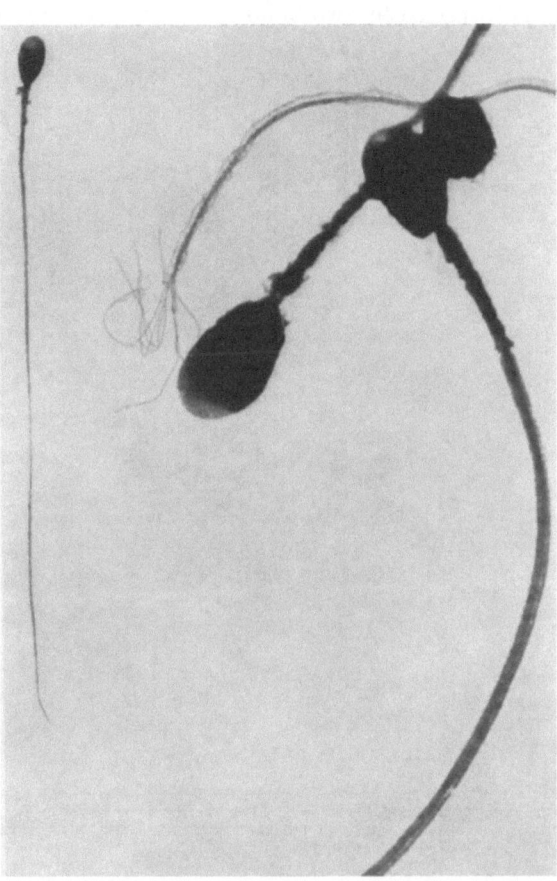

Fig. 19. *An electron photomicrograph of spermatozoön.* Note the portions of the caudal extremity the middle-piece. The ordinary at the posterior end of the middle-piece and the fine helix which surrounds the axial filament of the tail-piece. A nick at the side of the head reveals the site of the anterior margin of the nuclear shell. (Courtesy of ALBERT TYLER, Ph. D., Pasadena Institute of Technology, Pasadena, California, USA)

of the centriolar body become apparent in a number of conditions. In the miniature sperm or the so-called pin-head, the small mass which is regarded as the head actually consists only of the centriolar body. This appears as a small granule at the anterior end of the middle-piece and there is a complete absence of the nucleus and acrosome. Such cells may be highly motile. An enlargement of the centriolar body is frequently associated with a disturbance in the formation of the mitochondrial sheath of the middle-piece, with an abnormal lengthening of the neck-piece and with the abaxial attachment of the caudal appendage.

## b) Caudal appendage

The caudal appendage may be divided into four parts, the neck-piece, middle-piece, tail-piece and end-piece (Fig. 23).

*Neck-piece.* The neck-piece in most stained preparations appears as a lucid zone of about 0.5 microns long, lying between the caudal pole of the head and the middle-piece. Examined with the electron microscope, it is observed that it is traversed by two bundles of the axillary fibrillae which have arisen from the

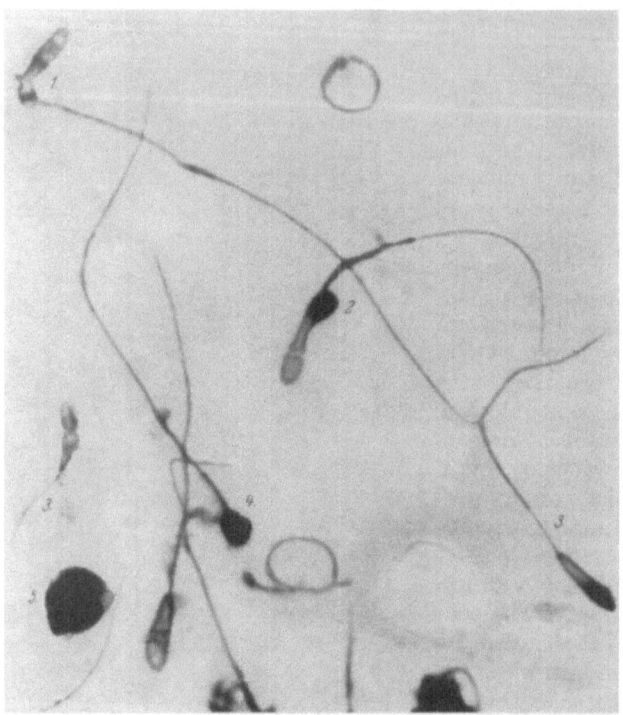

Fig. 20. *Nuclear abnormalities.* All of the spermatozoa in this specimen were abnormal. Note the narrowness and elongation of the nuclei (case 510). *1* Displaced nuclear shell, *2* cytoplasmic extrusion mass, *3* absence of mitochondrial sheath, *4* absence of acrosome, *5* immature sperm

lateral granules of the centriolar body and a single filament arising from the centrally situated centriolar granule. Surrounding these fasiculae, there exists a sheath which is not observed by ordinary microscopic methods because of its refractoriness to common stains, but may be visualized with the aid of the electron microscope. In some pathologic specimens, one observes a great lengthening of the neck-piece so that in locomotion, the head turns backward along the side of the body.

*Middle-piece.* The middle-piece is a thickened portion of the caudal extremity, lying between the neck anteriorly and the tail-piece posteriorly. Its diameter is about 0.3 microns, and its length is about the same as the head. The middle-piece is traversed through its entire length by a bundle of axillary filaments, which arise from the centriolar granules at the base of the head and terminate in the tail-piece (BRETSCHNEIDER, SCHNALL). The central axillary fibrillae are enclosed in a sheath, termed the mitochondrial sheath, composed of a spiral of two or three strands which make as many as eight to ten turns around its axis. Over the spirals, there is a thin covering of a cementing substance, and about the axillary filament, there is also a thin layer which seems to be a continuation of the sheath of the tail-piece.

*Tail-piece.* The tail-piece is the part of the caudal appendage which lies between the middle-piece anteriorly and the terminal filament posteriorly. It is ordinarily about eight to ten times the length of the head. It is composed of

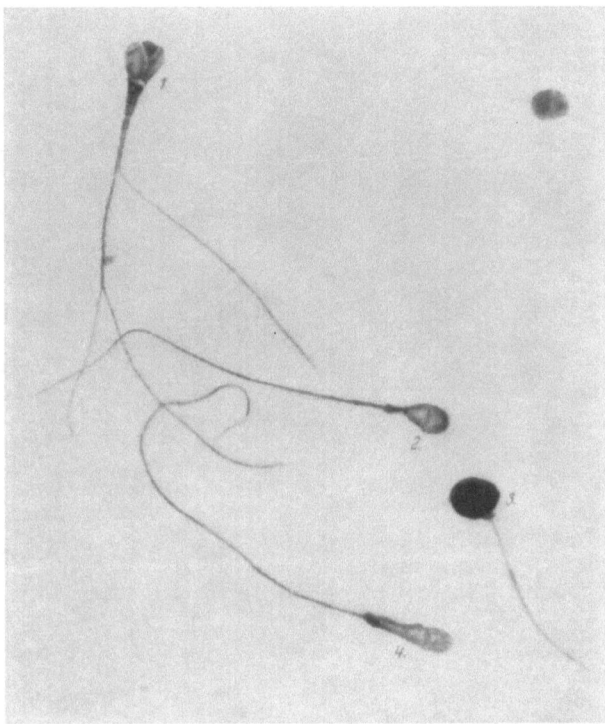

Fig. 21. *Acrosomic abnormalities.* Most of the spermatozoa of this population are deficient in acrosomic development, and consequently are smaller than normal. With some, there is a complete absence of the acrosome. Pairing of cells without an acrosome is common and is due to their failure to separate during the last stages of spermiogenesis. A single large immature type of cell is shown which stains dark because of its cytoplasmic covering

an axial fasiculus or core, containing nine or more fibrillae, which is surrounded by a cytoplasmic or cortical sheath. This sheath is largely composed of a helix of extremely fine fibrillae which spiral about the tail-piece for its entire length. Apparently it is the contraction of the mitochondrial spiral and the axillary filaments which is responsible for the motility of the sperm. The functional integrity of these seem to relate to the health of the centriolar bodies from which the fasiculus arises.

*End-piece.* The end-piece is the terminal segment of the caudal extremity. It is usually of about the same length as the head. There is ordinarily a thin cementing substance which binds together its axillary filaments so that under the oil immersion lens, it appears as a single filament. With specimens prepared for examination under the electron microscope, the cementing substance is frequently broken down, causing a separation of the individual fibrillae of the fasiculus so that one observes as many as nine to eleven fibrillae forming a tassel at the end of the tail-piece (Fig. 19, 24).

*Abnormalities of the caudal appendage.* Abnormalities of the caudal appendage usually occur in ratios of less than one per cent in the normal, fertile semen, but with the infertile may occur in much larger ratios. Such abnormalities seem to indicate a profound disturbance in spermiogenesis because when more than five to ten per cent of the sperm population is so involved, other pathology is also quite prevalent and the fertility of the individual is markedly impaired

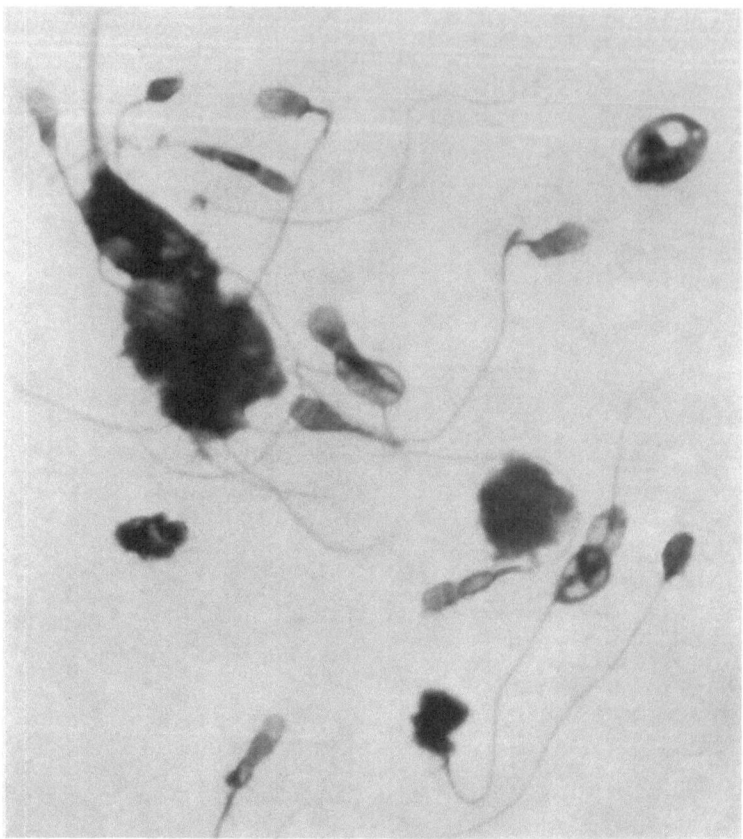

Fig. 22. *Pathologic nuclei with displacement of the nuclear shell.* When there is a very marked narrowing and elongation of the nucleus, its thin membranous covering, the nuclear shell, often slips caudalwards to form a bulbous mass at the caudal pole of the sperm. This mass is easily confused with a cytoplasmic extrusion mass or middle-piece anomaly but may easily be distinguished with a crystal violet-rose bengal stain, since cytoplasmic masses and middle-piece stain reddish, and the nuclear shell is colored blue

(WILLIAMS 1956). Most caudal appendage anomalies involve the mitochondrial sheath so that one observes a thickening of the middle-piece, or in others a bare axial filament. In about one per cent of male infertility, there exists a distinctive type of centriolar-mitochondrial disorder which is identified by immobility of most or all of the sperm population, an elongation and thickening of the middle-piece, a slight enlargement of the anterior end-knob, an elongation of the neck-piece, together with an abbreviated or absent tail-piece (WILLIAMS 1950). This signifies a progressive disorder of spermiogenesis, and as far as is known, it always leads to a progressive involvement of the entire sperm population with total and permanent sterility (Fig. 25, 26).

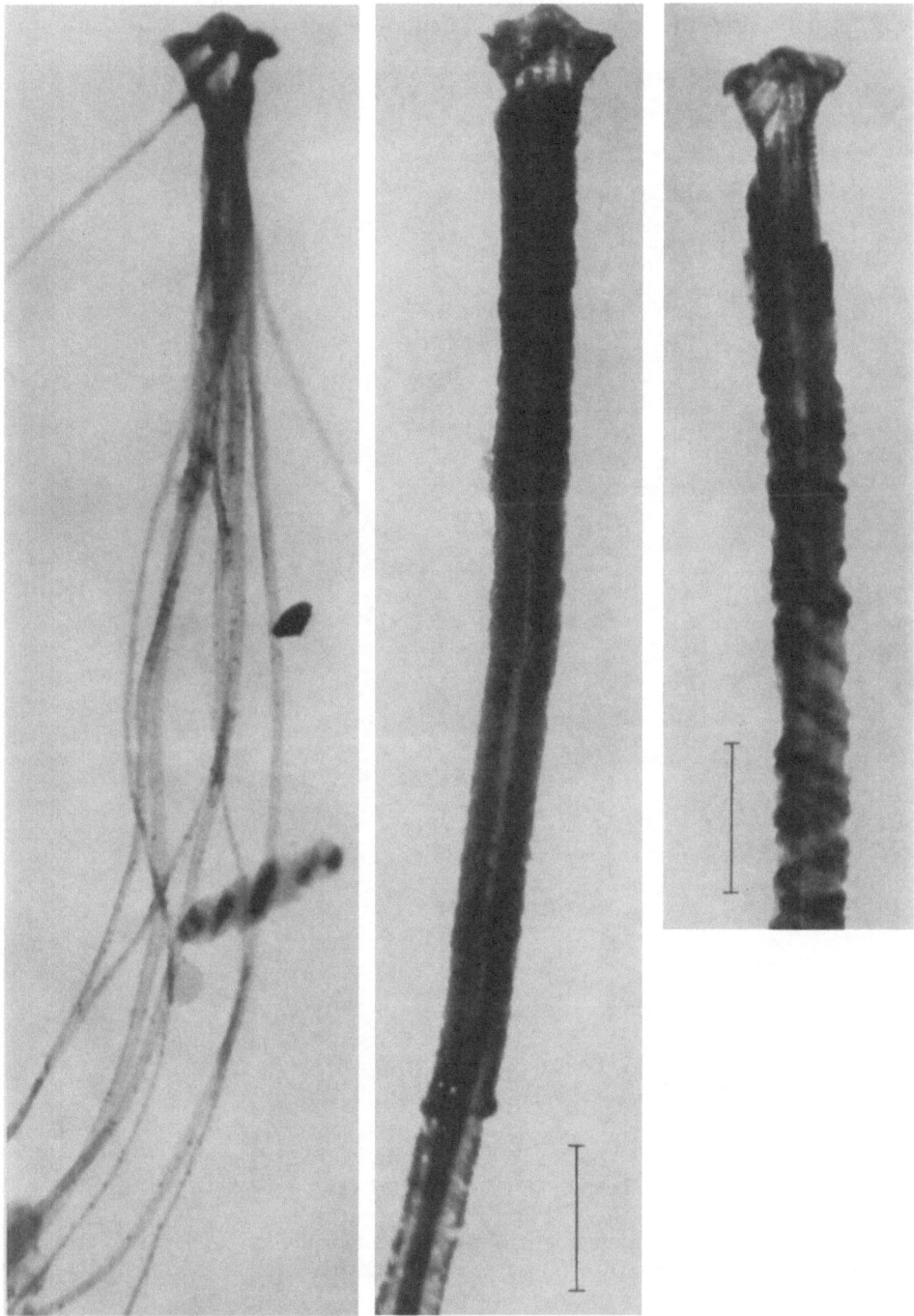

Fig. 23. *Electron photomicrograph of middle-piece of bovine spermatozoa.* Note segmental character of axillary fibrillae at neck region, that the axillary fibrillae arise from the proximal centriolar body and that there is a difference in the type of spiral filaments surrounding the middle-piece and tail-piece. The photomicrograph on the left reveals the individual fibrillae of the axillary filament which were separated by dissolving off the sheath of the middle-piece and tail-piece. 1) 16 000×; 2) and 3) 20 000×.
(Courtesy of Dr. L. H. BRETSCHNEIDER, Utrecht, Netherlands)

In some semen specimens, one observes a high incidence of coiled tails. This occurs frequently in association with immature spermatozoa, but more fre-

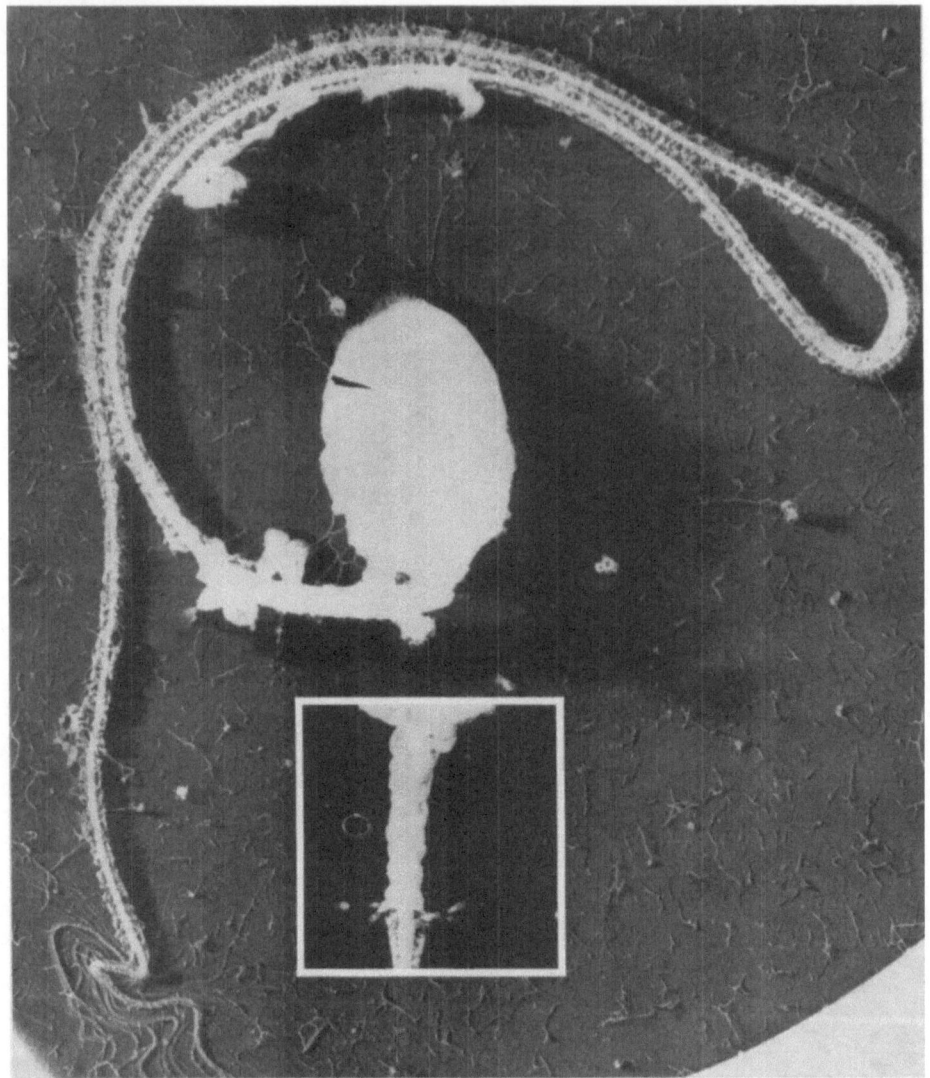

Fig. 24. *Human spermatozoon.* Note dense mitochondrial sheath of the middle-piece with the lateral undulations resulting from the dense filament which spirals about this segment of the caudal appendage. A nick in the cytoplasmic sheath separates the middle-piece from the main-piece which is surrounded for its entire length by a very fine, fibrillar helix. By courtesy of JORGEN SCHULTZ-LARSEN and RICHARDT HAMMEN, Copenhagen, Denmark

quently it seems to be independent of abnormal morphology and possibly exists because of a disturbance in osmotic pressure (EMMONS).

### c) Immature spermatozoa

Immature spermatozoa may be defined as those cells which have not yet passed through the final stages of spermiogenesis. Apparently, the final stage of the spermiogenesis consists of the extrusion of a small cytoplasmic droplet from the caudal pole of the head. This cytoplasmic mass is commonly observed attached around the middle-piece or at the distal pole of the head, and the spermatozoa may be quite fully developed in other respects. In the transition

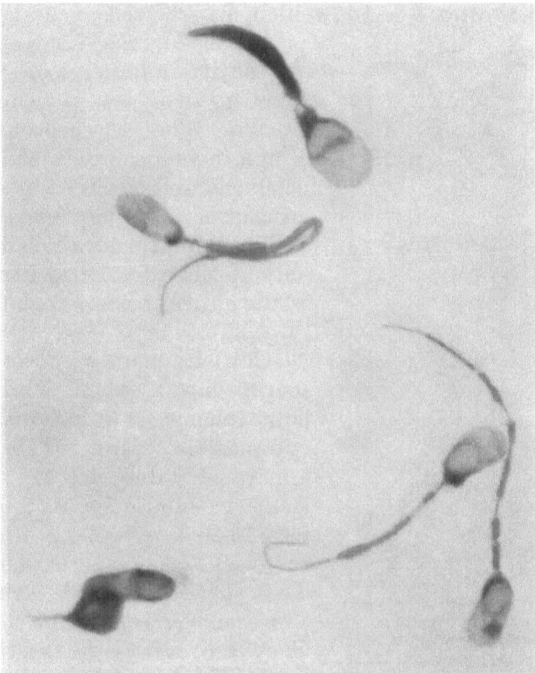

Abb. 25

Fig. 25. *Centriolar-mitochondrial disease of spermatozoa.* This abnormality generally involves the entire sperm population and causes complete immobility. The sperm head usually appears normal, but there is an enlargement of the proximal centriolar body, an elongation of the neck-piece, the mitochondrial sheath of the middle-piece is disorganized, there is commonly no evidence of a tail-piece but a bare end-piece is visible

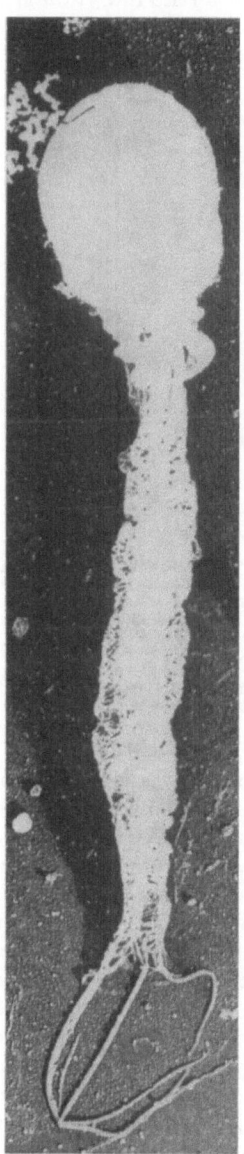

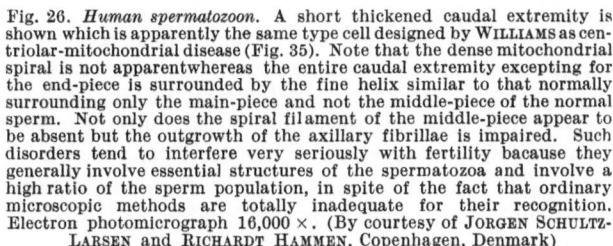

Fig. 26. *Human spermatozoon.* A short thickened caudal extremity is shown which is apparently the same type cell designed by WILLIAMS as centriolar-mitochondrial disease (Fig. 35). Note that the dense mitochondrial spiral is not apparent whereas the entire caudal extremity excepting for the end-piece is surrounded by the fine helix similar to that normally surrounding only the main-piece and not the middle-piece of the normal sperm. Not only does the spiral filament of the middle-piece appear to be absent but the outgrowth of the axillary fibrillae is impaired. Such disorders tend to interfere very seriously with fertility because they generally involve essential structures of the spermatozoa and involve a high ratio of the sperm population, in spite of the fact that ordinary microscopic methods are totally inadequate for their recognition. Electron photomicrograph 16,000 ×. (By courtesy of JORGEN SCHULTZ-LARSEN and RICHARDT HAMMEN, Copenhagen, Denmark)

Abb. 26

from the secondary spermatocyte stage to that of the mature spermatozoön, there is a marked loss of moisture from the nucleus. In consequence, the immature cell commonly possesses a much larger nucleus than the mature cell (Fig. 21, 27).

Extrusion of undifferentiated cytoplasm from the head of the sperm marks the final stage of spermiogenesis and signifies in general that the various intracellular changes of spermiogenesis affecting the nucleus, acroblast, mitochondria and centrioles, together with the budding out of the caudal appendage, have already transpired and that the cell has reached its mature stage. Small cytoplasmic rests, the remnants of these extrusions, are so common to the spermatozoa from fertile individuals that they can hardly be considered as pathologic. Larger cytoplasmic masses adhering to the neck region which may be nearly as large as the head, may surround the entire middle-piece and show no evidence of disintegration. When these occur in a high incidence, they should be considered as clinically significant because they represent a slight immaturity which may reduce the functional fitness of the entire sperm population (Fig, 27).

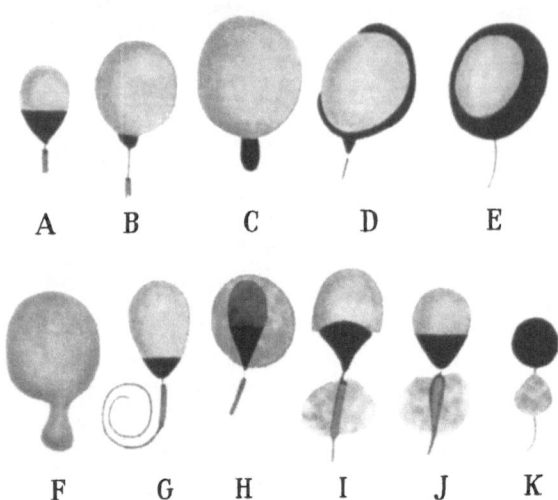

Fig. 27. *Immature types of spermatozoa* (drawings). If gametes in the spermatocyte stage are desquamated, they may appear in the seminal fluid. Desquamated spermatocytes occur in the semen very rarely and appear as illustrated in testicular biopsy specimens. Most immature cells in ejaculated semen are of the spermatid stage or exhibit incomplete cytoplasmic extrusions as here illustrated with different degrees of budding of the caudal appendage. These cells are usually larger in size than the mature spermatozoön because the latter loses in moisture and shrinks during spermiogenesis. A Normal; B—K Immature types

One frequently observes sperm heads which exhibit homogeneous staining with a cytoplasmic stain. This is apparently due to an extremely thin layer of undifferentiated cytoplasm which surrounds the sperm head. The specific clinical significance of such cells is not clear. They are, however, observed with greater frequency in association with coiled caudal appendages and immature cells, and in some instances, signify a state of immaturity. Such anomalies may be significant from the fertility viewpoint if a high ratio of the sperm population is so involved.

Most abnormalities which are observed in the ejaculated spermatozoa concern gametes which have passed through the various stages of spermiogenesis and are consequently abnormalities of the mature sperm. It is only in rare instances that one observes any considerable number of immature gametes in the ejaculated semen. These are distinguished from the mature cells principally by the larger size of their nuclei, the lack of a caudal appendage or its vestigeal development, the absence of an acrosome and the envelopment of the nucleus in a thick cytoplasmic covering which at times may present a double nucleus because of the arrest in the secondary spermatocyte stage. If the arrest of spermiogenesis occurs late in the process, one may observe considerable pyknosis of the nuclei which are either devoid of cytoplasm or surrounded with a cytoplasmic envelope without the development of an acrosome. With this type of disorder, a pairing of the spermatozoa is frequently observed because the cells do not separate following the final cell division in the spermatocyte stage (Fig. 20, 21).

### d) Relation of structure and function of the spermatozoön

It has previously been indicated that the spermatozoön possesses a very intricate structure. Likewise, intricate biochemic processes must operate in order that its viability, motility and fertilizing ability is maintained. As more is learned about spermatic cytology and physiology, it becomes increasingly apparent that the structural components of the sperm are all intimately concerned with its physiology. Male infertility will be better understood when it is realized that such structures as the acrosome, centriolar bodies, the mitochondrial sheath and other components not so readily discerned with the aid of the microscope, all have useful functions to perform. They are all concerned with the viability of the spermatozoön, with the chemical processes experienced by the spermatozoa, their ability to migrate, unite with the ovum, initiate its cell division and contribute the genetic anlaga of the male. The nature of the problem will also become more apparent when it is realized that many of the structural changes which are entirely too minute for recognition by ordinary microscopic means may indeed involve so large a proportion of the sperm population as to produce permanent and complete sterility.

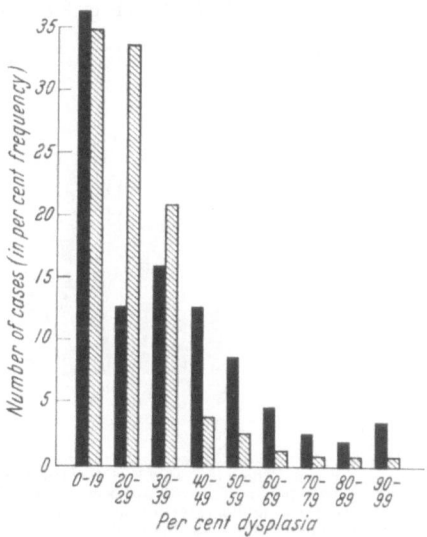

Fig. 28. *Relation of spermatic dysplasia to the incidence of conception.* Note that the ratio of conceptions drops off sharply when more than forty per cent of the spermatozoa are abnormal, but also that an occasional conception may occur when very few normal cells are present. 661 Sterile cases ▮▮▮ ; 157 Conceptions from intertile cases ▨

The purpose of a semen examination is to determine the availability of potentially fertile spermatozoa, and the examination is clinically valuable according to the accuracy with which the fertility may be thus anticipated. Very little difficulty is usually experienced in distinguishing the highly normal semen specimens (Fig. 16) from those which because of the absence of spermatozoa or the presence of a high ratio of faulty spermatozoa indicate an absolute sterility (Fig. 20, 21, 22, 25). Many cases with damage limited to only a portion of the sperm population require considerably more than a precursory view of a fresh semen specimen or a Sims test for recognition of the quality of the sperm population and its fertilizing ability.

Structural abnormalities of the spermatozoa are very common to the infertile, and in general, the higher the ratio of these abnormalities, the lower is the potential fertility of the individual. Thus semen specimens containing no more than forty to fifty per cent visibly abnormal spermia and with a high sperm concentration may in spite of the many normal appearing cells be absolutely infertile (Fig. 28). Clinical experience reveals a potential fertility of not over about five per cent if spermatic abnormalities involve more than forty per cent of the population, whereas an incidence of twenty per cent of pathologic spermatozoa may exert little or no influence upon fertility, provided that there is a high ratio of cells with high motility.

It may thus be inferred that the presence of a high ratio of visibly abnormal cells indicates in most instances that a much more extensive damage to the sperm population exists than is suggested by the observed abnormalities. When all the spermatozoa of a given population are of an abnormal structure or exhibit impaired motility, one can faithfully anticipate no conceptions, irrespective of the number of spermatozoa in the ejaculate. If, however, only an exceedingly small number of normal appearing cells are present, a conception is always possible, even though the probability of this occurring is very remote. The somewhat current idea of compensating for poor quality spermatozoa by increasing the number or concentration of faulty spermatozoa overlooks the common clinical experience that an increased supply of faulty spermatozoa almost always fails to increase potential fertility. Thus when a sperm population of one hundred million spermatozoa contains no cells capable of fertilizing an ovum, there is no reason to believe that two hundred million of the same quality will improve fertility (Fig. 29). The spermatozoa available for fertilization are largely those in the seminal fluid which contact the cervical mucus, and fertilization is related to the concentration of normal cells over a given area and not to the gross number of spermatozoa in the ejaculate. As the ratio of weak or pathologic cells in the ejaculate increases, the potential fertility therefore diminishes until eventually a point is reached when fertilization of the ovum is impossible. Clinically, it is evident that sterility frequently occurs in spite of the presence of millions of apparently normal appearing and normally active spermatozoa in the ejaculate (Fig. 28, 30).

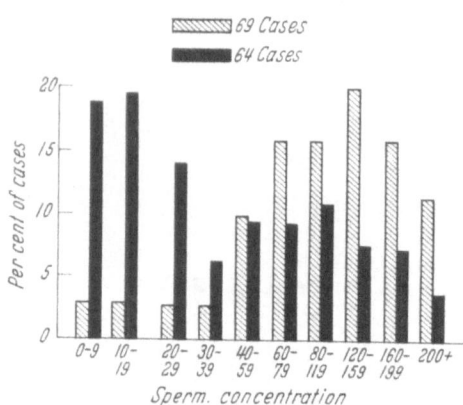

Fig. 29. *The relation of spermatic dysplasia to sperm concentration.* There is a very high incidence of pathologic sperm populations with a sperm concentration of less than thirty million per cubic millimeter. Also many sperm populations with high sperm concentrations are composed largely of pathologic spermatozoa.
69 Cases with dysplasia under 20%
64 Cases with dysplasia over 50%

On the other hand, a simple hypospermatogenesis which is not associated with a spermatic dysplasia does not seem to interfere too greatly with conception if a sufficient number of spermatozoa are present to cause a cervical insemination. The etiology, prognosis and therapy of male sterility will be made much clearer if basic spermatic pathology is not disregarded, and if differences in potential are recognized instead of attempting to draw a sharp line of demarcation between the normal and abnormal population, or between the fertile and infertile population. Some persons are highly fertile, others are absolutely sterile, but most of the so-called infertile group represent different degrees of potential fertility between these extremes.

## 2. Motility and viability

### a) Mechanism of motility

Motility is an inherent property of normal, mature spermatozoa. The life span of non-ejaculated spermatozoa is limited so that in the freshly ejaculated semen some dead cells are always observed and the rate of death increases rapidly subsequent to ejaculation. Motility of the spermatozoön is apparently accomplished similarly to that of a muscle fiber and possibly to that of cilia of ciliated cells; by means of a rearrangement of the protein molecule and a contraction of the fine fibrillae (SZYENT-GYORGI, HUXLEY). With the aid of an electron microscope, these fibrillae may be observed in the middle piece and tail piece of the spermatozoön (BRETSCHNEIDER, SCHNALL, SCHULTZ-LARSEN).

In order that sperm motility and the forces which interfere with motility may be better understood, one may well consider the analogous physiochemical and structural changes associated with muscle contraction. Thus, each muscle fiber is composed of a large number of longitudinal fibrillae which are of two types of fibrinous protein, myosin and actin. These are arranged in a regular, repeating pattern and in the same register, so that the analogous segments of the protein molecules of the different muscle fibrillae occur side by side. There exists during the resting stage a chemical connecting link between the proteinic fibrous molecules of myosin and actin, and the combination of these substances is termed actomyosin.

Under the influence of adenosine triplephosphate (A.T.P.), a molecular rearrangement breaks the bond between the actin and myosin molecules, permitting the myosin and actin fibrillae of the protein molecule to slip by each other and bring about a muscle contraction. Apparently, in this reaction, myosin works as an enzyme which is involved with the dephosphorylization of A.T.P., splitting it so as to form adenosine diphosphate (A.D.P.) which is later resynthesized to form A.T.P. This splitting of A.T.P. always occurs with muscle contraction and is associated with a molecular readjustment of the myosin and actin molecules. When the A.T.P. breakdown ceases, the reaction between the myosin and actin stops and no further contraction of the muscle is possible. It is now known that contractions of the muscle occur at the molecular level. Each enzyme site of the myosin molecule can take part in this reaction many times during each over-all contraction cycle, and thus much more work can be accomplished than would be possible with any single contraction.

Adenosine triplephosphate has been identified in the sperm by MANN and others, and it seems that the same general processes are at work with the sperm to cause its motility as applies to the muscle fiber (SIMMONET and BRUNAUD). In the process of the splitting of the adenosine triplephosphate, phosphocreatinin breaks down into creatin and phosphoric acid and is then resynthesized back into A.T.P. by energy derived largely from the anaerobic scission of glucose or fructose. By fructolysis or glycolysis, lactic acid is produced and energy is supplied for the resynthesis of phosphocreatinin into A.T.P. In so doing, in the case of a muscle, there is an aerobic oxidation of about one-fifth of the lactic acid, and this serves to reconvert four-fifths of the lactic acid into glycogen.

With spermatozoa, the process seems to be conducted on an anaerobic basis. Fructose or glycogen must be available as the source of energy for sperm motility and the resynthesis of A.T.P. As a result of this metabolism, a considerable amount of lactic acid and some hydrogen peroxide are produced, and these substances, if in sufficient concentration, are toxic to the spermatozoa. It has been demonstrated that fructolysis in the semen occurs at a rate which is proportionate to the number of live spermatozoa (BIRNBERG). Apparently the seminal fluid contains an amylase which is capable of converting glycogen to glucose. The presence of glycogen in various portions of the male and female tract under the influence of androgens or estrogens may constitute the principal source of energy.

In the case of activity of the caudal appendage of the spermatozoön, the contractile process is apparently similar to that which occurs with a muscle fiber, with similar component elements present, such as the molecular arrangement of the proteinic molecules and the fundamental chemical changes which are involved. Electron photomicrographs of the axillary fibrillae suggest a molecular arrangement which is in register as with the muscle fiber, and it has been shown that the energy for the contraction and scission of A.T.P. is likewise supplied by the oxidation of glucose or fructose. Apparently activity of the sperm is likewise dependent upon the interaction of A.T.P. and actomyosin.

Myosin and actin may be dissolved from the live muscle and then brought together to form actomyosin, thus artificially producing a fibrous protein which contracts as a muscle fiber under the influence of A.T.P. In the case of the striated muscle, this process is apparently set in motion by nerve stimulation through the end plate of the neuron, but the action with the artificially prepared fibrous protein shows that the process may be otherwise induced if the essential chemicals are present.

The triggering of the contractile mechanism of the sperm for inducing contractions appears to differ somewhat from that of the striated muscle, and results from the direct enzymic action between the myosin and A.T.P. Apparently this must initiate waves of contractions with very rapid changes from the contractile to the resting stage as the contractile impulse is carried along the proteinic segments of the myofibrils. The continuous activity of the sperm may thus result from brief refractory periods along the length of the fibrillae which would permit scission of A.T.P. and glycogen to be repeated rapidly along their course. Without the possibility of resynthesis of A.T.P. and without the energy for this, contractions of the fibrillae would have to cease.

The biochemical changes which bring about motility depend upon many different factors, such as the osmotic pressure of the seminal fluid, the hydrogen ion concentration, proteolytic and other enzymes, temperature, electrolyte balance, the isoelectric point, and the structure, health and age of the sperm. For instance, if there is an alteration in the electrolyte balance or in osmotic pressure, there may be a curling of the caudal extremities (EMMONS). Marked abnormalities in the structure of the caudal extremity commonly interfere with motility (WILLIAMS). Such structural abnormalities may be entirely too minute for observation other than with an electron microscope.

The helix of fine fibrillae surrounding the axillary fibrillae, and also the spiral of the middle piece, are not resolved excepting with the electron microscope, but there is ample evidence of their frequent disorganization. The development of the spiral fibrillae is closely related to the outcropping of the axial fibrillae from the centriolar bodies, and a disturbance in this process may involve and immobilize the entire sperm population. On the other hand, it is not infrequent that lesser disturbances in motility affect only a limited but fixed ratio of the sperm population and that this loss of motility is due to the faulty structure and the consequent physical incapability of reacting to the chemical stimulus necessary for motility. On the molecular level of cellular activity, the physical and functional properties thus merge.

It is improbable that an extrinsic factor can cause a pronounced loss in motility which involves only a limited segment of the sperm population. Under the influence of extrinsic factors, one would expect that the motility of the entire sperm population would be about equally reduced, in contrast to loss of vitality due to genetic factors.

By means of live-dead staining with eosin, one observes evidence that metabolism of the nucleus and acrosome ceases first, then that of the sheath of the caudal extremity and lastly that of the axillary filament and centriolar bodies. Clinically, it is observed that fertility is lost considerably in advance of the loss of mobility. The metabolic processes concerned with motility have only a limited dependence upon the condition of the nucleus and acrosome, but are closely related to the condition of the centriolar bodies and to the structure of the various portions of the caudal extremity.

The biochemical aspects of sperm motility offer an interesting field for speculation. The mechanism involved is indeed intricate. It is well to appreciate,

however, that the complicated biochemical changes are necessary for sperm motility and that these changes are associated not only with the chemical nature of the seminal fluid, but also with the structure of the sperm and the chemical nature of its component structures. It is hardly feasible at this time to forecast the fertilizing ability of spermatozoa by the chemical nature of the substratum or of the sperm, or by the products of its metabolism. It is not known whether chemical differences are sufficiently pronounced in the semen from the infertile and the fertile individual to permit their chemical differentiation. The principal differences which might be discerned are those resulting from metabolic and enzymic activity, which are parallel to the rate at which the spermatozoa perish under different influences and which would be indicated by failing motility.

### b) Migration or transport of spermatozoa

Considerable discussion has arisen from time to time as to the means of transport of spermatozoa into the uterus and through the fallopian tubes. Some authorities hold that uterine contractions transport the semen directly into the uterus and that the upward transport of the spermatozoa through the cervix and uterus does not depend upon the motility of the spermatozoa alone. In this respect, it is observed in women that seminal fluid is never found in the uterine cavity within the first few hours after coitus. By suction, one may obtain from the uterus a few drops of serosanguineous fluid which may contain a few spermatozoa of invariably high motility, whereas the spermatozoa in the cervical mucus and in the seminal fluid present variable ratios of immotile and abnormally formed cells according to the health of the cervical secretion and the fundamental health of the sperm populations from which they are derived.

Irrespective of the sperm concentration in the cervix, which may be as high as 200 spermia per high-power field, the uterine sampling rarely contains more than one to five spermatozoa per high-power field. If it were true that the seminal fluid enters the uterine cavity, we would occasionally find within the uterine cavity a much higher sperm concentration. We would also expect to find a ratio of dead spermia in the uterus comparable to that in the semen. This never occurs. Instead, one observes that all of the intrauterine spermatozoa appear normal and highly active. Apparently, the weak or dead spermatozoa do not pass through the internal cervical ring.

Furthermore, it is noted that spermatozoa with defective acrosomes are rarely observed in the cervical canal in spite of the fact that there may be a high incidence of such cells in the ejaculated semen, and in spite of the fact that such cells are usually of high motility. Various observers have pointed out that there is a higher ratio of normal cells in the cervical mucus than exists in the semen (COHEN, TEN BERGE). Any fluid entering the uterine cavity may easily pass through normally patent tubes under a very low positive pressure, as is experenced with uterotubal insufflations and salpingograms. Furthermore, the sampling of the uterine cavity after coitus never reveals free seminal fluid or a high sperm concentration. In many instances, any fluid entering the uterine cavity could easily pass through the tubes because of the very limited capacity of the uterine cavity and the widely patent tubal lumina.

By means of contraction and relaxation of the uterus during coitus, a partial recession of cervical mucus may occur and carry spermatozoa for a short distance into the cervical canal, but there is no tangible evidence that this mechanism is capable of drawing spermatozoa into the uterine cavity.

Because of the invariable bacterial contamination of semen and its action as a chemical irritant to the peritoneum, a high incidence of peritonitis should

16*

be inevitable if seminal fluid were introduced into the uterine cavity at the time of coitus. MOELLER and VANDEMARK have shown that bovine spermatozoa may travel by their own propulsion as rapidly as 6 cm. in ten minutes. In the human being, in vitro sperm specimens may migrate about as far as 0.5 cm. in ten minutes (ECHEADIA) and BELONOSCHKIN reports a migration of one centimeter in five minutes in the excised uterus. This migration is not necessarily in a stright line, but healthy spermia tend to migrate in the line of least resistance, which is toward the more favorable surroundings experienced with an upward migration, and not in the direction of the unfavorable acidity of the vagina. The transit rate is sufficiently rapid to permit the completion of the journey of about 6.5 cm. through the uterus in about two hours and through the fallopian tubes within four or five hours after coitus, by means of no other motivating force than that provided by the spermatozoa themselves.

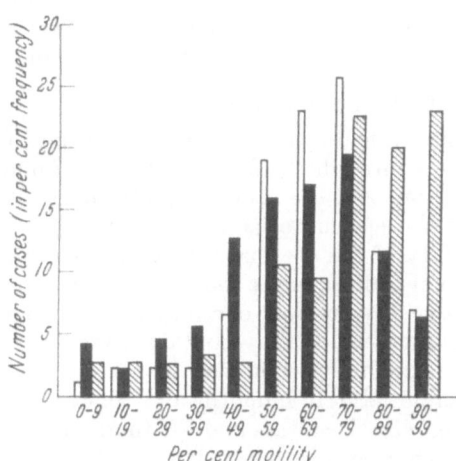

Fig. 30. *The relation of initial motility to fertility.* The percentage of conceptions is very low in the group of cases with immotility of more than fifty per cent of the spermatozoa.

150 Conceptions ▨, 389 general sterility cases ■, 86 conceptions from general sterility group ▢

Clinically, one ordinarily finds live spermatozoa in the uterine cavity within five hours after coitus, representing a minimum transit speed of at least 3 cm. in five hours or 0.6 cm. in one hour, a figure which is compatible with measured speeds of in vitro migration. Spermatozoa live in the uterine cavity for different periods of time in different animals. Thus, HAMMOND reports that the spermatozoa will survive all winter in the bat, sixteen days in the turkey, seven to eleven days in the duck, and only a few hours in the mouse. According to the writer's experience, it is uncommon to find any spermatozoa in the human uterus after thirty-six hours, but various reports have revealed that spermatozoa may be recovered from the fallopian tubes within one to two weeks.

## c) Relation of motility to morphology and fertility

A high motility of a definitely progressive nature is an inherent and essential property of fertile spermatozoa, but it should be realized that motile spermatozoa are not necessarily fertile. The ratio of motility, particularly of a highly migratory type, provides a rough index to the viability of the sperm population and its suitability for fertilizing the ovum, a property which is reduced as the ratio of immotile or weak spermatozoa rises (Fig. 30). There is a very decided reduction in fertility with the group of cases which persistently exhibit a sperm motility of less than 50 per cent. Some sperm populations with poor motility contain high ratios of morphologically abnormal spermia, and others are mostly composed of morphologically normal cells (Table 1). This lack of parallelism in the results of motility and cytologic examinations is observed so frequently that the omission of either type of examination can lead to important diagnostic errors. Actually, there is no uniform relationship between the incidence of motility and that of faulty structure. The sperm populations composed of highly motile spermia as well as those of low motility may be composed mostly of either structurally normal or structurally abnormal cells. With different

percentages of motility, the average percentage of abnormal spermia is about the same, but individual cases present wide variations in the incidence of morphologically abnormal cells at each motility level. Thus, the cases with motility ranging between 30 and 40 per cent may exhibit differences from 10 to 100 per cent of morphologically abnormal spermia, which cause wide individual differences in potential fertility.

The influence of structural defects upon motility is not uniform except in individual cases where the type of abnormality is a direct impediment to motility (Table 2). Thus one cannot justify the omission of either motility or morphologic examinations on the pretext that one can supplant the other in the recognition of a spermatic disorder.

When sperm populations are distributed into groups according to the percentage of structurally abnormal cells, it will be observed that the average ratio of motile cells is about the same with each group, irrespective of the per cent of abnormal cells. With a limited number of cases, one does find that immobility increases in proportion to the increase in the pathologic forms. This applies mostly to the group of cases which present sixty per cent or more pathologic spermatozoa. In general, however, motility and morphology are not interdependent, and the test for one provides no valid information concerning the other.

The significance of motility and morphology may be somewhat clarified by a consideration of some of the physiologic factors involved. The head of the spermatozoön, including the

Table 1. *Incidence of abnormal spermatic morphology as related to different ratios of motility (80 cases).*

| Per cent motile | Average per cent morphologically abnormal spermia | Different incidences of abnormal spermia |
|---|---|---|
| 0— 19 | 45.0 | 18 to 100% |
| 20— 39 | 42.5 | 11 to 90% |
| 40— 59 | 41.0 | 13 to 100% |
| 60— 79 | 47.5 | 35 to 80% |
| 80—100 | 43.0 | 43 to 50% |

If sperm populations are grouped together according to the per cent of motile spermatozoa, it will be observed that the ratio of structurally abnormal spermatozoa is about the same in each of the motility levels

Table 2. *Ratio of motility as dictated by different ratios of spermatic abnormalities (91 cases)*

| Per cent of abnormal spermatozoa | Average per cent motile | Differences in incidence of motility |
|---|---|---|
| 0— 19 | 34.5 | 13 to 48% |
| 20— 39 | 39.5 | 5 to 73% |
| 40— 59 | 41.5 | 6 to 90% |
| 60— 79 | 30.0 | 10 to 64% |
| 80—100 | 32.0 | 12 to 69% |

nucleus acrosome, galea capitis, and proximal centriolar body, are intimately associated with the fusion of the sperm with the ovum, the initiation of cell division, and the contribution of the male attributes to the fertilized ovum. The caudal extremity is principally concerned with motility, except that the centriolar bodies are intimately involved in the functional integrity of both nucleus and the caudal extremity. The acrosome is in some manner involved with directional mobility, since spermia with abnormal acrosomes rarely if ever migrate into the cervix and uterus.

It is then not realistic to consider that either cytology or motility is unimportant. With the more normal semen, 15 to 20 per cent of the spermatozoa are dead at the time of ejaculation, and thereafter they progressively perish. Individual spermatozoa of any given population exhibit different grades of vitality and survive for different lengths of time under the influence of different extrinsic and intrinsic factors. These factors when treated collectively will form the basis of the population potentiality. Clinically, however, fertility cannot be based on a formula by which one factor compensates for another, but rather by an estimation of the sum total spermatic damage as indicated by a variety of factors, which collectively destroy potential fertility according to the ratio of the involved population and the consequent laws of chance.

Most sterile sperm populations contain large numbers of spermia which appear microscopically normal in all respects. As previously pointed out, many structurally defective spermatozoa are highly motile.

Thus, the so-called "pinhead sperm", which consists of a caudal appendage to which only the proximal centriolar body is attached anteriorly and which possesses neither acrosome nor nucleus, may be very actively migratory, and also various nuclear or acrosomic defects may not reduce motility. On the other hand, a disturbance of the centriolar bodies or mitochondrial sheath of the middle piece causes complete immobility and early death of the spermatozoön even though the nucleus and acrosome appear normal.

The normal progressive mobility of spermatozoa seems to depend upon the functional integrity of the centriolar bodies, the axillary fibrillae, the mitochondrial sheath of the middle piece, and possibly also the fibrillae of the cortical sheath of the tail piece. The nucleus and the acrosome are not directly involved in this motility, except that when the nucleus perishes, cessation of metabolism of the caudal extremity and of motility will shortly follows this event.

### d) Factors reducing motility

If repeated examinations of freshly ejaculated semen reveal a high ratio of immotile cells which remains about the same with each ejaculation, it is very likely that the immobility is the result of a genetic damage to the primitive germinal epithelium. Frequently, however, the reduced motility is not on a fixed basis but is brought about by some transitory influence such as a general health factor, an acute illness, or an exhaustion of the seminal epithelium by excessive frequency of coitus. In some instances diminished motility is associated with an alteration in the physical characteristics of the seminal fluid, the fluid being too thick and viscid to permit normal sperm migration; or motility loss may arise from an alteration in the chemistry of the seminal fluid. If waning motility resulted from altered chemical or physical properties of the seminal fluid, one might expect that the deleterious factor, whatever it may be, would act simultaneously on the entire sperm population in contrast to the involvement of a definite fixed segment as is observed with primary spermatic disease.

Although the pH of the seminal fluid and of the secretion of the female genital tract exerts a considerable influence upon the ability of and duration of motility, actually the pH is so constantly at a normal figure that it does not ordinarily come into consideration in the evaluation of fertility. It is normal that there should be vaginal acidity with a pH of 4 to 5, and spermatozoa do not survive under such influence more than two to four hours. Because the pH of the semen ranges between 7.5 and 8.2, the vaginal acidity is temporarily neutralized; but this buffering effect usually endures not longer than about thirty minutes and is followed by the progressive death of the sperm population within the vagina. Actually, under normal circumstances, semen is deposited in contact with the cervical mucus with a pH of about 7.0 to 8. and the spermatozoa penetrate into the cervical mucus and migrate into the uterine cavity where the pH is about 8.

It is very seldom that the pH of the secretion of the vagina is more acid than normal, but an increased alkalinity because of various types of infection is quite common. A slightly acid vaginal mucus is one of Nature's provisions to hold in check the multiplication of bacteria, and is perfectly normal. Occasionally there occurs a slight reduction in the alkalinity of the cervical secretion, especially with a patulous cervix which is particularly exposed to the vaginal mucus. However this may be, an alteration in the pH of the semen or the secretions of the female tract plays an exceptionally small influence in the fertility problem except in those instances wherein the character of the secretion is altered by obvious disease. The addition of a properly buffered saline diluent may accelerate motility, but such treatment fails to restore fertility. The ratio and degree of motility of the in vitro specimen generally represent a stage in the progressive deterioration and death of the sperm population, and are associated with a corresponding reduction in metabolism of the different spermia, according to differences in their fundamental health.

### e) Aging and death of spermatozoa

At the completion of spermiogenesis, all of the spermatozoa are presumably alive, but they soon commence to perish at a rate commensurate with their fundamental health and the conditions under which they exist. Even before ejaculation, a variable number are continuously perishing and being replaced with more recently formed cells. In the human being, the number of dead cells at the time of ejaculation commonly amounts to as much as 18 to 20 per cent of the total, and this figure remains about the same for four to six hours after ejaculation, when the spermia begin to perish more rapidly. The spermatozoa of defective sperm populations commonly perish much more rapidly than those of healthy populations. Weak motility is an invariable indication that the weak spermatozoa will soon be dead and that another observation made a little later will reveal a much higher proportion of dead spermatozoa. As semen ages, there is usually a period of several days during which the live segment of the population, as indicated by the Blom live-dead stain, is larger than the motile group, thus indicating that many of the live spermatozoa have lost their motility[1]. Repeated observations on semen specimens retained in the refrigerator at 40⁰ F. furnish evidence that diminished motility

Table 3. *Sperm survival in vitro after 24 hours refrigeration* (161 cases).

| Initial motility | Percentage of dead spermatozoa after 24 hours[1] |
|---|---|
| 10—29 | 52% |
| 30—49 | 40% |
| 50—69 | 34% |
| 70—90 | 24% |

As many as twenty-five per cent of the spermatozoa of healthy sperm populations will be alive and motile twenty four hours after ejaculation. The number of dead or immotile spermatozoa at the end of 24 hours is usually closely related to the per cent of initial motility. The lower the initial motility, the more rapidly will the sperm population perish.

signifies imminent death of the cells so involved and a progressive deterioration of the sperm population as a whole (Table 3).

When semen is examined for live and dead spermatozoa, it will usually be found that all of the spermatozoa of poor-quality populations will perish several days sooner than the spermia of healthy populations. Thus the record of the initial motility and the percentage of dead cells twenty-four hours later will usually provide as reliable an index of sperm viability as if more frequent observations were made. From these two observations, one obtains an indication of the progressive death or vitality of the sperm population without the influence of extrinsic factors which often invalidate observations after the first twenty-four hours.

When in vitro semen specimens are kept at a temperature above 80⁰ F., a rapid decline in motility is to be anticipated because of hastened enzymic

---

[1] Blom stain reveals frequently that immotile cells are not actually dead.

and metabolic activity plus the toxic effect of bacterial multiplication, whereas if the semen is retained in the refrigerator at a temperature of about 40° F., it is not uncommon to find a few of the cells showing life for as long as ten days. The spermatozoa of some animals, notably bovine, seem to survive almost indefinitely if kept frozen with carbon dioxide ice in a properly buffered diluent.

## 3. Sperm concentration

Low sperm concentrations are observed in association with various factors such as a hypoplasia of the germinal epithelium, a pathologic germinal epithelium which in consequence is incapable of a normal rate of spermiogenesis, exhaustion of the germinal epithelium arising from excessive sexual activity and various extrinsic factors such as acute or chronic illnesses, especially those with high fever which may at least temporarily reduce the rate of spermiogenesis and consequently the sperm concentration in the ejaculated semen.

Individuals are endowed with different sized testes possessing different amounts of germinal epithelium. This causes marked differences in spermatogenic potential. In general, the functional fitness of the sperm population diminishes as the incidence of pathology increases until eventually either the complete absence of spermatozoa or the presence of wholly abnormal or immotile spermatozoa renders fertilization impossible. A relatively small sperm population may at times be composed of relatively healthy and fertile spermatozoa, whereas a large sperm population composed of mostly pathologic cells may be sterile. Sperm populations with concentrations of under twenty thousand to thirty thousand per cu.mm. are much more liable to be infertile than the larger populations because of the greater likelihood of a high incidence of pathologic spermatozoa; but the health and fertilizing ability of different sized sperm populations varies so widely that the sperm concentration in itself provides a very unreliable index to fertility.

The sperm concentration with both fertile and infertile individuals exhibits a wide range of variability, but with a given individual commonly assumes a more or less fixed level. Wide fluctuations in concentration may occur because of such factors as the general health, the character of the germinal epithelium or frequency of sexual activity. In general, the more pathologic sperm populations show the greatest variability in concentration in different samplings. Low sperm concentrations are very commonly associated with testes of a subnormal size or abnormal consistency.

In many dissertations upon the subject of male infertility, principal emphasis is accorded to the sperm concentration in the ejaculated semen and therapy which is intended to increase the number of spermatozoa. In this respect, one might well consider a few basic physiological factors involved with fertilization.

*Relation of sperm concentration to sperm migration and conception.* The number of spermatozoa ordinarily entering the cervical canal is determined largely by the number of healthy spermatozoa contacting the cervical mucus within the first few minutes after coitus. Soon thereafter death of the vaginal spermatozoa ensues because of the unfavorable influence of the vaginal acidity and bacterial multiplication. The holding of semen within the vagina more than fifteen to thirty minutes after coitus seems to accomplish no useful purpose because of the unfavorable circumstances which cause them to perish or lose their vitality. Apparently, the gross number of spermatozoa does not decide the magnitude of sperm migration but rather the number of healthy cells which contact the cervical mucus immediately after coitus. Otherwise, one would expect much higher sperm concentrations in those cases where conception occurs. Conceptions are not, however, ordinarily associated with high intra-cervical sperm concentrations (Fig. 31).

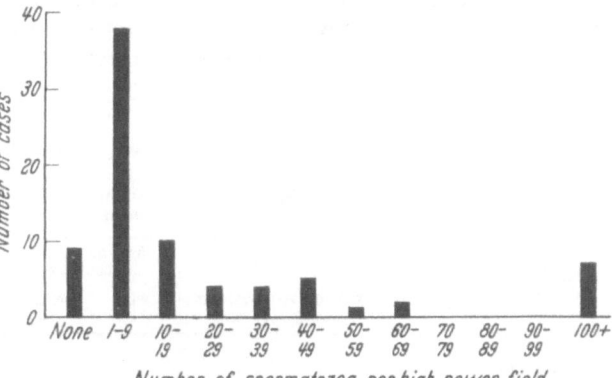

Under normal circumstances, even with the highly fertile, a relatively small number of spermatozoa migrate into the cervical canal. Only a very small proportion of those gaining entrance into the cervix will pass the barrier of the internal cervical ring and pass into the uterus. Considerable discussion has centered about the factor of sperm concentration in its relation to infertility.

Fig. 31. *The relation of intra-cervical sperm concentration to fertility.* In this group of eighty consecutive conceptions, over fifty per cent presented in the cervical mucus a sperm concentration of less than ten cells per high power field. Since many infertile cases present high intra-cervical sperm concentration, the number of intracervical spermatozoa per se provides a very unreliable criterion by which potential fertility of the male may be stimatede

At least statistically, the fertility of an individual is not greatly impaired by sperm concentration alone provided that there are enough healthy spermatozoa to cause cervical insemination. With the concentration of under twenty thousand per cu.mm. the impairment is usually related more to the relatively high incidence of pathologic or weak spermatozoa than to the failure of cervical insemination, excepting in the cases with concentrations of under five to ten thousand per cu.mm., when the chances for cervical insemination may be considerably reduced (Fig. 32).

When it happens that conception fails as a result of normal relations, it is indeed exceedingly rare that an increase in the number of spermatozoa by means of a cervical cap insemination, intra-cervical or intra-uterine insemination, or by other means, will cause conceptions. WILLIAMS (1953) has reported four conceptions out of one hundred fifty cases where the husband's semen was used. About half of these one hundred fifty cases had abnormal sperm populations, but all four conceptions occurred from cases with normal semen which should

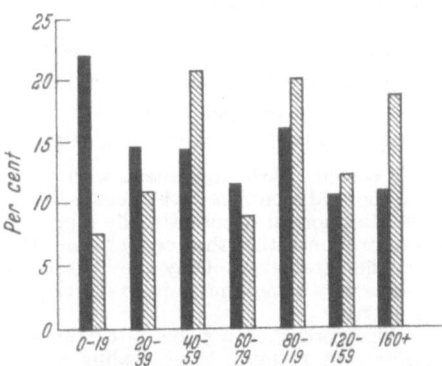

Fig. 32. *The relation in sperm concentration in semen to the incidence of conception.* Note that the ratio of conceptions is not influenced materially by the sperm concentration in the ejaculated semen. The ratio of conceptions is often influenced by the female factor which serves to reduce fertility in the higher registers of sperm concentration. There is an especially high incidence of cases in the infertility group where the sperm concentration is under twenty million per cubic centimeter. In this group, there is a particularly high incidence of pathologic spermatozoa which serve to lower fertility.

500 Infertility cases. Sperm concentration ▬▬, Percent of total conceptions ▨▨

have been successful by natural means. In these particular cases, it seemed evident that the prolongation of cervical contact of the semen failed to improve the rate of conception. These results are in very marked contrast to the results with artificial insemination with high potency donor semen where one expects a prompt conception in about fifty per cent of the cases.

One might assume that there would be an increased cervical concentration of spermatozoa if semen were held in contact with the external os for an increased length of time, and protected from the acidity of the vagina. This may be accomplished by the use of a cervical cap and to a lesser extent by assuming a knee-chest position after coitus. It is noted, however, in most instances where the cervical cap is used that the cervical concentration of spermatozoa is decreased rather than increased and that the ratio of conceptions is not increased by its use (Table 4).

Table 4. *The effect of Prolonged Contact of Semen with the External Cervical Os.* (50 Infertility cases)

| cervical sperm concentration | Conceptions | | Average sperm concentration | |
|---|---|---|---|---|
| | with cervical cap | without cap | with cap | without cap |
| Cervical sperm concentration increased after use of cervical cap. . . . . | 20 | 0 | 7 | 62 | 12 |
| Cervical sperm concentration decreased after cervical cap insemination . | 30 | 1 | 5 | 31 | 84 |
| Total inseminated both with and without cap . | 50 | 1 | 12 | 57 | 43 |

When a paucity of spermia is associated with a fundamental disorder of spermiogenesis, very little or no improvement in fertility can be anticipated from any type of therapy, but in many instances, the low sperm concentrations present no fundamental disorder of the spermatozoa and consequently it does not interfere seriously with fertility. Even if the sperm concentration is below twenty thousand per cu.mm., one may anticipate a conception rate of about five to ten per cent if the concentration of normal spermia is sufficiently great to cause a cervical insemination (Fig. 30).

If semen is held in contact with the cervix with a cervical cap so that it is protected from the acid secretion of the vagina, the intra-cervical sperm concentration is usually lower than after normal coitus. Usually a post-coital examination will reveal a much higher sperm concentration within the cervical canal than occurs in the cervical mucus which is sampled from the external os. Only the healthier spermatozoa migrate into the cervical canal, and of these only a small proportion are capable of migration past the internal cervical ring into the uterus.

Oligospermia or a paucity of the spermatozoa in the ejaculate has received special attention by many of those dealing with the male infertility problem. This term is rather ambiguous, since it signifies to different observers widely different meanings. Thus, in analysis of reports of sixty-four doctors dealing with the androgen rebound therapy, GETZOFF (1955) reports that oligospermia signified with different physicians, various sperm concentrations ranging from only a few spermia per. cu. mm. up to seventy thousand per cu. mm., and that much of the therapy was given to cases which by clinical experience could not be considered as of impaired fertility on the basis of sperm concentration. It therefore seems desirable to indicate the sperm concentration in precise terms rather than by the use of a term with such widely different meanings.

Experience reveals that a vast number of spermatozoa are required under normal circumstances to provide a single sperm which is suitable for fertilization. In the case of spermatic disease, the number of spermatozoa required to provide this single fertile cell is not the same as exists under normal conditions; and with the infertile case, there is no known mathematical relationship between the number of sperm present, the number of motile sperm and the incidence of fertile sperm. The assumption that there is such a relationship detracts markedly from the accuracy of prognosis.

A very informative study concerning male fertility has been conducted in connection with artificial insemination of cattle which are of considerable comparative value from the viewpoint of human infertility. These studies are of particular value because with bulls, it is possible to determine the percentage of conceptions per insemination with a given seminal picture, a feature which is not possible with human. Semen from a highly fertile bull may be diluted with an extender to as much as 1:100 or 1:200, with the result that $1/_{100}$ to $1/_{200}$ part of the diluted semen will exhibit essentially the same fertilizing ability as if the entire ejaculate were used. It thus becomes possible with highly fertile semen to obtain over one hundred conceptions from a single ejaculate.

Various types of semen extenders have been used in connection with artificial inseminations of cattle, so as to produce the most favorable circumstance for survival and the maintenance of fertility. The following extender is being currently used by the New York Artificial Breeder's Co-operative, Inc., where extensive artificial inseminations are being carried out (DUNN).

Weigh out all buffer ingredients *(except citric acid)* into cylinder or calibrated flask. Add about $1/_3$ of final volume of boiling glass-distilled water. Quickly add room temperature distilled water to near complete volume. Set cylinder or flask in cold running tap water. When buffer is cool, add citric acid and make up to final volume. *(Store in dark at room temperature no longer than 1 week.)*

Extender is prepared by adding 20 parts of yolk to 80 parts of buffer. Streptomycin and penicillin are added to give 1,000 units/ml. of extender.

When semen is to be retained in deep freeze, glycerine is usually ad-

Table 5. *Preparation of Foote's cue extender* (DUNN)
*Grams of constituents for cue buffer*

| Chemical | Brand | 100 ml. | 1,000 ml. |
|---|---|---|---|
| Sodium citrate-2 $H_2O$ . | Baker & Adamson | 1.45 | 14.5 |
| Potassium chloride . . | Mallinckrodt | .4 | 4.0 |
| Sulfanilamide . . . . | Merck | .3 | 3.0 |
| Dextrose anhydrous (granular) (Glucose) | Mallinchrodt | .3 | 3.0 |
| Glycine (amiboacetic acid) . . . . . . . | Nutritional Biochemical Corp. (Cleveland, Ohio) | .937 | 9.37 |
| Sodium bicarbonate . | Mallinckrodt | .21 | 2.1 |

*Before final volume is reached add:*

| | | | |
|---|---|---|---|
| Acid citric. . . . . . | Mallinckrodt | .1 | 1.0 |

Cue extender: 80 parts buffer / 20 parts yolk / (1,000 units of penicillin / streptomycin / ml.
pH buffer = 6.5—6.8.
pH extender = 6.6—6.8.

ded in a dilution of 10 per cent to lessen the damage to the spermatozoa during the freezing and thawing processes (POLGE). The semen from a highly fertile bull may have a conception rate of as high as 80 per cent without freezing, and loses only about 10 per cent in the ratio of conceptonis as a result of the freezing process at a temperature of —79 degrees Centigrade.

DUNN states: "With some bulls the number of live spermia per insemination can be dropped to as low as 5 million and still have a good conception rate but we only use such an extension when an emergency arises. Our dilution or extension rate is based on number of live sperm per insemination. This varies with the concentration and motility of each ejaculate. For example, if the ejaculate contains 2 billion sperm per ml. and 60% are motile, there would be 1,200,000 live sperm per ml. and this would give an extension rate of 1:120 for 10 million live sperm per insemination, which is our standard for normal operations. In general we might say that the extension rate would be in the range of 1:80 to 1:100."

Although the semen from a highly fertile animal may be diluted as much as 1:100 without impairing its fertilizing ability, it is nevertheless apparent that most of the spermatozoa in the highly fertile sperm populations are actually incapable of fertilizing an ovum, and that as many as ten million spermia per cu. cc. are ordinarily required to provide a single fertile spermatozoön. It may be argued that the ovum must be bombarded by a vast number of spermatozoa so that the ovum be penetrated by a single spermatozoön, but this lacks reality because of the fact that even with the sperm populations of highest fertility, only a very few of the spermatozoa are capable of migration through the cervix, uterus and the tubes. Regardless as to whether there is an artificial intra-cervical insemination, or coitus, very few spermatozoa will survive in the cervical canal or migrate into the uterus. With human infertility, we are not, as with cattle, dealing with the dilution of highly fertile sperm populations; but rather with sperm populations of various sizes in which the ratio of fertile spermia has already fallen below the critical level which will permit fertilization. In the bovine species with high fertility, the critical number of motile spermatozoa required for insemination without reduction of fertility is about ten million. On the other hand, with human infertility, the gross number of motile spermia which are required to provide a single fertile cell is often many times greater than when a normal fertile population is involved.

It is possible that the use of semen extenders with highly fertile human specimens might provide multiple conceptions from a single ejaculate as in the case of the bovine species; but it is quite a different problem in human when dealing with an infertile sperm population where the availability of normal, motile spermatozoa has already dropped below the critical level, irrespective of the sperm concentration. If we consider then that a large segment of male infertility results from a genetically faulty germ plasm, and that only the portion of the semen which contacts the cervical mucus can provide the spermia essential for fertilization, it becomes quite evident that alterations in numbers or motility may not be very helpful in overcoming the infertility arising from a fundamentally pathologic sperm population.

# B. Diagnosis

## I. Anamnesis and physical examination

It has been pointed out previously that male infertility may result directly or indirectly from various factors. In some instances, a semen analysis alone will indicate absolute infertility but more frequently, an insight into the potential fertility will be enhanced by information gained from a comprehensive anamnesis, physical examination and various laboratory procedures.

Consistency and comprehensiveness of infertility investigations will be favored by the adoption of a record system which can be routinely employed with all cases, making such modifications as may be dictated by individual circumstances. The anamnesis should include various items which may either directly or indirectly affect reproductive function, such as genetic factors, somatic disease, psychosomatic and functional factors, various types of pathology of the generative organs and of the germ plasm (BAYLE et GOUYOU, BELONOSCHKIN, HELLINGA, PALMER, WILLIAMS 1944).

As a matter of efficiency, the routine record form for anamnesis and physical examination should be limited to items of information that are considered as essential to most infertility investigations and not encumbered with irrelevant, unusuable information (Table 6). A systematic, general physical examination of the male partner, including all systems, should be routine with most infertility cases, and investigations should not be limited to a precursory semen analysis or an examination of the generative organs as is so frequently done. Items of endocrine interest, such as body conformation, disproportion in skeletal development, voice, skin texture and hair distribution, and items pertaining to secondary sex characteristics should be noted as a possible clue to a glandular

*Table 6*
*Anamnesis*

Date

Name                                    Occupation

   Address                              Telephone Number

Age

*Previous Sterility Investigations and Treatment*

*Marital History*

   Number of years married
   Number of pregnancies
   Number of normal deliveries
   Number of miscarriages
   Number of years without contraceptives
   Previous marriage of wife        Result
   Previous marriage of husband     Result

*Etiologic Factors*

   Industrial hazards, including toxic factors
   General infections            General            Focal
   Operations
   Systems
        Gastro-intestinal
        Cardio-respiratory
        Urologic
        Nervous
   Sexual History
        Number of days between relations
            First year married        Past year
        Inflammations and infections of generative organs
   Miscellaneous Factors
        Tobacco                   Diet
        Alcoholic beverages       Exercise
   Family History
        Health and age of father, or if deceased, the cause of death
        Health and age of mother, or if deceased, the cause of death
        Total number of aunts and uncles
        Total number married
        Total number with families
   Past History
   Present Complaints

*Physical Examination*

Temperature        Pulse          Blood pressure
   Height          Weight         Present          Previous
   General appearance
   Skin                           Chest
   Ears                           Lungs
   Nose                           Heart
   Throat                         Abdomen
   Eyes                           Rectum
   Mouth                          Neurologic
   Neck                           Skeletal abnormalities
   Generative Organs
        Pubic hair growth
        Phalus
        Right testis — size and consistency
        Left testis — size and consistency
        Right epididymis
        Left epididymis
        Spermatic cords
        Inguinal rings
        Prostate

imbalance. It is important that any doctor dealing with marital infertility should exhibit an interest in the general health of his patients if he is to enjoy their confidence and co-operation. This phase of the infertility problem is too frequently overlooked and leads to examinations whose scope is much too limited.

## II. Examination of the generative organs

In the examination of the generative organs, one commences with a general inspection, the amount and distribution of pubic hair, the development of the phalus, its size, any abnormalities such as hypospadius or epispadius and the status of the foreskin. The testes are then measured in centimeters and palpated to determine their consistency, differentiating the flabbiness of a hypoplastic testis or the firmness of a fibrosed testicle from the normal resilient consistency of normal testicular tissue. The size of the normal functioning human testicle varies with different individuals between about $4^1/_2$ to 6 cm. There is considerable variation in the size of normal functioning testicles, but if the testis measures less than 4 cm., a permanently lowered sperm concentration or azoospermia may be anticipated. One must be warned, however, that testes of slightly subnormal size are occasionally capable of forming a sufficient number of normal cells, and that the functional fitness of the germinal epithelium should always be measured by a semen analysis. A testicular hypoplasia is, however, in general to be considered as the clinical expression of a germinal hypoplasia, and the small testes are usually very poorly endowed with germinal epithelium. A testicular fibrosis may, however, serve to maintain a testis of essentially normal size in spite of a germinal hypoplasia.

After examination of the testes, the globus major and the globus minor of the epididymis are examined for evidence of induration, which is commonly bilateral and leads particularly to an obstruction of the globus minor. Most obstructive lesions of the epididymis are due to Neisserian infection and do not affect the size or consistency of the testes. Therefore a palpable induration of the epididymis or vas, with a testicle of normal size and consistency, together with a history of urethritis, is strongly suggestive that an azoospermia is due to obstruction and not to a germinal disorder; whereas an azoospermia associated with hypoplastic testes or testes of abnormal consistency, commonly suggests that azoospermia is caused by a germinal hypoplasia or aplasia. The spermatic cord is next examined and particularly the accessible portion of the vasa deferentia from the region of the superior pole of the testes, and then the inguinal rings for evidence of inguinal hernia.

A congenital absence of the epididymes or vasa deferentia may occasionally be revealed, or an induration of the vasa deferentia. Varicoceles are very frequently encountered, particularly on the left side. Commonly, the larger varicoceles are associated with an atrophy of the testis on the involved side, and if the condition is bilateral, may assume clinical significance because of the resulting circulatory disturbance of the testes. In most instances, a closure of the vas may be determined only by exposing the vas at the level of the superior pole of the testis, and injecting it by means of a small hypodermic needle with a saline solution or a solution of methylene blue which may be recovered from the posterior urethra if the vas is patent. The status of the vasa deferentia may also be demonstrated by injecting them with a radio-opaque media such as Diadrast and visualizing by means of x-ray. In the latter case, if the needle is directed proximally, the fine tubules of the globus major and minor may be visualized, and if directed distally, the entire length of the patent vas deferens can be visualized. The proof of the patency of the vasa deferentia should always precede an epididymo-vasotomy, as well as proof of the capability of normal spermiogenesis (BRODNY, BOREAU).

A digital rectal examination is now made of the prostate gland, noting its size, consistency and comparative tenderness of the two lobes. It is then massaged, commencing at the apex of each lobe and directing the massage towards its inferior end so as to strip it of possible secretion and force the secretion into the urethra. During the massage, the patient is directed to hold a microscope slide at the tip of the penis to collect any fluid expressed from the prostate. Usually, two to four drops of the fluid will be recovered. The prostatic fluid which is overlaid with a cover-glass is examined under the microscope for white blood cells or other formed elements. In healthy cases, not more than ten to fifteen white blood cells per high power field are encountered, but in others, as many as several hundred cells may be observed. When no fluid is obtained from a highly sensitive gland, its massage a few days later may produce an abundance of leukocytes. It is commonly considered that an altered secretion of the prostate gland may affect the vitality of the spermatozoa, and therefore this examination has become more or less routine with fertility studies; but from the viewpoint of the diagnosis of infertility, prostatic disease plays a rather minor role. Those with the complaint of infertility are generally not of the age group in which a prostatic hypertrophy occurs. A patient with an acute prostatitis or a urethritis usually consults a doctor because of the urologic complaint and not because of infertility. The presence of many leukocytes in the seminal fluid is not known to affect the vitality of the spermatozoa to a significant degree, but one cannot overlook the possibility that any inflammatory exudates may alter the character of the prostatic secretion and consequently lower sperm viability. Although with such cases, massage or antibiotics do not materially affect the leukocyte content or perceptibly increase fertility, it does seem reasonable to consider that a high leukocyte component in the prostatic fluid should be considered as pathologic and justify occasional prostatic massages. This should not be carried out solely under the pretext that it will definitely improve fertility, but rather under the general principle that it may be beneficial to a chronic passive congestion of the prostate and general health.

Very little is known concerning the evaluation of the condition of the seminal vesicles in connection with infertility studies. Enlarged tender vesicles are not readily distinguished by rectal palpation and their secretion is usually not obtained in a sufficient amount for differentiation from that of the prostate. Furthermore, cases with significant pathology of either the prostate or seminal vesicles which cause clinical symptoms are not apt to be interested in the infertility problem until relieved of their vesiculitis or prostatitis.

## III. General laboratory examinations

Because the general health of the individual may affect his procreative ability in various ways, it is well that a few routine laboratory examinations should be made, such as a blood count, urine analysis, determination of the basal metabolic rate, microscopic examination of the prostatic fluid, and other types of examinations according to special indications. Ordinarily the blood examination includes a red blood count, hemoglobin, white blood count, differential and occasionally a sedimentation rate if there is clinical evidence of any chronic infection. In a limited number of cases, one finds a significantly lowered basal metabolic rate. The determination of the basal metabolic rate with a metabolator is highly satisfactory for the diagnosis of a lowered metabolic rate, and for regulating thyroid administration.

Highly consistent results will be obtained with a metabolator if the machine is handled by an experienced technician who follows the standard rules and precautions pertaining to such tests, and if the nervous element is brought under control with a small dose of a barbiturate at bedtime the night before the test and repeated the following morning about two hours before the test. If the nervous factor is not controlled and inconsistent results are obtained after rest and a barbiturate, a protein-bound-iodine or radio-active iodine absorption test should be run, especially when there is a question of hyperthyroidism; but the latter is indeed uncommon amongst the infertility group of patients. A lowered basal metabolic rate which is not less than about minus twenty per cent and which is without clinical evidences of hypothyroidism, seems to exert no deleterious effect upon reproduction.

Contrary to frequently expressed opinions, a basal metabolic determination with infertility studies is usually just as reliable as protein bound iodine or $I^{131}$ absorption tests. If the basal metabolic rate is elevated, or if nervousness interferes with the basal metabolic determination, the results may be rechecked with other tests, but this is usually not necessary. Most infertility cases are euthyroid and with this group, as with those having a reduced basal metabolic rate, the basal metabolism usually furnishes a very satisfactory guide for the regulation of thyroid therapy and in addition is usually less expensive for the patient.

In cases of glycosuria or nutritional disturbances, blood sugar determinations are in order. If the blood or urine examinations suggest other pathology, such further examinations as may be indicated as a means of restoring the patient to good health should be applied.

# IV. Semen analysis

A careful semen analysis is by far the most important element in the diagnosis and prognosis of male infertility, and no infertile mating can be considered as adequately studied if this phase of the investigation is omitted. Comprehensive semen examinations are, however, often neglected by gynecologists and urologists because of the belief that equivalent information may be otherwise more easily obtained by a hurriedly conducted estimation of the sperm concentration, a Sims-Huhner test or perhaps a testicular biopsy. Such items as a lack of knowledge of spermatic cytology, sperm staining methods, inadequate microscopic methods have contributed to reduce the accuracy of diagnosis and prognosis of male infertility.

The maintenance of a given sperm concentration in the seminal fluid after different periods of sexual abstinence furnishes a fairly reliable index to the ability of the germinal epithelium to form a sufficient number of spermatozoa, particularly if considered in connection with the history of sex activity and the general health. The degree and duration of motility under uniform conditions provides evidence of sperm vitality. Examination of a stained semen smear for morphologic defects reveals the fundamental ability of the germinal epithelium to form spermatozoa which are structurally suitable for fertilization. The volume and consistency of the ejaculate and its cellular content gives evidence of the function of the accessory glands and the possible influence which they may exert on the biochemistry of the semen. Potential fertility is decided largely by the quality or general health of the ejaculated sperm population, provided that it contains enough spermatozoa to cause cervical insemination.

By means of the examination of the fresh semen specimen alone, the more normal semen is readily distinguished by the exceptionally high concentration of normally formed, motile spermia migrating rapidly in a microscopic field which is exceptionally clear, and free from formed elements other than the spermatozoa; whereas with abnormal semen, there is commonly a reduced motility, a paucity of spermatozoa, a high prevalence of abnormal forms, and frequently the presence of much detritus, and often crystals. It is, however, only with the extremely normal and the highly pathologic cases that the differential picture and the consequent prognosis is so clear cut.

During the past two decades, certain rather routine procedures in semen examination have been evolved for the purpose of avoiding technical errors and attaining a more precise evaluation of the number and quality of the ejaculated spermatozoa. This requires strict attention to the proper collection and preservation of semen before examination, uniform procedure for motility examinations and the employment of staining techniques which permit the recognition of spermatic abnormalities.

## 1. Collection and care of semen specimen

All specimens of semen for laboratory examination should be collected in a clean, dry, glass container, then tightly sealed, kept at essentially sixty to seventy degrees Fahrenheit, and delivered for examination within three to four hours after collection. Either a withdrawal sample or a sample obtained by masturbation is satisfactory[1]. The semen is usually collected after a sexual abstinence of three or four days. When longevity studies are to be made, it is best that the semen should be transferred promptly after collection to a small vial of not more than eight to ten cubic centimeters capacity to avoid undue exposure to the air and drying that may destroy some of the cells and cause false readings. The first portion of the ejaculate is invariably richer in spermatozoa than that which follows, and thus the sperm concentration may be reduced if any of the first portion is lost. In some cases, it will be well to collect specimens at different intervals of sexual continence to determine the effect of increased frequency of coitus upon the rate of spermiogenesis. Thus with the more severe germinal disorders, an interval of one or two days between relations may cause a sharp depression in the concentration and quality of the ejaculated spermatozoa which is not experienced to a like degree with normal spermiogenesis.

## 2. Preservation of semen

The semen specimen to be subjected to the examinations as hereafter outlined should be retained in a refrigerator at about forty degrees Fahrenheit as soon as it has been examined for the inital motility and sperm concentration. Longevity examinations by means of the Blom Stain are made from this refrigerated specimen. An antibiotic, such as streptomycin may be added to impede bacterial multiplication, and the properly preserved fluid specimens may remain suitable for cytologic examination for several weeks.

---

[1] According to the tenets of the Catholic Church, it is not permissible to collect a semen specimen for diagnostic examination either by means of relations and withdrawal, or by masturbation. The writer is advised, however, that it is permissible to collect the specimen with the aid of the Doyle Cervical Spoon. This instrument is placed in the vagina by the patient just before coitus, with the expanded spoon portion lying posterior to the cervix. Immediately following coitus, the cervical spoon with the contained semen is withdrawn by the recumbent patient and its contents transferred to a clean glass vial. This usually provides a very satisfactory specimen for examination.

## 3. Examination of gross semen specimen[1]

One should note and record the volume, opacity and viscosity, since when abnormal in these respects, an alteration in the number or quality of the spermatozoa is more likely to occur (Table 7).

Table 7. *Record of seminal findings.* The record of seminal findings should include information concerning the physical properties of the seminal fluid, spermatic morphology and sperm viability

| Semen Examination | Date |
|---|---|
| Name_____ Addr._____ | |
| Vol._____cc.   Dnsty_____ m. | Special Group Characteristic |
| **Cytology** I. Normal _____% | |
| II. Abn. Nuclei _____% | |
| III. Abn. Acrosomia _____% | |
| IV. Miscell. (over) _____% | |
| **Longevity**     Motility    Grade    Dead | |
| 2 hrs._____% _____ _____% | |
| 9 hrs._____% _____ _____% | |
| 1 d _____% _____ _____% | Detritus:   0   1   2   3   4 |
| .... d _____% _____ _____% | |
| .... d _____% _____ _____% | Total Abn.    % |
| | Prognosis |
| Rel. _____ A.M.    Rec'd. _____ A.M. | Misc. Cytologic Abnormalities |
| _____ days since last coitus | 1. Unclassified _____ |
| Viscosity_____ | 2. Megalosperm_____ |
| Opacity_____ | 3. Centrosomic_____ |
| Color _____ | |
| Cyto, Extr. _____ | 4. Middle-piece |
|        Per H.P.F. | |
| W. B. C._____ | 5. Undiff. cytopl._____ |
| Crystals_____ |      Amorph. _____ |
| Prostatic Bodies_____ |      Extrusions _____ |
| | 6. Immature |
| Total Cells Classified: | Total Misc. Abn.    =   % |
| Referred by | |
| Address | |

[1] For characteristic of normal semen and spermatozoa, see section on the character of semen.

# 4. Motility

Various methods for determining and recording sperm motility have been devised, but description will here be limited to the more simplified procedures which can be readily carried out in the average physician's office under the duress of a clinical practice. It should be realized when making motility examinations that the percentage of dead or immotile cells and the relative activity of the live segment represents merely a stage in the progressive death of the sperm population at a given interval after ejaculation unless their metabolism is suppressed. If motility examinations are to be of value in the estimation of the sperm vitality, they should be conducted under constant conditions, as to temperature and the length of time transpiring since ejaculation. Because only a small proportion of a normal ejaculate remains long in effective contact with the cervical mucus, the number of vigorous, healthy spermia which immediately contact the cervical mucus at the time of coitus may be very significant.

## Technique

a. Place a small semen drop on the middle of a microscope slide and overlay with a cover-glass rimmed with petrolatum, thus hermetically sealing the semen between the cover-glass and the microscope slide.

b. Examine under the high dry objective with a $10 \times$ ocular, noting the general appearance of the microscopic field, the relative number of cells, the general motility of the population as a whole, the presence of detritus, crystals, leukocytes or other cellular matter. From this cover-glass preparation, an estimation of the sperm concentration should be made and a note of the approximate ratio of highly motile, progressive motility and clumping of spermatozoa. The latter is associated as a rule with either a general weakness of the sperm population or faulty physical properties of the seminal fluid.

c. Reduce the thickness of the semen film to essentially a single optical plane by pressure on a piece of filter paper placed over the cover-glass. Reduce the size of the optical field by the use of an ocular diaphragm[1] with an aperture of about 3 mm. and then enumerate the motile and immotile spermatozoa in a sufficient number of the reduced microscopic fields to attain a constant figure. Usually the enumeration of about one hundred fifty cells will suffice, but with a very uneven distribution of the motile and immotile cells, a larger number may need to be counted to produce an accurate figure.

The motility status of a sperm population may be signified by recording the percentage of motile cells, their relative degree of activity and the percentage which are actively migratory. Thus different degrees of motility may indicate a progressive deterioration of a sperm population. To obtain consistent and comparable results, the initial motility observation should be made within two to three hours after ejaculation, with a semen sample retained at a temperature of sixty to seventy degrees Fahrenheit.

The ratio of motile cells may also be determined from a semen specimen diluted with Ringer's or Locke's solution and placed in a hematocytometer counting chamber. Usually a dilution of $1:10$ is satisfactory, although with a low sperm concentration a lesser dilution should be used. The dilution may be made with a blood diluting pipette or by gross dilution, adding sufficient Locke's solution to 0.5 cc. semen in a graduated cylinder to effect the required dilution. One first counts the number of immotile cells in five squares of the hemato-

---

[1] An ocular diaphragm may be made by cutting out a disc of thin cardboard of the size to fit the inside of the ocular and perforating the disc with a hole of the desired size.

cytometer as is done when making a red blood count. Then all the spermatozoa
are killed by heat or formaldehyde and the total number of spermatozoa are
counted in the squares that were previously enumerated. The difference between
the total count after all the cells have been killed and the count of the immotile
cells before the application of heat represents the segment killed by heat or
formaldehyde, or the number of motile cells. This method of determining the
percentage of motile cells is highly accurate. From these figures, one may
calculate:

1. The sperm concentration (Number of spermia per cu. mm.)[1]
2. The ratio of motile cells.
4. The total motile cells per cc.[2]
4. The total motile cells in the ejaculate. (Multiply the number of motile
cells per cc. by the number of cc. in the ejaculate).
5. The total number of spermia per ejaculate. (Multiply number of cells
per cc. by the number of cc. of ejaculate.)

## 5. Longevity

Information concerning the longevity of spermatozoa may be obtained
either by repeated observations on motility or by the live-dead staining of
interval samplings from a specimen kept in the refrigerator. For such observations, the same sealed cover-glass preparation may be used as was employed in
the original motility examination and retained in the refrigerator at about forty
to forty-five degrees Fahrenheit between observations. It is warmed to about
ninety degrees Fahrenheit before examination. A record of the ratio and degree
of motility may be made at twenty four hours and repeated at other intervals if
considered desirable. The cover-glass preparation should be thinned to about
a single optical plane to avoid counting errors. In poor quality semen, most
or all motility may cease within twenty-four hours; but with the healthier
specimens, as many as twenty to twenty-five per cent of the population will
survive for one day and a few cells may survive as long as eight to ten days. Usually
a motility observation at two to four hours and another at twenty-four hours
is adequate, since these two observations serve to establish the survival trend.

Longevity may also be gauged with the aid of the Blom eosin-nigrosin live-
dead staining method, as described under sperm stains. Live spermatozoa do
not absorb the stain whereas dead spermia stain with eosin. The results of this
staining method coincide closely with the motility observations during the first
four hours after ejaculation, but after this, one commonly observes that many
live spermia as indicated by the Blom method have lost their motility prior to
their death.

## 6. Sperm concentration

From the cover-glass preparation previously prepared for the motility
examination, a rough estimation of the sperm concentration is made as a guide
in diluting the semen for the actual count. If a high sperm concentration is
present, make a dilution of 1:10 or even 1:20, but if there is a paucity of spermia,
a lesser dilution should be made.

a. For a 1:10 dilution, add 0.5 cc. of semen with a pipette to a 5 cc. graduated
cylinder. Fill to the 5 cc. mark with a 0.5% chloramine[2] solution or other

---

[1] Refer to section on Sperm Concentration for method of calculation of sperm concentration.

[2] Abbott Laboratories — "Chlorozene" (paratoluene sodium sulfachloramid).

satisfactory diluent. This serves to kill the spermatozoa and liquefy the mucus so as to cause a more even distribution of the spermia in the counting chamber. If a greater or lesser dilution is desired, the amount of semen or of chloramine solution may be varied [1].

b. Add the thoroughly mixed sperm suspension to blood counting chamber with the aid of a dropper pipette.

c. Count the spermatozoa in five squares as is done in making a red blood count.

d. The number of spermatozoa per cubic millimeter equals: Number of spermia counted $\times$ dilution $\times 5 \times 10$.

Most determinations of sperm concentration are made with a 1:10 dilution, counting five small squares of the hematocytometer. In this case, the sum total of spermia per millimeter equals the number counted multiplied by 500; or if the dilution is 1:20, multiply by 1,000. If it is desired to express the sperm concentration in terms of the number per cubic centimeter instead of per cubic millimeter, add three ciphers to the above figure.

To facilitate the count of low sperm concentrations, the semen may be introduced into a counting chamber without dilution, the cells then killed by heat or formaldehyde and counted. If no spermia are to be found in the cover-glass preparation, it is desirable to centrifuge the specimen and examine the sediment since cases may prove fertile even though the spermia occur in such small numbers that they are missed without centrifugation. If there are no spermatozoa or so few that they are found with difficulty, the ultimate prognosis is, however, essentially hopeless, irrespective of therapy.

## 7. Spermatic cytology

### a) Preparation of semen smear for staining

Place a small drop of semen near the end of a microscope slide and with another slide held at about forty-five degrees to the first, pull the semen drop from one end to the other of the slide as is done in making a blood smear, thus producing a thin, even spread. Dry the smear quickly, either by waving it in the air or with mild heat. Slides so prepared are satisfactory for use with various stains not having a strong affinity for the mucus of the semen. If the mucus is intensely stained, it clouds the image of the spermatozoa and the mucus should be removed before staining.

With some special differential sperm stains, it is preferable to remove the mucus from the semen film before the stain is applied. This can be accomplished by overlaying the film with a 0.5% chloramine solution for a period of five to thirty seconds, washing briefly and gently with water, and then drying so as to refix to the slide any loosened spermia. If the mucus does not interfere with the staining procedure used, or if very few spermia are present, this step should be omitted.

---

[1] The use of a white blood pipette lacks adaptability in providing for different dilutions, and produces undue sampling errors when working with thick, viscid semen, or where the cells have undergone considerable clumping. Bulk dilution reduces somewhat this technical error. If the semen dilution for sperm concentration is made in a graduated centrifuge tube, one may withdraw the sample for the determination of the sperm concentration and then immediately centrifuge the tube and make a smear for cytologic study from the mucus-free sediment. By so doing, one may obtain mucus-free semen smears, which can be stained to produce remarkably clear microscopic fields.

## b) Selection of sperm staining method

A great many different types of semen stains may be employed, but description will here be limited to a few which, because of their simplicity, have been found especially suitable for clinical studies. Tissue stains and various types of hematologic stains are generally not satisfactory for staining spermatozoa because they fail to adequately differentiate different spermatic structures. Many mistakes in the clinical evaluation of semen arise from the failure to employ a differential staining technique and microscopic method which will permit the identification of structural abnormalities. Unfortunately during the past twenty-five years, only a relatively few persons studying infertility have paid any attention to spermatic cytology and cytogenesis other than that the sperm is perhaps large, small, narrow, pear-shaped or round. Thus reports on spermatic structure are often very uninformative and meaningless.

The application of special sperm stains and the microscopic examination for cytologic defects requires but a few minutes time and is technically so simple that any doctor equipped with a good microscope and the knowledge of its proper use, can conduct this phase of the examination in his private office. A description of the more simple staining methods follows:

*Crystal violet and Rose Bengal sperm staining method* (WILLIAMS 1934):

1. Cover a heat-fixed, mucus-free semen smear with crystal violet solution (0.25% aqueous) for three to four minutes.

2. Wash briefly with water and then with 95 per cent alcohol until any unfixed stain has been removed. Permit slide to dry. Avoid loosening spermatozoa from slide when washing with water by gently adding a few drops of water at a time to one end of the slide and tipping the slide so as to cause the wash fluid to run slowly off the opposite end.

3. Cover with one per cent aqueous solution of rose bengal stain for twenty to twenty-five seconds.

4. Wash with water, dry and examine under oil immersion lens.

The crystal violet-Rose Bengal staining method is highly differential and aids in the identification of a wide variety of spermatic abnormalities, including those of cytoplasmic origin. Because of its simplicity, quickness of application and easy availability, it is very satisfactory for routine clinical studies. The nuclear area retains the bluish coloration, the acrosome and the caudal appendage is of a reddish hue, and the centriolar bodies stain a somewhat deeper red (Fig. 33).

*Wollschwarz, methylene blue, Rose Bengal sperm staining method* (WILLIAMS 1934):

1. Apply Wollschwarz[1] stain to semen smear for three or four minutes. Chloramine treated semen smears are preferred but often a clear image is possible without removal of the mucus. The Wollschwarz sulphuric stain is prepared as follows:

| | |
|---|---|
| Wollschwarz[1] . . . . . . . . . . . . . . | 1.0 gm. |
| Sulphuric acid 2% . . . . . . . . . . | 1.6 cc. |
| Distilled water q. s. . . . . . . . . . . | 100.0 cc. |

2. Wash with water.

3. Cover film with Loeffler's methylene blue diluted 1:15 with water, for eight to twelve seconds. Reduce or lenghten staining time with methylene blue to alter intensity of staining.

---

[1] Wollschwarz or Wool Black may be purchased under the following names:
Calcocid Fast Black 2B: American Cyanamid Company, Calco Chemical Division.
Coomassie Fast Black B: National Aniline Division, Allied Chemical & Dye Corp.
Milling Fast Black 2B: Nyanga Color and Chemical Company, Inc.
Sulfoncyaninschwarz BB konz.: "Bayer" Leverkusen.

4. Wash with water.

5. Counterstain with one per cent aqueous rose bengal stain for twenty-five seconds.

Anomalies of the middle-piece may be clearly defined and enumerated by the use of a Wollschwarz dye which stains the caudal extremity a dark gray or black, whereas the nucleus is stained a yellowish or olive color, and the acrosome stains a reddish hue.

This is one of the most highly differential sperm stains, and is to be preferred to all others that the author has used. It is quickly and easily applied, provides

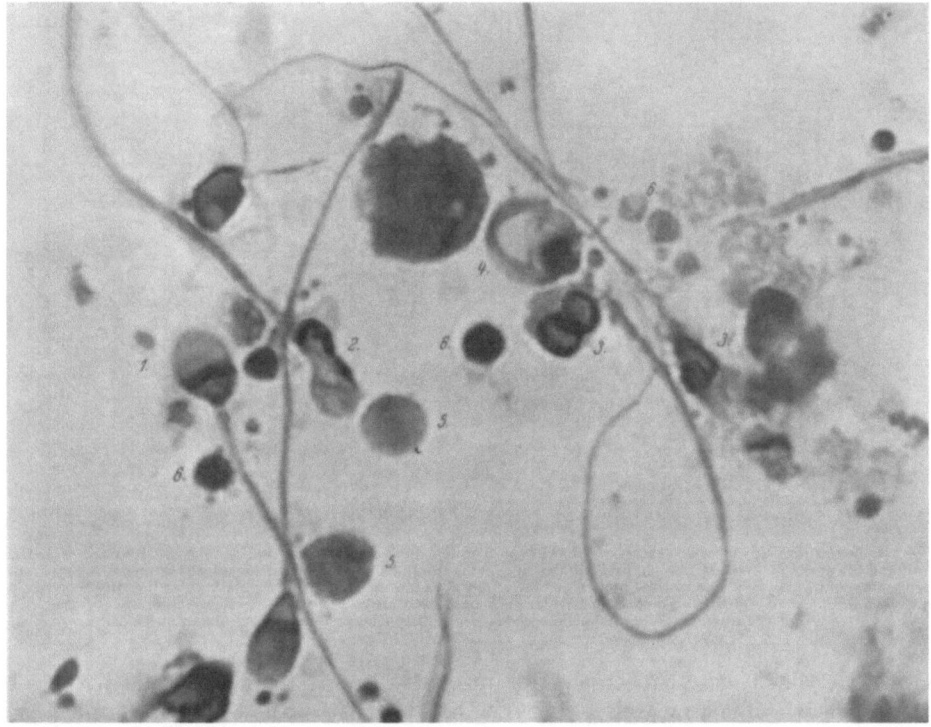

Fig. 33. *Semen smear stained with crystal violet and rose bengal.* One may distinguish with this stain the nucleus, acrosome, cytoplasmic extrusion masses and various abnormalities of the caudal appendage. Most of the spermatozoa of this specimen are abnormal, and there is an abundance of free cytoplasmic globules which are a frequent concomitant of faulty spermiogenesis. *1* Normal sperm, *2* abnormal nucleus, *3* paired spermia without acrosomia, *4* coiled caudal appendage, *5* large cytoplasmic globule, *6* cytoplasmic extrusion mass

good contrasts and is highly satisfactory for photomicrography. This staining method possesses some particularly desirable qualities, especially its differential features for various structures of cytoplasmic origin.

*Blom eosin-nigrosin staining method* (Blom 1950, Williams and Pollak 1950):

1. Place three small drops respectively of 10 per cent aqueous nigrosin, 5 per cent aqueous bluish eosin, and of semen, about one centimeter apart on a microscope slide. The nigrosin drop should usually be slightly larger than the other two drops, and the semen droplet should be larger with a paucity of spermatozoa than with a high sperm concentration.

2. Using a glass rod, mix the semen and eosin droplets together thoroughly to form a homogeneous mixture and then stir the nigrosin droplet into the mixture. The mixing process should not last longer than fifteen to twenty seconds.

3. When the entire mixture is homogeneous, make a smooth, even film or spread over the microscope slide with a glass rod held flatwise to the slide.

4. Dry the film quickly with a mild heat.

The eosin-nigrosin stain furnishes a highly accurate method to distinguish live from dead spermatozoa (Fig. 34). The spermatozoa staining red with the eosin were dead at the time of staining whereas the unstained cells were alive at that time. The smear is best examined under the oil immersion lens with a 10× or 15× ocular. The fluid semen specimen for the eosin-nigrosin staining is retained in the refrigerator in a tightly stoppered vial and observations made

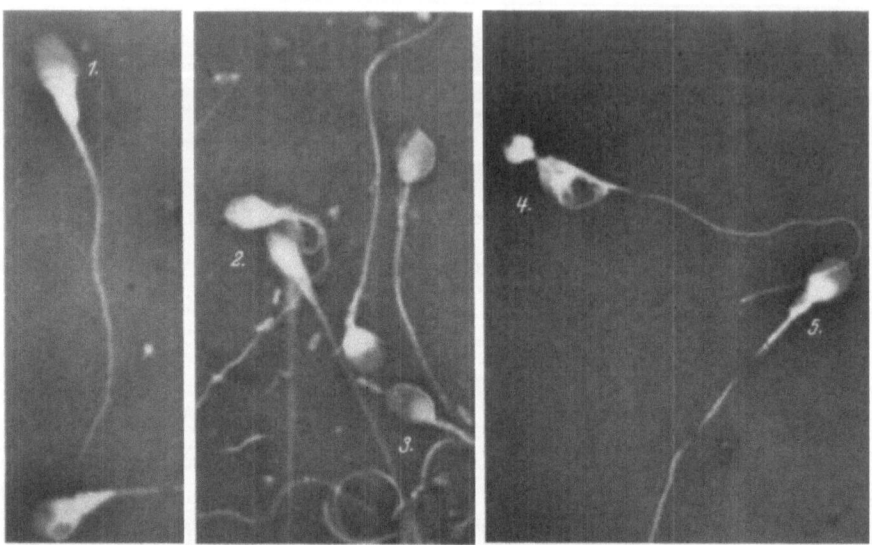

Fig. 34. *Eosin-nigrosin live-dead sperm stain* (blom). The live spermatozoa do not stain with the eosin and the dead sperms stain reddish with eosin and appear darker in the photograph. Live spermatozoa and dead spermatozoa may thus be very accurately distinguished. The staining method reveals that motility often ceases a considerable length of time before metabolism of the cell completely stops. *1* Live spermatozoön, *2* live spermatozoön with abnormal nucleus, *3* dead spermatozoön, *4* absence of acrosome, *5* cytoplasmic extrusion.

on the live-dead ratio at convenient intervals. Of particular interest with this staining method is the ability to recognize the live cells which lack motility, the production of a fairly permanent record of the ratio of live and dead spermatozoa, and the facility with which one may distinguish whether cells with normal or abnormal morphology are dead or alive at given intervals after ejaculation.

When there is a question of the presence of immature gametes, hematoxylin-eosin staining may be very helpful. Good differentiation may be attained by applying a one per cent Harris hematoxylin for three minutes and counterstaining with a one per cent aqueous eosin or Rose Bengal for one to two minutes. Thus small rounded immature gametes fringed with a cytoplasmic layer may be readily distinguished from tissue cells, and a variety of different immature sperm types may be identified.

### c) The microscopic examination of stained semen smears

The microscopic examination of stained semen smears should always be carried out with the aid of an oil immersion objective under a magnification of 1,500 to 2,000 diameters to permit the identification and enumeration of spermatic pathology. This entails the employment of an adequate source of light and attention to developing the best resolving power of which the microscope is capable. Unless the semen smear is properly stained, adequate magnification is not possible. The use of an apochromatic lens system and a binocular microscope is preferable.

The general characteristics of a sperm population may usually be satisfactorily portrayed by the classification of two hundred to three hundred spermia into four groups, based on cellular structure, viz:

1) Normal morphology (Fig. 16).
2) Abnormal nuclei (Fig. 20).
3) Abnormal acrosomia (Fig. 21).
4) Miscellaneous anomalies (Fig. 18).

Into Group 4, one classifies the various bizarre sperm types which occur more or less infrequently and which do not fit into the first three groups. With highly fertile males, the ratio of cells falling into Group 4 rarely exceeds five per cent of the sperm population. Occasionally, however, an unusually high incidence of some anomaly classified in this group renders it clinically very significant (Fig. 25). Nuclear and acrosomic anomalies may be readily observed and enumerated by any clinical observer with ordinary microscopic equipment. When describing or classifying various spermatic anomalies, it is highly desirable to adhere to standard cytologic nomenclature and avoid the specially manufactured terminologies which are so common to literature on infertility.

Aside from spermatic abnormalities, special note should be made of extraneous cellular material, cytoplasmic extrusion masses, and detritus in the semen smear, since such may be of considerable significance[1].

The cytologic picture of the sperm population is usually very constant for a given individual over a period of many years and a single, carefully executed cytologic analysis will usually suffice for estimating the fundamental character of the germ plasm.

The true diagnosis of infertility may be completely missed when an investigator fails to study semen preparations which have been stained in a manner to permit identification of common spermatic anomalies.

# V. Special tests or examinations

## 1. Hormone assays

Hormones of testicular or anterior pituitary origin are excreted in the urine where they may be detected by urinary hormone assays. By this means, a primary testicular failure may be distinguished from a secondary testicular failure. In the former, the assay will reveal a decrease in the 17-Ketosteroids with an increase in the pituitary gonadotropic principles, whereas in association with anterior pituitary failure, there is a decrease in' pituitary gonadotropes which in turn depresses Leydig cell activity. This reduces to a variable degree the urinary 17-Ketosteroids. Then with a diminished androgen elaboration, this may result in a disturbance of the germinal epithelium, causing a germinal

---

[1] Cytoplasmic extrusion droplets are commonly less than half the size of the sperm head when observed free in the seminal fluid. They may be readily identified in the stained preparations by their strong affinity to cytoplasmic stains, such as Rose Bengal. The cytoplasmic droplets appear identical in most cases to the cytoplasmic extrusion masses so commonly observed about the middle-piece. In case that the Blom live-dead stain is used, the cytoplasmic extrusion masses which have not yet separated from the live spermatozoa will fail to take the eosin stain, thus revealing that they are under the influence of sperm metabolism, but when they are free in the seminal fluid, they exhibit a strong affinity for the eosin.

hypoplasia or aplasia and consequently hypospermatogenesis or aspermatogenesis. Often the results of urinary assays are very inconclusive because of
the wide variations in 17-Ketosteroids which can occur without clinical significance.

The presence of urinary 17-Ketosteroids may be determined by the effects
of the urinary hormones on the growth of a capon's comb or by colorimetric
methods. The identification of anterior-pituitary gonadotropic hormones is
commonly accomplished by means of determining the ability of the urinary
hormones to cause follicular maturation or growth of the generative tract of
test animals. For technical details concerning urinary hormone assays and their
interpretation, the reader is referred to a standard work on endocrinology.
Either with a primary testicular failure such as occurs with eunuchoidism or
with secondary failure associated with anterior pituitary failure, a bio-assay
will reveal a reduction or absence of 17-Ketosteroids. The normal 17-Keto-
steroid for the male averages about 13 mg. in 24 hours, of which about 8 mg.
is of adrenal and 5 mg. of testicular origin (REIFENSTEIN). It is noted, however,
that the 17-Ketosteroids range between 6.7 and 27.2 mg. per day with normal
men, and unless the ketosteroids are extremely low such as might occur in
clinical hypogonadism or clinical evidences of anterior pituitary failure, that
the 17-Ketosteroid determination possesses very little or no value in sterility
diagnosis.

The normal value for F.S.H. in man is 6 to 50 mouse units a day. There
is ordinarily an increased F.S.H. titre in the case of hypogonadism with a lowered
17-Ketosteroid, whereas with anterior pituitary failure, there is a diminished
F.S.H. Actually, however, hormonal assays in cases of male infertility possess
little value because the wide normal variability in titres interfere with their
evaluation, and because the cases with endocrine stigmata and decidedly abnormal assays commonly provide a type of germinal epithelium which is not
amenable to therapy. Such cases may almost invariably be recognized by signs
and symptoms of endocrine pathology plus the seminal findings which serve
to negate the clinical value of hormone assays. The clinical value of such assays
is not sufficiently evident to justify their routine inclusion in clinical investigations of infertility. The use of endocrine products, either androgen, or gonadotropins of placental or anterior-pituitary origin have so far proven essentially
worthless in promoting or improving spermiogenesis and potential fertility,
whether the failure is of endocrine or genetic etiology. As far as is known, the
spermatic disorders encountered in the study of infertile marriages are very
rarely of endocrine etiology. In cases where major endocrine stigmata are
present, it is generally the rule that the damage to the germinal epithelium is
far beyond repair as indicated by the physical status of the testes and the absence
of or character of the spermatozoa in the seminal fluid. Thus until hormone
assays can be employed to produce a more reliable prognosis, such assays should
remain on the research and academic level, and not be employed to produce
unjustifiable expense to the patient.

## 2. Testicular biopsy

In general, a testicular biopsy possesses a very limited diagnostic value with
infertility studies, excepting as a means of distinguishing between epididymal
obstruction and germinal aplasia or hypoplasia. If spermatozoa are present
in the ejaculate, a semen examination will reveal much better than a testicular
biopsy the quality of the ejaculated spermatozoa. When spermiogenesis is so

impaired that no spermia are present in the ejaculate, the sterility with few exceptions will be absolute, irrespective of the histologic picture observed with testicular biopsies. Clinically, a hypoplasia of the germinal epithelium causes a reduction of sperm concentration in the ejaculate, and conversely, we may expect a germinal hypoplasia and a reduction in the volume and activity of the germinal epithelium whenever there exists a fixed lowering of sperm concentration in the ejaculate. The value of testicular biopsies is essentially limited to a group of less than one half of one per cent of the infertile marriages wherein there is the possibility of surgery to correct an epididymal obstruction and with which it must be known in advance that the germinal epithelium is capable of normal spermiogenesis. When the testes are atrophic and the seminal fluid is without spermatozoa, one may be reasonably assured that there is a germinal aplasia or hypoplasia, and that nothing of clinical value to the patient will result from a testicular biopsy.

Those who are concerned with the clinical phases of male infertility generally attach very little value to the routine clinical application of testicular biopsies. Thus GETZOFF (1957) reports attending a meeting of about eight hundred and fifty urologists at which only two of this number considered a testicular biopsy of any value in general infertility studies.

*Technique of testicular biopsy* (CHARNY):

*Anesthesia.* Pentabarbital or spinal anesthesia may be employed to relax the cremaster muscle and lessen sensation of the tunica albuginea. In some instances, the scrotum and tunica albuginea may be infiltrated with one per cent novocaine at the site of the biopsy and provide sufficient anesthesia.

*Technique.* Grasp the testis to be biopsied between the thumb and first finger, stretching the scrotum tightly over its greater curvature and make an incision with a sharp scalpel through the scrotum and tunica vaginalis, down to the tunica albuginea. Care should always be taken to avoid the lesser curvature and any injury to the epididymis. It is best to retract the scrotum and tunica vaginalis with mosquito forceps or a special small spring retractor so as to bring the tunica albuginea clearly into view over an area of about five-eights inch long. With the scrotum and tunica vaginalis thus retracted, an incision about one-quarter to three-eights inch in length is made through the tunica albuginea, whereupon by continued pressure on the testis, a small bead of the yellowish matrix of the testis is caused to bulge through the incision. Then by using a small curved iris forceps, a small specimen of the matrix of the testis is obtained and immediately transferred to Bouin's solution for fixing. This specimen need be no larger than 0.5 cm. in diameter. The incision through the scrotum should be directed parallel to the veins to prevent bleeding. After obtaining the biopsy, the tunica albuginea will require no suturing. Any bleeding blood vessels in the tunica vaginalis should be closed with No. 000 catgut suture, and the incision in the scrotum closed with two or three interrupted silk sutures (Fig. 35).

# 3. Post-coital examinations

Post-coital or Sims-Huhner tests for sperm survival in the vaginal and cervical mucus are commonly a part of the diagnostic study of marital infertility. Their purpose as generally applied is to reveal the fertility status of the male partner, and by many, it is believed that this type of test reveals more accurately the fertility status than can be accomplished with any type of a direct examination of the semen. This is because of the belief by some that motile spermia arefertile á priori.

To be informative as to the ability of sperm survival and migration in the female tract, sampling should not be made until at least five hours after coitus and thus permit spermatozoa to perish either because of their intrinsic weakness or because of the continued unfavorable influence of the cervical secretion. Normal ovulation-type cervical mucus will continue to harbor healthy strong spermatozoa for as long as thirty-six hours after coitus, and many times for a much longer period of time. If the sperm concentration in the mid-cervix is

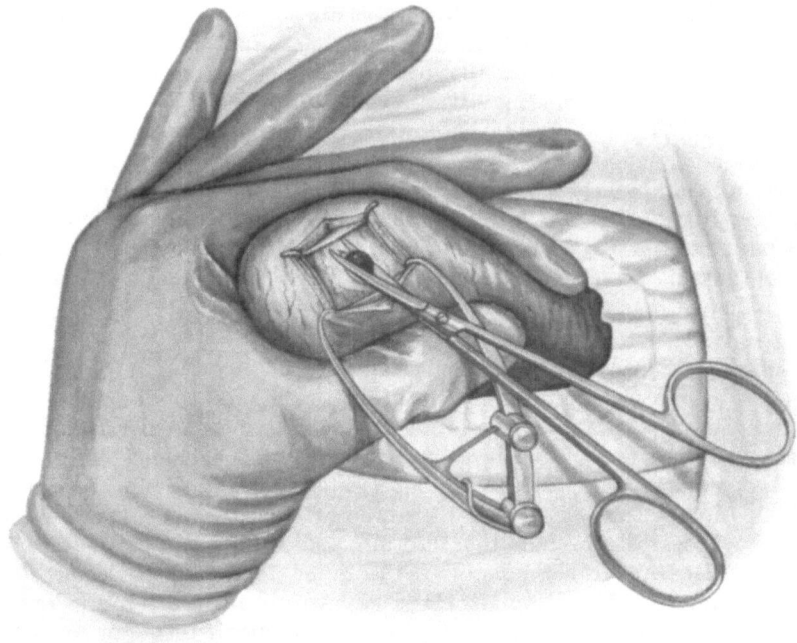

Fig. 35. *Biopsy of testis.* The scrotum and tunica vaginalis have been incised, exposing the tunica albuginea which has been punctured to permit a small mass of matrix to bulge through the opening. This is snipped off with a fine pair of curved forceps, bleeders tied off and the wound in the scrotum closed with interrupted sutures. (Courtesy of LEWIS MICHELSON, M. D. San Francisco, California, U.S.A.)

as high as fifteen to twenty spermatozoa per high power field, one may expect under normal conditions to find as many as one to five highly motile spermatozoa per h. p. f. in fluid withdrawn from the uterus.

When the male is aspermic, post-coital examinations are without any useful purpose whatsoever. With either normal or pathologic sperm populations, live spermatozoa may be found in the vagina immediately after coitus, but even the more healthy spermatozoa ordinarily die within the first four hours after coitus (WEISMAN 1941). Thus the finding of live spermatozoa immediately after coitus, or the failure to find any live spermatozoa in the vagina five hours after coitus has no special clinical significance. If some device is used to prevent the spilling of the semen from the vagina after coitus, then one will find a larger number of dead spermatozoa.

The sampling of mucus from the cervix is accomplished in two stages, first a sampling from the region of the external os, where some of the mucus partially exposed to the acidity of the vagina is removed and transferred to a glass slide with a thumb forceps, and the second sampling from the mid-cervix with a curved glass cannula to which a Luer syringe is attached to produce suction. Before introducing the tip of the glass cannula into the cervical canal, the mucus is removed from the external os so that it is not mixed with the mucus from deeper within the cervical canal. The sperm concentration within the cervical canal is almost invariably greater than that at the external os which is partially exposed to the acidity of the vagina. One may observe as many as two hundred to three hundred spermia per high power field or even more, but most conceptions occur with those cases where the sperm concentration is not over ten to twenty cells per high power field. Indeed with many cases, irrespective of sperm concentration in the semen and in the cervix, or irrespective of fertility, not more than zero to five spermia are found per high power field in the uterine sampling. It therefore appears that conception is the result of a few healthy spermatozoa, rather than the result of a mass migration. An exceptionally high cervical concentration of spermatozoa does not seem to represent a normal status, but rather an excessive accumulation of spermatozoa in the cervical canal results either because of a weakness of the spermatozoa, or an abormality of the cervical secretion in the region of the internal os which creates an effective barrier to further sperm migration. At the internal os there does exist a natural barrier, but this barrier is increased under the influence of pathology in the cervix. At any rate, the excessively high sperm concentrations in the cervical canal fail to produce correspondingly high intra-uterine sperm concentrations or a correspondingly high incidence of conceptions.

The failure to find live spermatozoa in the cervical canal or the finding of an excessive sperm concentration which is incapable of further migration is merely a challenge to better diagnostic methods so as to ascertain whether the fault lies with the secretions of the female, with the condition of the spermatozoa or both. As commonly applied, however, post-coital examinations are often employed to circumvent the necessity of a semen examination, and in so doing, there comes about a disregard of spermatic pathology and of the physiology of the female tract and the physiology of sperm migration. The underlying factors which predicate motility or immotility, or the presence or absence of spermatozoa, are often not investigated or recognized.

The sampling of the uterine cavity for spermatozoa was apparently first introduced by WEISMAN (1940). Preliminary to this test, the mucus from the cervical canal is removed by means of a cotton swab and by suction with a cannula. A disinfectant, such as Schiller's solution, can be then introduced into the cervical canal to destroy any spermatozoa in that location, and swabbed with cotton to remove any excess iodine. The cannula is then introduced into the uterine cavity. In this manner, fluid from the uterus can be obtained without any carryover from the cervix. There is no free fluid in the uterine cavity, but by this method, a few drops of a sero-sanguinous fluid derived from the endometrium and often a little fragment of endometrium is obtained. If any live spermatozoa are found in the cervical canal, one may find as many as one to five per high power field in the uterine cavity. The intra-uterine spermia are invariably of high motility, but even with the highly fertile cases, very few spermatozoa may migrate into the uterine cavity, and these may be missed in the sampling. Without ovulation-type mucus present in the cervical canal, the intra-uterine spermatozoa are usually not found.

If it were true that an abundance of live motile intra-cervical spermatozoa signified a reasonably high fertility or that the failure to find a considerable number of live spermatozoa in the cervical canal at a given interval after coitus signified sterility, then post-coital examinations would gain in value. Clinical observations reveal, however, that this is not the case (WILLIAMS 1953, 1957) and it seems desirable that a more precise knowledge should be attained concerning the underlying factors which predicate sperm survival.

### 4. Mucus penetration tests

Mucus penetration tests are for the purpose of determining the ability of spermatozoa to penetrate the cervical mucus. This is best performed by placing a drop of mucus obtained from the mid-cervix by suction on a microscope slide, overlaying it with a cover-glass and then contacting the mucus with a small drop of semen. Under normal circumstances, spermatozoa will soon commence penetrating the cervical mucus from the area of contact. One observes first a few spermatozoa breaking through the barrier between the two fluids, and where the barrier is broken, other spermia follow through the break, channeling through the mucus in long strings until finally the entire mucus drop is heavily loaded throughout with active spermatozoa.

Under abnormal circumstances, due either to abnormal mucus or abnormal spermatozoa, penetration is limited and spermia may penetrate only slightly and perish; or there may be no penetration whatsoever.

The lack of penetration will occasionally occur when the mucus and semen appear quite normal, but the failure is more apt to be associated with an abnormality of the mucus or of the sperm population. Cross matching by using a known normal semen against questionable mucus or employing proven normal mucus against questionable semen, may serve to fix the fault on one or the other partner when pathology of the semen or mucus is not apparent.

# C. Therapy of male infertility

The treatment of male infertility has in general been highly unsatisfactory, both because so large a ratio of it results from intractable germinal disease of genetic origin and because diagnostic methods are so frequently inadequate for its recognition. Indeed, there is a relatively small segment of male infertility which is due to other than germinal factors. Thus the proper handling of male infertility is very often merely a problem of a sound prognosis and is not greatly concerned with therapy. This prognosis may, however, be difficult because of the uncertainty that the observed abnormalities are adequate to explain the reproductive failure and because the prognosis is so greatly influenced by unrecognized, obscure female pathology which may be the primary factor. About sixty per cent of male partners to barren marriages present seminal pictures in which an altered sperm concentration, motility and morphology is insufficient to reasonably interfere with fertility. Of the remaining forty per cent, about one fourth, or ten per cent of the total infertility is azoospermic. An additional ten to fifteen per cent will commonly exhibit either an extremely low sperm motility or an extremely high ratio of structurally abnormal cells which render them essentially as sterile as if no spermatozoa at all were present. This leaves a group of about fifteen to twenty per cent of the male partners in infertile marriages with different degrees of reduced fertility potentials of which some are permanently sterile and others may improve sufficiently to permit conception. Useful therapy for male infertility applies largely to this group with widely different fertility potentials, and not to the more normal group or to the segment wherein spermatic disease or azoospermia obviates successful therapy. It is, however, important that various prophylactic measures shall apply to the healthy appearing group of cases so as to favor in this group the maintenance of the highest possible fertility.

Therapy of male sterility is influenced to a considerable degree by difference in concept of its etiology and the particular criteria by which it may be identified. There has been a rather widespread tendency to consider spermatic disease as innocuous from the viewpoint of infertility and thus to justify the omission of semen examinations in clinical studies. Thus LANE-ROBERTS states: "It would be a grave error to regard abnormal spermatogenesis, however precisely defined, as one of the primary conditions causing sterility." He considers faulty spermiogenesis as the end product of a number of disorders, each of which needs its own special therapy. This viewpoint seems to be at considerable variance with the observations by many clinical observers who report a striking correlation between the quality of spermatozoa that the individual is capable of producing and his fundamental fertility. It is a concept which tends to invalidate routine semen examinations as commonly employed as the basis for the recognition and prognosis of spermatic disorders and to reveal the fundamental ability of normal spermiogenesis. The gynecologist may justify this omission because he is supposed to be concerned only with the female. The urologist is often more interested in urology per se and not with spermatic disorders. The dogma of the Roman Catholic Church often forbids those of Catholic faith from collecting semen for examination otherwise than from the vagina after coitus, and thereby interferes with the reliability of diagnosis and prognosis of male infertility.

The presence of spermatic abnormalities is regarded by many as merely incidental and of insufficient clinical significance to justify a cytologic evaluation of the sperm population. This is evidenced by the infrequency of cytologic evaluations by those investigating marital infertility. Thus MACLEOD (1957) states: "We have suggested that abnormal sperm morphology per se is not a deciding factor, but that the poor morphology is related to motility and that failure of abnormal spermatozoa to reach the ovum is the cause of sterility in such cases." Male sterility is thus conceived as due to the failure of abnormal spermatozoa to reach the ovum. The possibility that a normal nucleus, acrosome and centriolar bodies being in any way involved in the fertilization of the ovum is thus discarded. This concept of the dissociation of spermatic structure and function although lacking in factual criteria either from the cytologic viewpoint or clinically, has nevertheless brought about a considerable disregard of the role played by faulty sperm populations in the etiology of male infertility.

During the past twenty-five years, the clinical handling of the male infertility problem has in general been highly unsatisfactory, partly because its refractory character is so often disregarded, partly due to the omission of diagnostic studies which might permit its recognition and partly because of the widespread belief that fertility is decided primarily by the size of the sperm population rather than its quality. Very minor population deviations from the normal which are difficult or impossible to distinguish, may decide the fertility status of the male and render it exceedingly difficult to accurately evaluate the effects of therapy.

The value of therapy may however be indicated by comparing the incidence of conception following therapy with the incidence of conception in a properly selected control series which has not received therapy. This is rarely accomplished. The effect of therapy may also be indicated by observing changes, if any, in different seminal factors which are commonly associated with male infertility.

# I. Therapy directed at seminal factors
## 1. Seminal volume

In general, the volume of the ejaculate is fixed by the functional development of the accessory sexual glands, together with the secretion from the epididymides and the activity of the seminiferous tubules, and is not influenced by medications. In some instances, a small seminal volume results from a genital hypoplasia. Aspermia, or a complete lack of semen, is extremely uncommon with marital infertility and generally exists only when a severe genital hypoplasia prevents the function of the accessory sexual glands. There is no valid therapy for this condition from the viewpoint of infertility. In other instances, a hyperplasia or hyperfunction of the accessory glands causes an increase in seminal volume which may be as great as 8 to 10 cc. A volume of under 2 cc. or over 8 cc. is generally associated with low fertility. Therapy of these cases with either a high or low volume has been very unsatisfactory. An excessive frequency of coitus may cause a temporary reduction in the volume of the ejaculate as also psychic factors which interfere with a full ejaculation. The seminal volume which is normal to the individual is commonly restored within twenty-four to forty-eight hours after coitus. Thus under ordinary circumstances, no great variation in the seminal volume is observed. If, however, the seminal volume is too small to permit cervical insemination and contains a reasonably normal sperm population, one may mix the semen with a semen diluent for a homo-insemination. The failure of intra-cervical survival in these cases is, however, usually due to the high ratio of pathologic spermia, which renders therapy valueless. With a semen volume as high as 8 to 10 cc., the sperm concentration may be as great as 100 m. per cu.mm. thus bringing about an excessive strain upon the germinal epithelium in maintaining this high sperm concentration. Presumably, the excessive spermatogenesis is lessened by widening the interval between relations and thus slowing spermatogenesis. This brings about a greater maturity of the ejaculated spermia. In practice, however, this does not seem to increase fertility.

Within a wide range of variability, the seminal volume exerts in itself no influence on fertility, provided that the volume is sufficient for cervical insemination. PERLMAN (1958) has recently pointed out with a small series of cases that a reduction in seminal volume occurred after the administration of Meticorten (prednisone) and suggests that the increased volume may be due to an increased androgen elaboration associated with a high gonadotrope titre. Two of his four cases conceived after reduction of semen volume. The number of cases observed is too small to be clinically significant were it not for the fact that conceptions are so uncommon with this type of case.

## 2. Sperm concentration

Without any therapy, wide fluctuations in sperm concentration may amount to as much as 20 m. to 50 m. in the different samplings from the same individual, and particularly those with low fertility. These wide natural variations should not be confused with the possible effects of therapy. It is the general rule with infertility, as with other branches of medicine, that the overworked, defective organ can be best conserved by rest. Thus to prevent exhaustion of the defective germ plasm and further reduction in sperm concentration, sexual activity should be restricted. If as much as four to five days elapse between relations, it is often observed that a uniformly higher sperm concentration is maintained than that associated with a greater frequency. This is especially true when there is a faulty sperm population, because in such cases, the germ plasm is commonly less capable of a normal rate of spermiogenesis.

Because of a somewhat common belief that the number of spermia or their concentration in the seminal fluid is usually the primary etiologic factor in male sterility, many methods have been introduced during the past few years for the purpose of increasing the number of available spermia. The following are some of the methods which have been employed:

*Endocrine therapy.* Androgen therapy and the so-called rebound phenomenon has been recommended and used with large numbers of cases. It consists of the administration of sufficient androgen to depress or eliminate spermatogenesis. After withdrawal of the androgen therapy, there occurs with some cases a rate of spermatogenesis which exceeds that observed prior to therapy. This procedure has failed to increase the ratio of conceptions and it is generally considered that the danger of permanent injury to the germinal epithelium of the individual with essentially normal androgen elaboration far outweighs any possible benefit that might be derived from the use of testosterone. Pituitary and placental gonadotropins have also been employed rather frequently for many years, but as yet, no substantial evidence of significant improvement in spermatogensis and fertility has been observed following their use. They may, however, as with androgen therapy, injure the germinal epithelium and still further depress spermiogenesis.

*Increased frequency of relations.* Patients are occasionally advised to compensate for a sperm deficit by increasing the frequency of relations. This tends to produce a sexual overload, exhausting the already defective germinal epithelium and greatly reducing potential fertility, rather than increasing it.

*Intra-cervical insemination.* An increased number of spermatozoa may be provided by intra-cervical insemination with the husband's semen, but there is no evidence of an increase in conception rate thereby (WILLIAMS 1953). In the case of artificial insemination in breeding of cattle, an exceptionally high ratio of highly fertile spermatozoa permits the dilution of semen with semen dilutors and its division into as many as one hundred parts, with each part maintaining essentially the same fertility potential as the original undiluted specimen. On the other hand, with human infertility where there are commonly few or no normal fertile spermatozoa to contact the cervical mucus, no such dilution is possible without still further lowering an already extremely low fertility potential. With a relatively small ratio of potentially fertile spermatozoa present in the semen, clinical experience indicates that the addition of a few hundred million more defective spermatozoa will result in no recognizable improvement of fertility potential.

*Concentration by centrifugation.* Semen with an increased sperm concentration may be obtained either by centrifugation or by the use of the first portion of the ejaculate, and the woman inseminated either intra-cervically or with the aid of a plastic cervical cap. The method fails with the infertile male because the quality of the sperm population remains unchanged.

The futility of attempting to overcome male infertility by increasing the number of spermatozoa from an infertile individual is quite evident. Excepting those cases with aspermia, azoospermia and oligospermia, hundreds of millions of spermatozoa are commonly made available week after week for perhaps several years without a fertilization. Under these circumstances, if any fertile spermia were present, some of them should eventually contact a fertilizable ovum, but it happens that in spite of the hundreds of millions of spermatozoa

and their opportunity for migration, that no fertile spermia are present. It is
further noted that the number of spermatozoa which survive in the female tract
after homo-inseminations is on the average no greater than that from natural
intercourse, thus indicating with inferior sperm that very few of the spermatozoa
are actually capable of surviving in the female genital tract irrespective of the
circumstances. It is not surprising therefore that the addition of a few hundred
million faulty spermatozoa to the vagina, cervix or even injected into the
uterine cavity, will not increase perceptibly the fertility potential. This circumstance is quite different than pertains to a highly fertile male with a superfluity
of normal, healthy, fertile spermatozoa which requires only a small segment
of the sperm population for the necessary fertile spermatozoa.

*Maintenance of vaginal or cervical pool of semen for an extended period of
time after coitus.* For many years, advice has been given to maintain a vaginal
semen pool for extended periods of time by elevating the buttocks after coitus
to prevent the loss of seminal fluid. More recently the use of a vaginal obturator
has been recommended for this purpose so that the seminal fluid can be held
in the vaginal cavity for several hours, irrespective of the position of the patient.
Such methods are very appealing to patients because they are so often greatly
concerned about the loss of semen immediately after coitus. It happens, however,
that spermatozoa retained in the vaginal cavity will normally perish within
two to five hours, and the semen decomposes. It is the apparently healthy
spermatozoa which contact the mucus at the external os during the first few
minutes after coitus which usually cause fertilizations. These quickly penetrate
into the more favorable media of cervical mucus where they may survive,
whereas those remaining in the vagina will quickly perish. Measures to bring
about the retention of dead or devitalized spermatozoa and decomposing semen
in the vagina do not seem to be a practical solution to either male or female
infertility problems. If a cervical cap is used to hold the semen against the
cervix, then the cervical mucus with some bacteriostatic action serves to prolong
the life of the spermatozoa and limit the bacterial decomposition for a period
of as long as forty-eight hours. At the same time, the cervical cap serves to
keep the entire semen specimen in actual contact with the external os and
protected from the harmful influences of vaginal acidity; but even this method
fails in most cases to increase the number of spermatozoa migrating into the
cervical canal and fails to increase the conception rate above that which would
have occurred with normal coitus.

There seems to be no reliable evidence that fertility can be improved by
increasing the number of faulty spermatozoa, regardless of the method employed.
This is further borne out by the clinical experience that homo-inseminations
with semen containing high ratios of pathologic spermatozoa will almost invariably fail to cause conceptions, whereas with both man and animals, a high
ratio of conception results from artificial inseminations with healthy semen.

## 3. Motility

Motility is not synonymous with fertility as is amply demonstrated by the
observation that most infertile males, unless azoospermic, will present large
numbers of highly motile cells in spite of their infertility. No type of therapy is
apt to prove of any benefit if the immobility is based upon demonstrable cytologic abberations of the spermatozoa. Some cases present a low motility which
is not constant and which may be influenced by variations in somatic health
and sexual activity; but when repeated semen examinations reveal a **constantly**

high ratio of immotile or feebly motile cells, there may be a genetic etiology which precludes improved fertility from any type of therapy.

Many empiric remedies have been introduced from time to time for the purpose of improving sperm motility. The use of buffered glucose solutions and special semen dilutors or extenders such as used with artificial insemination with animals have been employed for many years upon the presumption that lowered motility and reduced fertility are related to some chemical factors in the seminal fluid or vagina. Although the lowering of sperm vitality by chemical factors cannot be dismissed, the ability of these diluents or nutritive agents to increase fertility has not yet been established even though motility may temporarily improve when used either as a pre-coital vaginal douche or for the dilution of a vitro semen specimen prior to artificial insemination.

A semen diluter cannot, however, be expected to effectively alter the intrinsic nature of a spermatic disorder nor the character of the cervical secretion through which the spermatozoa must travel. The same may be said in general about other medicinal agents or gland products given for the specific purpose of increasing motility and thereby fertility. On the other hand, if the anamnesis reveals excessive sexual activity, there is always the possibility that a reduction in the sexual overload by widening the interval between relations may improve the quality of the spermatozoa and consequently the potential fertility, and there is also the possibility that an improved somatic health may favor an improvement in the vitality of the spermia.

## 4. Cytologic abnormalities

Cytologic abnormalities of spermatozoa are almost always of genetic origin and become of increasing clinical significance as their ratio in the sperm population increases. Conceptions are exceedingly rare if the spermatic abnormalities involve as much as 80 per cent of the sperm population, in spite of the presence of millions of apparently normal spermatozoa. Unless, however, all of the spermia appear pathologic, there is always the possibility that a fertile sperm might become available even though this chance is very poor. Because of the intrinsic nature of the morphologic anomalies of spermia, there is apparently no type of therapy which can materially influence the type or ratio of pathologic spermatozoa. The frequent claims of ability to alter the cytologic characteristics of spermatozoa have not been verified. The low fertility resulting from a high incidence of spermatic anomalies serves to eliminate a breeding animal such as a bull and end its career, whereas with man, it commonly perpetuates his low fertility.

## 5. Pyospermia

Pyospermia, as encountered in connection with infertility studies, usually arises either from chronic prostatitis or a chronic passive congestion of the prostate. It is rarely associated with either a specific or non-specific urethritis. When present, the treatment is according to the general urologic principles which need not be covered in this section on infertility. A high leukocyte content in the prostatic fluid is frequently encountered when investigating male fertility. This serves to increase the number of leukocytes in the ejaculated semen. The use of antibiotics is usually of little or no value. Occasional prostatic massages may reduce the leukocytic content of the prostatic fluid, but usually the improvement is temporary.

18*

Unless associated with infection, the presence of leukocytes in the semen or in the prostatic fluid seems to exert very little influence upon fertility (GET-ZOFF 1958). It is, however, considered a sound clinical practice to occasionally massage the prostate gland so as to rid it of an excessive accumulation of purulent secretion. There is always the possibility that an abnormal secretion from the accessory glands may alter the chemical properties of the seminal fluid suffi-ciently to lower sperm viability. In this case, we would expect a uniform devitaliza-tion of the entire sperm population instead of a reduced motility which involves only a limited segment of the sperm population.

## 6. Consistency of the seminal fluid

The consistency of the seminal fluid is determined by the several structures which contribute to it, such as the seminiferous tubules, epididymides, prostate and the seminal vesicles. As far as is known, the character of the secretion from these structures cannot readily be altered to any significant degree by therapy. Moreover, it happens that there is a very close correlation between the character of spermatogenesis and the physical properties of the seminal fluid to the extent that thin watery semen, or thick viscid semen is commonly associated with ab-normal sperm populations. When this is the case, any correction of the physical properties will serve no useful purpose. If the semen is so thick and gelatinous as to interfere with sperm migration from it into the cervical mucus, one may employ a semen dilutor such as a homogenized milk with 5% to 10% glycerol added, or egg yolk extender[1], and in this way bring about a dispersion of the spermatozoa. This may be used as a vaginal injection just prior to relations or added to vitro semen specimens for intra-cervical injection. It is not likely, however, that this type of therapy will possess any value unless it is first shown that the sperm population is essentially normal.

## II. Failure of cervical insemination

The failure of cervical insemination may be due to various factors, such as inability of intromission, hypospadius, epispadius, the paucity of spermatozoa in the ejaculate, the inability to consummate relations because of impotency or premature ejaculation. If the sperm population is apparently normal and no post-coital spermia are in the cervical canal, it should be determined whether intromission has actually occurred. The phalus may fail to enter the vagina either because of an imperforate hymen or spasm of the bulbocavernosus muscle of the female. This may usually be corrected by stretching or incision of the hymen or if due merely to spasm, by stretching of the bulbocavernosus muscle. In some instances wherein coitus is essentially impossible because of spasm of the bulbocavernosus muscle, the daily insertion of a finger by the patient in the posterior commissure of the vulva and pressing forceably posteriorly until the muscle relaxes, will usually obtain sufficient dilatation within a few days to permit normal coitus.

When a semen examination reveals very few or no normal spermia, a cervical insemination is not be expected and any therapy aside from a hetero-insemination may be of little or no value. If cervical insemination fails because of premature ejaculation, abnormalities of the phalus or with cases of impotency who ejaculate semen without an erection, then, a homo-insemination at the fertile phase of the cycle may be indicated.

---

[1] *Egg yolk extender:* Egg yolk 25.0 cc., Glycerol 6.5 cc., Sodium citrate 6.5 cc., Aqua q. s. 100.0 cc., Add Streptomycin 200 to 500 units per cc.

## III. Somatic health

It has already been pointed out that the viability of ejaculated spermatozoa may occasionally be improved by various factors, amongst which is the maintenance of a high state of general health, and the correction of any pathology which may interfere with normal sexual function. Proper rest, recreation, exercise and nutrition, and relief from nervous tensions may all have their place in the general health program. Any disorders such as anemia, diabetes, hypoglycemia, hypothyroidism and various types of infection, either focal or general, should be brought under control whenever encountered. It is commonly considered that anything which favors good health may indirectly improve the vitality of the spermatozoa, and factors favoring poor health, may indirectly reduce the quality of the spermatozoa and their fertilizing ability even though microscopically demonstrable changes in the sperm population are not apparent. Much effort will, however, be wasted on therapy if it is attempted to cause the germinal epithelium to accomplish something for which it is not genetically endowed, or by evading general health factors which may cause transitory infertility. Thus various metabolic disorders, overweight and underweight, the excessive use of liquor or tobacco, overwork, sedentary occupations and many other factors may contribute to ill health and indirectly involve the health of the gametes. Infertility associated with occupational factors may be occasionally recognized and corrected.

If a general health study of each male partner is included as a part of every sterility survey, one will find that there will be much less difficulty in making more complete studies and in receiving the full-wholehearted support of the husband as well as the wife. A considerable increase in both the sperm motility and concentration is frequently observed with patients undergoing general infertility studies, a circumstance which is related to psychosomatic factors as well as to the general health. In the breeding of lower animals, it is recognized that the male maintains a higher potential fertility if his general health is satisfactory and he is not driven to excessive sexual activity. These factors are regarded very closely by live stock breeders but commonly disregarded in the human race which is so commonly given to sedentary occupations, poor eating habits and sexual activity which is far in excess to normal tolerance.

It is seldom that specific genital infections are encountered with cases seeking medical care for infertility, but if so, they should be adequately treated prior to any special examinations or therapy for infertility. Any infection causing a high fever may temporarily reduce spermiogenesis and fertility.

In the cases of mumps orchitis, prompt confinement to bed and cold compresses to the testes may serve to reduce the swelling of the testes. The necrosis of the seminal tubules is probably in part due to the exudate in the stroma of the testes which creates considerable pressure under the unyielding tunica albuginea and a consequent circulatory disturbance. Good results have also been reported from the use of diethylstilbesterol, mg. I qid or prednisone 20—30 mg. daily in the control of the inflammatory reaction in the testes. Multiple incisions of the tunica vaginalis have also been employed in an effort to relieve pressure and conserve the germinal epithelium. If not promptly treated, about fifty per cent of the involved testes will subsequently atrophy.

## IV. Functional factors

Functional factors in male sterility concern more particularly the ability of normal copulation and the results of excessive sexual activity. Some individuals experience difficulty in performing the sexual act under compunction, such as may arise when directed to have relations at some specific time of the menstrual cycle. They may miss the fertile phase of the cycle in consequence. Others, because of an excessive sex drive or an excessive desire for a family, are led erroneously to the belief that frequency of relations can compensate for a lowered fertility. It is therefore desirable to discuss the problem of frequency of relations with both partners so that they understand the possible detrimental influence of a sexual overload, particularly in association with a faulty germinal epithelium. In general, we might expect a healthy man, endowed with normal germinal epithelium, to tolerate sexual relations about every four days without danger of affecting the quality of the germinal epithelium and the spermatozoa which it produces. Thus, according to the laws of chance and without paying any attention to the possible fertile day of the cycle, a conception is almost bound to occur within three to four months with a coital frequency of about four days, provided that both partners are highly fertile.

Impotentia is mostly considered as a functional episode (see previous section on impotentia), and although generally of neurogenic or psychogenic origin, it does not ordinarily respond to psychosomatic or other types of therapy. In some instances, it is possible to obtain ejaculated semen, although an inadequate erection does not permit coitus. In these cases, homo-insemination may cause a fertilization. It is not possible to obtain a semen specimen from most cases of impotency, and then the only possible means for obtaining a conception is by artificial insemination with foreign donor semen.

## V. Endocrine therapy

With few exceptions, such outstanding endocrinopathies as myxedema, Fröhlich's syndrome and eunuchoidism are associated with an intractable germinal hypoplasia or aplasia, and even before puberty, the germinal epithelium is injured far beyond the possibility of repair by any type of therapy. Cases with outstanding clinical evidence of disorders of the glands of internal secretion do not commonly come under the purvue of those dealing with marital infertility. This is largely because the permanent character of their endocrine disturbance, such as the lack of testicular development or of the normal secondary sexual attributes, favors celibacy. Their problem then assumes a more purely endocrine nature, and their fertility may not come into serious consideration.

The endocrine aspects of male infertility have been badly misrepresented, first by falsely attributing various abnormalities of the germinal epithelium to glandular disturbances, and secondly by attributing conceptions to empiric glandular therapy without the use of clinical control series so as to reveal whether the conceptions occur because of the therapy or in spite of it.

*Gonadotropins.* Gonadotropic and 17-Ketosteroid assays made in connection with germinal disorders will usually reveal that such cases are endocrinologically normal. Neither the cytologic changes of the gametes or histology of the germinal epithelium are commonly pathogenomic of any particular endocrine disturbance. A vast amount of completely worthless endocrine therapy has arisen partly because of the faulty assumption of the glandular etiology of germinal disorders and partly because of the belief that genetic potentialities of spermatozoa may be altered by glandular therapy. The administration of gland products to cases without endocrine disturbances seems to lack any ethical justification. A few instances have been reported in which an improvement in spermiogenesis and conception has followed the use of gonadotropins or androgens, but the smallness

of the series, the lack of adequate clinical control groups and the lack of cytologic evaluation before and after the therapy leaves the validity of many of
these reports open to considerable doubt.

*Androgen therapy.* If sufficient androgen is given to a male who delivers
spermatozoa in his ejaculate, there may be a reduction or cessation of spermiogenesis. Commonly, 25 mg. of methyl testosterone administered daily over a
period of two to four weeks will accomplish this. Then if administration is discontinued, some will return to their pretreatment sperm concentration and
others will continue to produce spermatozoa at a lesser rate than before. The
administration of androgens has been carried out principally with two types of
cases, first those with a eunuchoid habitus with which it is valuable in overcoming the lack of normal secondary sex attributes, and secondly with cases
wherein there is a germinal hypoplasia and a consequent paucity of spermatozoa
in the ejaculate. The administration of testosterone to the eunuchoid male is
essentially without any value from the fertility viewpoint, because the germinal
aplasia or hypoplasia is usually already beyond repair at the time of puberty.
A few cases, however, have been reported wherein androgen has been administered
to the eunuchoid with a remarkable improvement in spermatogenesis, followed
by conception. Such cases are, however, very rare. Most cases with germinal
aplasia or hypoplasia are, however, endocrinologically normal and the administration of the male sex hormone to these may very readily exceed normal requirements, depress spermatogenesis and do more harm than good. Sometimes the
injury is transitory and at other times rather permanent. Because it was observed
that some of the individuals so treated eventually experienced an increased rate
of spermiogenesis after cessation of androgen therapy, and a few conceptions
followed, it was assumed by some that this type of treatment possessed certain
therapeutic merits. A study of the records of androgen therapy reveals, however,
that most of the conceptions occur amongst the cases with sperm concentrations
between 20 and 40 m., a sperm concentration which is not sufficiently reduced to
account for the failures in conception. GETZOFF (1956) has analyzed the results
of androgen therapy as reported by 64 different observers. The sperm concentrations of the treated cases ranged from a very few spermia per cubic centimeter
up to 70 million spermia per cubic centimeter. In this group which totaled
840 cases, there were 56 or 6.6 per cent conceptions after androgen therapy.
Most of these had sperm concentrations ranging between 10 and 40 million per
cubic centimeter, a concentration which under ordinary clinical conditions
without endocrine therapy would give a conception expectancy of about 10 to
20 per cent, in contrast to the 6.6 per cent after androgen therapy. In this group
of 840 androgen treated cases, the therapy of only 39 was based on a endocrine
diagnosis, as provided by hormone assays or the recognition of endocrine stigmata. These results from androgen therapy seem to provide no ethical
justification for this type of therapy, especially since it may be detrimental to
many cases and fails to increase the fertility of the others. Krishna Rao states
"It has been our experience that in cases with which the density was below ten
million per cubic centimeter that the response (with testosterone) was either
poor or nil." In the series analyzed by GETZOFF, conceptions occurred mostly
with cases having a sperm count of over ten million per cubic centimeter and who
were endocrinologically normal.

Although an increased sperm motility has been reported following the use
of both androgens and gonadotropins, their ability to increase fertility has not
been adequately confirmed excepting with a very few cases exhibiting proven
glandular deficiencies. According to clinical observers, both androgens and

gonadotropins are capable of bringing about considerable damage to the germinal epithelium and the risks resulting from their use seem to contra-indicate their use with individuals without a proven glandular imbalance. As a general rule, germinal pathology associated with a marked endocrine imbalance tends to be permanent and causes an irreversible, intractable pathology of the germinal epithelium.

*Thyroid therapy.* Although thyroid therapy has been widely used throughout the world for both male and female sterility, its precise therapeutic value for infertility has not been adequately documented. Thyroid therapy has very frequently been empiric, without regard to the metabolic requirements of the patients and without any knowledge of its effect upon fertility potential. This practice is apparently related to a long-standing and somewhat common belief inherited from the past that the important item in the treatment of both male and female infertility is some type of stimulation which would increase gameto-genesis or favor increased sexual activity. Therefore, any line of therapy which promises some stimulating or energy-producing effect is easily accepted as a part of an anti-infertility program. In consequence, a large number of patients will have gone through a regimen of thyroid therapy before any diagnostic examinations have been made to determine thyroid function or the cause of the reproductive failure.

A basal metabolic rate of as low as minus 20 per cent is ordinarily tolerated without any loss of reproductive function and with these cases, no benefit will be derived from the administration of thyroid extract. However, when the basal metabolic rate is much lower than minus 20 per cent, the deficit may be significant and the patient may benefit from thyroid medication. Apparently, however, any benefit is secondary to an improvement in general health and no significant changes are ordinarily distinguished in the sperm populations after thyroid medication.

Thyroid therapy if medically indicated should be administered in an amount sufficient to elevate the basal metabolic rate to about the normal level. Extreme thyroid disorders such as Graves disease or myxedema are rarely encountered amongst infertile marriages, but if present, should be brought under control prior to any further infertility studies. One grain of thyroid extract will usually elevate the basal metabolic rate about 6 to 7 per cent with a 150 pound individual. There seems to be no advantage in elevating the rate entirely to the normal level since this is not necessary for the general health and normal reproductive function. By keeping the metabolic rate slightly lower than normal, there is a less danger of overdosage.

If thyroid extract is administered, it is well that the patient should record his pulse rate daily before taking his thyroid dosage and to at once discontinue the thyroid extract if the pulse rate should rise above about 85 per minute, or if nervousness, or other unfavorable symptoms appear. Thyroid extract may be contraindicated with cardiac disease, hypertension and other disorders. If a large dose of thyroid is prescribed, the basal metabolism should be repeated after a period of three or four weeks of administration to determine that the proper dosage is being given.

# VI. Surgery

Surgery to correct male infertility is indicated most frequently by an obstruction of the fine tubules of the globus minor of the epididymis. This occurs almost invariably as a complication of Neisserian infection and involves less than 0.5

per cent of the male partners of infertile marriages in those communities where effective venereal disease control measures have been in operation. When control measures are not in operation, the incidence of epididymitis is much higher.

The correction of epididymal obstruction is accomplished by an anastomosis of the globus major with the adjacent segment of the vas deferens, so as to by-pass the globus minor and create a channel for the passage of spermatozoa from the testes. As a prerequisite for a successful anastomosis, it must be established that the germinal epithelium is capable of normal spermiogenesis, that spermatozoa are present in the tubules of the globus major, that there is no obstruction in the globus major and that there is no obstruction in the vas deferens peripheral to the site of anastomosis. The ability of normal spermatogenesis is established by means of the examination of a testicular biopsy specimen taken in advance of a proposed epididymo-vasotomy.

When performing an epididymo-vasotomy, the globus major and the vas deferens are exposed by means of an incision through the scrotum at the superior pole of the testicle. First, a small incision is made in the globus major at the point selected for the anastomosis and fluid from this site is examined at once for spermatozoa. Unless spermatozoa can be obtained, there is no need for proceeding further with the operation. The vas deferens is exposed and a small longitudinal incision of the proper length for anastomosis is made in it. A small, blunt hypodermic needle is then introduced into the lumen of the vas in a peripheral direction and a small amount of a solution of an analine dye such as methylene blue introduced to determine its patency. If patent, the dye will readily pass through the vas and may be recovered through an indwelling urethral catheter. Then if the vas deferens is patent, and spermatozoa have been recoverd from the incision in the globus major, the incised area of the epididymis and the opening in the vas may be brought together and sutured. A small caliber silver wire, or a nylon or polyethylene splint may be inserted through the site of the anastomosis so as to better assure that an opening between the vas and the epididymis shall remain patent until healing is complete. One end of the splint is inserted for 2 or 3 inches into the vas and the other brought out through the scrotum so that it may be removed after ten to fifteen days without further surgery (MICHELSON, BAYLE).

Epididymovasotomies have attained only limited success. BAYLE reports finding spermatozoa in the seminal fluid in about 40 per cent of the cases operated by him and a few others report similar ratios of patency. In most instances, however, the end results are very poor, since conception will fail with most of the cases with which surgery is apparently successful. Because of the expense of the procedure and the relatively poor end-results in terms of ultimate fertility, adoption or artificial insemination with foreign donor semen is usually preferable to surgery; but individual circumstances in some cases may render an epididymo-vasotomy the most desirable solution for their infertility problem.

Various types of pathology of the generative organs may give rise to surgical procedures for their relief, but in many, the type of pathology may obviate the possibility of the restoration of fertility. The surgical correction of a hydrocele or varicocele may not only improve the circulation of the testicle but also favors the reduction of the temperature of the testicle and thus creates a more favorable circumstance for spermiogenesis.

Occasionally, a surgeon is called upon to repair an impatency of the vas due either to trauma, the deliberate section of the vas for purposes of sterilization or because of the accidental severance of the vas during a herniorrhaphy or varicocelectomy. An end to end anastomosis is then often very successful, provided that the severed ends may be brought together. The use of a nylon splint may improve the chances of success in such operations. Various congenital anomalies such as failure of testicular descent, absence of the seminal vesicles, vas or epididymis and failure of union of the epididymis do not usually lend themselves to surgical correction in so far as prospective fertility is concerned (HANLEY).

# VII. Artificial insemination

Artificial insemination signifies a mechanical insemination without recourse to coitus. It may be a homo-insemination, with semen from the lawful spouse, or may be a hetero-insemination with semen derived from a foreign donor. Provided that the semen is normal, a homo-insemination may be indicated when a natural insemination is not possible because of some insurmountable difficulty with coitus, such as premature ejaculation, epispadius or hypospadius which obviates the possibility of natural intra-vaginal insemination, or when impotency renders intromission impossible. With some impotency cases, the failure of erection does not prevent ejaculation, and accordingly, semen may be available for homo-insemination, should such be desired. Homo-insemination with semen which has failed to produce a conception after normal coitus is usually worthless from the viewpoint of fertilization, but a homo-insemination may be indicated in certain cases to by-pass a cervical barrier arising from a destruction of the endocervical epithelium or due to an excessively thick cervical secretion through which the spermatozoa are unable to migrate.

In the absence of any religious deterrents, a hetero-insemination may be indicated principally if the husband is adjudged sterile or essentially sterile although the wife is normal, or when conception from spermia of the husband is contraindicated because of an Rh incompatability or the danger of the transmission of some hereditary defect from the husband to the offspring. Although the practice of artificial inseminations has been criticized on various grounds, its employment the world over has increased very rapidly. The potential field for hetero-inseminations becomes apparent when one considers that about one-fifth of the male partners of infertile marriages are either absolutely sterile, or essentially so. A large segment of the female partners desire a child to which they themselves have given birth. This viewpoint is often shared by their husbands, and when it comes to a final decision, they will value a child from their wife more than an adopted child to which their relationship is not so close. When absolute male sterility exists, the couple is thus presented with one of four decisions (1) adoption, (2) artificial insemination with foreign donor semen, (3) to divorce and seek a fertile mate and (4) to dismiss the idea of having a family and occupy their interests and thoughts with other matters. The strength of the philogenetic impulse, together with the mutual love, respect and consideration of husband and wife for emotions and desires of the other, will provide a decision as to which course will best fulfill their desire for a successful and happy married life.

In most civilized communities, moral ideas and practice do not condone either illegitimate conception by mating with other than the spouse, or divorce as a means of satisfying the philogenic desires of a woman. It is those individuals with a strong aversion towards of these solutions who request artificial insemination as the solution to their matrimonial problems.

## 1. Initial arrangements or requirements of artificial insemination

Preliminary to undertaking an artificial insemination, there are a number of steps which should be taken so as to make certain that the procedure is to be properly carried out and fulfills the desires and requirements of the couple. Its various aspects should be freely discussed with both husband and wife together, and not separately. It is well that the requirements for adoption and artificial insemination be discussed and the advantages and disadvantages of each pointed out. For instance, in many communities, there is a paucity of babies available for adoption. Most of the available babies are derived from illegitimate conceptions and often little is known of their true parents, especially of the father and of their hereditary potentialities. A high-class adoption agency will do the best they can to select a baby which has a background and physical characteristics similar to that of the foster parents, but the degree to which this can be accomplished is many times quite limited because of the sparcity of babies and the competency of the agency. There are usually several times the number of applicants than available babies and many desiring to adopt will be unable to do so. In many instances, a baby will not be furnished to a mixed marriage where those of different religions or races intermarry. This is based on the consideration that a better home and better opportunity in life is commonly better assured if both parents are of the same race or religion. This, however, is not always true.

An adopted child should eventually be informed of the fact that he or she is adopted. In contrast, the child conceived by artificial insemination is to be considered as the child of its legal father and mother. It is rightfully a confidential procedure and the sacred and ethical responsibility of the doctor and also of the couple that it be kept so. An artificial insemination is not performed merely because a woman desires a baby, but rather to unite and perpetuate a family unit with strongly bound ties. This is often accomplished best by a child that the mother truly feels to be her own.

When artificial inseminations are performed, it is ordinarily required that nothing shall be said by either husband or wife which would in any way even intimate any question of the fertility of the husband. The couple is warned that even their parents must not under any circumstances have any knowledge of an artificial insemination or of suspected infertility. When a conception occurs, the wife is referred for obstetrical care to an obstetrician who has no knowledge of the artificial insemination. No difficulty will be experienced in maintaining this confidence if it be made a condition for conducting the procedure. Although the patient receives a description of the characteristics of the donor, the donor's identity is never known by the recipient or the recipient's identity by the donor. It is also the hard and fast rule that a donor shall never know whether any conceptions have been derived from his semen.

## 2. Selection of donor for artificial insemination

When selecting a semen donor, there are a number of factors which should be considered.

a. The physical characteristics should be similar to those of the husband, and the hereditary background should favor the transmission of these characteristics. Therefore, one must be as much interested in the characteristics of the donor's parents as those of the donor.

b. The mental characteristics and aptitude should be of a high order, and an effort should always be made to use donors who are mentally and physically superior to the husband of the recipient. This is often not possible because of the extremely high-class husbands which are commonly encountered in the group requesting artificial insemination. In general, mating of the human race is but a random, hit and miss affair, with very little opportunity for race improvement by means of mating inferior females with superior males and thus improve the general quality of the population. The general practice is that individuals of somewhat similar qualifications mate with each other. Those of different mental and aptitude levels tend to find a mate of their own level. Thus the general population characteristics remain rather constant and inasmuch as artificial insemination deals largely with the upper intelligence stratum of the population, the chances of providing donors who are greatly superior to the recipient can be accomplished to only a very limited degree. The problem of obtaining a donor with a high-class genetic background is, however, extremely important because any couple desiring artificial insemination, also desires a superior child. Thus every possible effort should be made that the semen is derived from an individual with unquestioned high mental, moral, physical and sexual status.

c. Artificial inseminations do not seem to be as effective in causing conceptions as natural relations, and repeated inseminations may be necessary before conception occurs. Careful attention must be given to the general health status of the donor, avoidance of any sexual excesses and the condition of the sperm population which he ejaculates. Since there is marked difference in the fertility potential with individuals possessing similar seminal characteristics, an already proven highly fertile donor is always advantageous. Such proven donors are often not available in sufficient numbers and it becomes necessary to use the semen from unmarried college students, house officers at hospitals and others whose fertility has not yet been proven. It is then necessary when evaluating potential fertility, to rely to a considerable extent upon a thorough semen analysis.

### 3. Health of female partner

It is usually justifiable to consider the wife as fertile as any other woman who has not been exposed to pregnancy, provided a brief pelvic examination and anamnesis are negative. If conception fails after two or three inseminations, a more detailed examination of the wife is in order to identify any factors which might interfere with conception.

### 4. Appointment for artificial insemination

Inasmuch as there are only a few days during a given menstrual cycle when fertilization is possible, it is important that the time of ovulation shall be determined as accurately as possible and the insemination performed at this period. A study of fertilizations in relation to the basal body temperature changes reveals that about fifty per cent of all conceptions occur on the day of the low basal body temperature just preceding a sustained rise, commonly termed the day of ovulation shift. Most of the other conceptions occur in the two days preceding or following the day of temperature shift. Therefore, a record of the basal body temperatures for two or three cycles will provide a reasonably satisfactory method by which one may time the insemination to the most fertile phase of the cycle. If the basal temperature does not clearly reveal the day of shift or if the day of shift varies greatly from cycle to cycle, it is quite likely that ovulation is abnormal and the chance for fertilization is greatly diminished. It is usually desirable to perform the first insemination on the day of temperature shift. If that is unsuccessful, the insemination is repeated the next cycle a day or two before the temperature shift and again the day after the ovulation shift. Any subsequent inseminations should be timed to the fertile phase of the cycle. The time of ovulation and the most favorable time for an insemination may also be determined by the physical characteristics of the cervical mucus, the glycogen content of the cervical mucus and the examination of vaginal smears for cornification.

Wholesale artificial inseminations, using the semen of individuals with proven high fertilizing ability, and divided for the insemination amongst a number of different women on a given day may be highly satisfactory from the viewpoint of the number of fertilizations obtained, but it invites a disregard of the hereditary background of the given individual. It would be very difficult to obtain several women, ovulating on a given day, with husbands so nearly alike that a single donor would be genetically suitable for all.

Before an appointment for an artificial insemination is given, the expected time of ovulation must have been established, one or more suitable donors agreed upon by both husband and wife, and assurances that both husband and wife are completely in accord with the proposed artificial insemination. An appointment is then given for the fertile phase of the cycle, about two weeks in advance of that event. The selected donor is immediately advised so as to make certain of his availability at the appointed time. Both the recipient and the donor are instructed to verify the appointment the morning of the day for which the appointment is given. The husband of the recipient should always be present at time of an artificial insemination and be a party to it. This is a phase which is at times neglected and if so, invites misunderstandings and paves the way for legal difficulties. Having the husband merely sign a statement of permission is not enough. There are apparently no laws governing artificial inseminations per se, but if done dishonestly or in a manner to deceive either husband or wife, it may invite severe legal difficulties. Such complications may, however, be easily avoided by any doctor if normal ethical professional relations are maintained with his patients and he respects the rights and privileges and best interests of both husband and wife.

The donor is usually given an appointment to deliver the semen specimen a few minutes after the appointment for the recipient, so as to make certain that there is no delay in the use of the semen which might reduce sperm fertility. Arrangements must always be made so that the donor and recipient have no opportunity of meeting or determining the identity of each other.

## 5. Collection of semen for use with artificial insemination

Semen for use with artificial insemination is preferably obtained by friction without coitus, and collected directly into a sterile wide-mouth jar. When married donors are used, a withdrawal specimen may be used, but this method is not generally advised because of the greater possibility of contamination of the semen. If married, the donors must be warned to have no relations for three or four days prior to the semen collection and no extra-marital relations. Unmarried donors must have no sexual activity other than the providing of the semen specimens and under no circumstances must donors be used if they cannot be relied upon to not engage in promiscuous sexual relations. One must deal only with individuals who are reliable and willing to adhere to proscribed safeguards.

Inasmuch as certain deteriorative processes in the semen commence soon after the ejaculation, it is best to not attempt the preservation of the semen but instead to use it soon enough that these deteriorative changes are of no consequence. Although various diluents and deep freezing have been successfully employed to conserve fertility of spermatozoa of domestic animals for long periods of time, this has not been successfully accomplished in man excepting as reported with a few isolated cases whose validity is open to some question. Artificial inseminations may be of considerable expense to the patient and every effort should be made that the condition of the wife, the quality of the spermatozoa and the proper timing of insemination are such as to provide the best possible opportunity for success.

## 6. Technique for artificial insemination

a. Recipient is placed in position of dorsal recumbency.

b. Insert Graves bivalve speculum and bring cervical cone into view.

c. Note is made of the condition of the intra-cervical mucus and ovulation dilatation of cervix.

d. Connect a sterile, dry glass cannula with a curved tip to a Luer syringe with the aid of an adaptor and short piece of rubber tubing. Draw into the tip of the cannula about 0.5 cc. of semen and insert the tip of the cannula about $1/_2$ to 1 cm. inside of the cervical canal. Have the husband press the syringe so that he forces about $1/_2$ cc. of the semen into the cervical canal. This puts him in the position that he can honestly sign a statement that he has himself inseminated his wife. The plunger of the syringe is then pushed back and forth a few times so as to thoroughly mix the seminal fluid with the intra-cervical mucus. The buttocks of the patient are then elevated a few inches and an additional 2 to 3 cc. of semen are injected about the cervix so that as the speculum is withdrawn, the cervical cone remains in the semen pool.

e. The patient maintains this position for a period of thirty to forty minutes.

Several other procedures for insemination have been used, with varying success. A plastic cervical cap may be applied to the cervix after the intra-cervical injection. In this position, it can be easily filled with seminal fluid with the aid of a small curved cannula attached to a syringe. The tip of the cannula is guided in between the cervical cap and the cervix, and the semen injected in the cap. The cap is held in position by suction and retains the semen in close contact with the cervical canal as long as desired. This is a convenient method, since it requires only a few moments and the patient can arise and be on her way at once, with the semen remaining in contact with the cervix. HAMAN (1954) reports a conception rate of 83.3% with cervical cap insemination with high grade donor semen, as compared to 56 per cent conceptions following intra-cervical and intravaginal inseminations.

Spermia may remain highly motile in a cervical cap for over twenty-four hours whereas intravaginal spermia perish in one to five hours. Some of those performing artificial inseminations make it the practice to inject a few drops of semen directly into the uterine cavity and report favorable results. One must bear in mind, however, that normal spermatozoa have no difficulty in traversing the length of the cervix, uterus and Fallopian tubes. To insert semen above the cervical barrier into the uterine cavity must necessarily invite the hazard of introducing infection through the tubes into the peritoneal cavity. This method should not be employed excepting in those cases in which one has reason to believe that there is an impediment to sperm migration past the internal cervical ring. Then the amount of semen used should be limited to not more than 0.1 or 0.2 cc. If one merely injects semen into the vagina so that it reaches the external os, comparable to what is ordinarily accomplished with normal coitus, a considerable number of conceptions may be anticipated; but with artificial insemination, where much is at stake, it seems best to make certain that the semen actually contacts the endocervical mucus. In case that a cervical cap is employed, it should be removed in about five hours, since after this time, it can serve no useful purpose.

## 7. Legal aspects of artificial insemination

It is desirable that certain steps be taken to safeguard particularly the wife, baby and the doctor involved. This protection commences with a thorough discussion of the problem in advance with both husband and wife and to ascertain definitely that both of them are in complete accord. It is necessary that the husband shall feel that he has a part in the process and that he is not being overlooked or discarded. Some doctors have required the signing of legal papers giving permission to have the procedure performed. Others have insisted on the filing of adoption papers. The simplest method is apparently to have the husband partake in the procedure and to sign a statement to the effect that he inseminated his wife, and to have his wife witness the signature (Fig. 36).

---

This is to certify that I this day _____ 195__.

inseminated my wife _____
                              (insert name of wife)


Signature of husband _____

Witnessed by _____
                              (signature of wife)

---

Fig. 36. *Affidavit covering artificial inseminations when foreign donor semen is used.* This form is to be signed by both husband and wife at the time of the artificial insemination, and as the basis for this, the husband is required to push the plunger of the syringe holding the semen so that he actually inseminates his wife

The introduction of legal papers or complicated forms into the situation only serves to suggest that the doctor is attempting to protect himself or his patients from something which he considers immoral or illegal. It seems clear that no doctor should undertake any activity which he might view in that light. On the other hand, most of the patients requesting artificial insemination are the highest class, respected citizens, and mostly with strong church affiliations. They are happily married and desire to keep their married life on a high plane. The woman is not interested in an illicit conception and she is not interested in another mate. The husband is naturally much disturbed over the fact that he cannot impregnate his wife, but he desires his wife to be happy and under these circumstances, he often desires a child from his wife more than a child by adoption which he believes he could never consider as much his own as one born of his wife. It is with this background that many couples insist on artificial insemination with foreign donor semen, because they know the background of the donor, and they relish the fact that the child will have at least the background of the wife.

The force of circumstances and time may often alter the viewpoint of a couple on their desire for artificial insemination. Temporarily, they may believe that adoption would be a satisfactory substitute for a child of their own, but later find that it does not do so. In other instances, they favor artificial insemination because a mixed religion prevents them from obtaining a child by adoption. Regardless of the process by which the couple comes by their decision, the factors which initiate legal and moral conflicts are eliminated if they both are in full accord.

There exists a considerable difference of opinion concerning moral and legal aspects of artificial insemination. It is certainly within the province of the doctor to give his patients an insight into the scientific and technical aspects of the subject. He should make certain that there are no unresolved emotional conflicts. If he believes that either party is in any way opposed to artificial insemination, he should not be a party to it. Many patients are guided by very erroneous ideas concerning artificial insemination, which if corrected will completely change their opinions on the subject. Thus some will have the idea that the donor would know their identity, or that their personal affairs would become public property.

## 8. Obstetric care of patient conceived from an artificial insemination

One of the most important factors in the successful results with artificial insemination is to respect the position of the husband as the acknowledged father of the unborn child. This requires that he be made a part of the procedure and every one whom he contacts will regard him as the biologic parent. If the husband does not desire to be so regarded, an artificial insemination should under no circumstances be performed. This commences with the initial interview, is continued by requiring his participation in all the artificial inseminations and then a signed statement that he inseminated his wife and finally that obstetrical care to his wife be given by an obstetrician who has no knowedge of the infertility of the husband. Thus no records on the procedure are made available to anyone, including other doctors, or any social or legal agencies. By this means, experience reveals that normal relations are maintained between both husband and wife, so that the husband feels no different towards his wife than any other husband whose wife is to give birth to a child. The general experience is that when a couple is so treated in a perfectly normal matter-of-fact professional manner, that any significant emotional conflicts are avoided, and that the husband regards the newborn child with the same filial affection as if it had been conceived from his own spermatozoa. Emotional conflicts may, however, be introduced if the doctor takes the viewpoint that they are dealing with a subject which is taboo and which is contrary to normal, ethical and legal standards; and prepares elaborate papers and takes legal measures to protect them from these hypothetical difficulties which would not be produced if he had not departed from the normal confidential ethical basis of doctor-patient relationship.

## 9. Objections to artificial inseminations

In recent years, considerable discussion has occurred as to the propriety of artifical inseminations on various grounds, such as professional, ethical, moral, legal, religious and the possible emotional conflicts which might accrue to the husband and wife because of conception from foreign donor semen.

## a) Legal factors

Since there has been no law passed governing artificial insemination and no courts have passed upon its legality as such, there is no ground for considering its legality at this time. In most civilized countries, a child born in wedlock is the legal offspring of the couple, if there is possible cohabitation by husband and wife during the period of conception. Courts in the future, as at present, cannot be expected to be used as an instrument to bastardize a child born in wedlock from a legally married woman.

Occasional legal conflicts have arisen because inseminations were done in a manner to deceive one or the other partner, because there was a lack of accord between the couple, or professional ethics or standards had been disregarded. They have not been based on interpretation of any laws pertaining to artificial inseminations. Various attempts have been made to consider artificial insemination as adultery. Yet, law, the Bible and the generally accepted definition of the word "adultery" all consider this term as referring to actual extra-marital sexual relations, which does not occur with artificial insemination. Therefore, judicial opinions adjudging artificial insemination as adultery merely express the personal opinion of the spokesman and possess no factual support in law. Isolated personal opinions in redefining the term adultery cannot alter its meaning as defined by law and common usage over a period of many hundreds of years. The legal situation may be aptly summed up by the opinion of Superior Court Judge Elva N. Holmgren who states "When a child is born within a marriage by whatever method, there is a legal presumption that both marriage partners are its parents" (HAMAN 1957).

Obviously, almost any law which could be written governing artificial insemination would require for compliance an abrogation of information of a very confidential nature, would gravitate against the sanctity of marriage, the family unit as the cornerstone of our civilization, and encourage divorce because of infertility. To legislate against the philogenetic instinct of male woman might encourage illegitimacy, since it would disparage the fulfillment of the greatest value of life of many women who find themselves married to an infertile husband. This is a difficult problem for any legal solution because it involves principally our best citizens, mostly with strong church affiliations and who seek artificial insemination because they wish a family of their own and because they have strong moral and ethical objections to either divorce or extra-marital contact for this accomplishment.

## b) Professional viewpoint and ethics

From the viewpoint of the physician, it is clear that his primary duty is to his patients and their welfare is in accordance with the highest precepts of society. In so doing, it is incumbent upon him that he should do nothing which might be considered as illegal or immoral. With respect to artificial insemination, if such be against his moral, religious or ethical principles, it is clear that he should have no part in it. It must be pointed out, however, that moral ideas and practice are not established by common law, or edicts by church or state, but rather develop according to what is found most valuable to a civilization. The State and the courts then codify these ideas and aid in their general acceptance. In this respect, it is very unlikely that any court, any law, or any edict or religious faith can convince many women who really desire motherhood that they shall be denied that privilege, or that they should resort to divorce or illegitimacy for its attainment. It is hardly possible with thinking people to redefine the word adultery to mean other than extra-marital sexual relations, and most doctors will fail to convince a healthy young woman who sincerely desires a child that there is an acceptable substitute for motherhood.

### c) Religious factors

The attitude of the Church towards AID* largely centers about a difference of opinion as to the definition of adultery. Spokesmen for various protestant churches generally consider that adultery consists in having extra-marital sexual relations. Inasmuch as AID is without any such relations, and is often done by the husband, it is considered that the biologic phases of reproduction by AID do not involve any factor of disloyalty with the husband, does not consistute adultery in any sense of the meaning of the word and is not contrary to acceptable social, legal, ethical and moral standards or against the will of God or the doctrines of the Christian Church.

On the other hand, the Roman Catholic Church considers AID in the light of an adulterous act and against the natural laws which God has made. It is intended that reproduction of the human race is to be carried on in accordance to these natural laws and that it is not within the right of man to interfere with their operation. As a result, the obtaining of semen by masturbation apart from intercourse lacks the approval of the Catholic Church. Because of this natural law as laid down by God and to which the Church subscribes, biologic activity and personal intercourse cannot be dealt with separately, and even though conception occurs without extra-marital relations, it cannot be considered otherwise than of an adulterous nature (Gibbons, Pius XII). The Roman Catholic Church takes the attitude that it is right and just that any measures possible be carried out for the treatment of infertility, either male or female. Sexual relationship and the mutual love expressed in the act is essential to married life and excepting for impotency wherein sexual relations are not possible and wherein marriage cannot be consummated, divorce is not permissible. In consequence, it then becomes the will of God that barrenness must be accepted if the male partner is sterile. It is not the unqualified right of the individual to have children excepting in accordance with these natural laws, and if this be denied because of incurable sterility of the husband, they must accept the childlessness as the will of God. In the case of complete impotency, nullification of a marriage would be justifiable because it would interfere with natural law and the consummation of the marriage.

The more liberal elements of the Jewish Church see nothing objectionable in AID. The Orthodox Jewish Church will permit artificial insemination only under certain circumstances which, however, require a special dispensation from the Rabbinical authority (Schnall).

### d) Emotional factors and the attitude of the intertile couple

Emotional factors arising from AID may involve the patients because of the belief that they may be doing something illegal, the fact that their mutual marital relationship might be caused to suffer, fear that the procedure might not be kept confidential, fear that the donor would know of their identity and make trouble for them later on, or the fear that they would be breaking some religious or moral law. Usually when the procedure is explained, the reasons for these tensions will disappear. Apparently, the two greatest causes for emotional disturbances is that the means of conception will not be entirely

---

* AIH-Homo insemination, AID artificial insemination with foreign dopor semen.

confidential and secondly, the fear on the part of the wife that the husband's feeling towards the child and herself would not be that expected from a normal father. It is the rule that these fears are dispelled if the procedure is discussed in the various aspects with the husband and wife together. Occasionally, the husband will assume the attitude that if his wife cannot become pregnant by spermatozoa from him, that he is completely opposed to her conception. Less frequently, the wife will concur in this attitude, but these cases do not commonly inquire about AID and there is little means of knowing their frequency. However, such an uncompromising attitude on the part of an absolutely sterile husband is often not conducive to continued harmonious marital relations. When AID is contemplated, it is very necessary that the attitude of both husband and wife should be determined by means of a frank discussion of the entire problem and that this discussion be carried on with husband and wife together and not separately. This provides an opportunity to observe the reaction between the two and the nature of their conflicts. It furnishes an opportucity for the wife to bring out her opinions and to determine how her husband reacts to them. Occasionally, the young wife will react very violently when she finds her husband desires to condemn her to barrenness when the cause of the reproductive failure lies wholly with him.

There arises also the question as to the emotional reaction towards the baby and towards her husband as the result of insemination with spermatozoa from another man. This does not seem to produce any disturbing factor provided that the insemination is agreed to by the husband. The wife looks forward to the baby as her own regardless of the identity of the biologic father, and with the same filial affection and devotion. Experience with the handling of marital infertility reveals that essentially 100 per cent of them desire conception by natural means with spermatozoa from their own husbands; but if this is not possible, a very large proportion of them see no objection to conception by artificial insemination with donor semen. In an effort to bring out the attitude of this group of patients, concerning artificial insemination with foreign donor semen, a series of questions were put to patients being examined for fertility, some of whom had sterile husbands and others who were experiencing difficulty in conception but with husbands who were considered to be fertile. The following questions were asked:

1. If your husband were totally sterile, would you desire to become pregnant from spermatozoa from another man by artificial insemination, provided that this had the approval of your husband and that the semen was derived from a high-class individual?

2. What would be your attitude towards a baby so conceived? Would you feel towards it the same as if conceived from spermatozoa from your husband?

3. What would be your principal objection to the procedure?

4. Do you believe that your husband would love and cherish a baby which is half yours and the other half from a high-class individual as much as a baby by adoption where little is known of the background of either of its progenators?

5. Do you believe that your husband would prefer that you remain without a child unless it could be conceived by his own spermatozoa?

It was thought desirable to obtain the opinions and attitude of the individuals who are actually faced with the infertility problem since it is these individuals who produce the problem and who are most vitally concerned with it. The attorney may express the legal viewpoint, the clergy the moral and ethical precepts according to their view, the teaching of the Church or according to ecclesiastic law. The geneticist may have reservations on the ability of proper selection of donors and recipients, etc., but in the long run, it is the unfortunate infertile couple whose future is at stake, and whose opinions and rights in a civilized community must be respected.

The discussion of the moral and ethical aspects of artificial insemination with infertile patients brought out several rather pertinent observations, viz.

Most of the women questioned expressed the viewpoint that she would prefer impregnation with spermatozoa from her husband, but that if this were not possible, that it really made little difference whose spermia caused the fertilization of the ovum, provided that the artificial insemination had the approval of her husband, did not jeopardize their ethical relationship and provided that the spermatozoa were derived from another male of high quality, both mentally and physically and of similar characteristics to her husband. They would love and cherish such a baby just the same as if her husband's semen partook in its genesis because "After all, it would be my baby and that is what I want."

Their principal fear was the possibility that the husbands might feel badly hurt because the baby was not conceived from his spermatozoa and in consequence, a loss of ego. Further, it was feared that he might feel estranged with both wife and baby because he was not the biologic father. They were generally not sure whether their husband would wish for them to remain barren rather than to become pregnant from spermatozoa derived from another individual.

The questioning of husbands brought out very frequently the feeling that they would prefer a baby which was at least half theirs because of being born from his wife and that he believed that he would love a baby so obtained much more than an adopted baby which would be unrelated to both of them. Some expressed the view that if his wife could not be pregnant by him that he would insist that she remain barren. Obviously, in some of these instances, the marriage existed as a one-sided institution for satisfaction of the ego of the male partner. When there was a strong philogenetic impulse by the wife, this attitude often was not conducive to a harmonious marital relationship. In a very few instances, the views expressed by the husband were so at variance with those of the wife that it would be dangerous to proceed with artificial insemination. However, in a number of cases, the point of view of the husband changed after a lapse of two or three years when it was found that conception had not occurred by natural meaus and that for some reason adoption was impossible. It became recognized by the husband that there was a certain void in his family life which he could not repair otherwise than by artificial insemination. Then his attitude towards artificial insemination changed, and the couple reached a better mutual understanding as to how they could make their marriage more satisfactory. It has seemed very apparent with most infertility cases, first that nothing must be done which will in any manner jeopardize their marriage. In most instances wherein the sterility is entirely due to the male, the husband will accept, love and cherish a child from his wife more than any other, irrespective of the fact that the conception was not derived from his own spermia.

It has been previously pointed out that the Roman Catholic Church, the high Episcopal and some branches of the Jewish Church are opposed to artificial insemination because of the belief that it is at variance with their religious teaching, the dogma of their church and the will of God. One may expect that members of churches which are opposed to artificial insemination will respect the doctrines and teaching of their church. For this reason, it generally is considered that the subject of artificial insemination must first be brought into discussion by the patient and that the doctor must maintain an entirely neutral interest in it, clarifying misconceptions when they arise but never attempting to impose his views on others. With a known member of the Catholic Church, it is well to mention that they get in touch with the parish priest if the husband is sterile and if they desire to adopt. No mention should be made of artificial insemination as a means of having a family.

A strong religious faith may be much stronger than emotional desires which are precipitated by the philogenetic impulse of a woman. Then it becomes possible for an individual to compensate for childlessness which is not otherwise of easy accomplishment. With others, this adjustment may not be so easily accomplished and the desire for motherhood continues to dominate their thoughts.

## 10. Genetic aspects of artificial insemination

Although the genetic aspects of artificial insemination place considerable responsibility upon the involved physician, these difficulties have been greatly exaggerated. With the ordinary care which any physician can exercise, there seems to be no unreasonable liability in bringing about genetic or hereditary abnormalities, but rather the reverse by means of the selection of normal, healthy donors without apparent genetic faults in their background.

When a physician selects a donor with similar physical characteristics to that of the husband, an individual of high mental caliber with forebears who have demonstrated aptitude for the above average business or professional ability, that there are no known hereditary abnormalities of the family of the donor that, the general apperance and stamina of the donor is of a quality which will justify perpetuation, and that there is good general health, freedom from disease and freedom from genetic disorders of the germinal cells, then the doctor has certainly done his part in providing the best possible quality of a baby and done much more than accomplished by natural selection.

It must be realized that the young woman who selects a man for her spouse, the city clerk who issues a marriage license and the minister who marries them, require none of these safeguards concerning the husband, as pertains to AID. It will not be possible for a doctor to make a detailed genetic study of each donor extending back several generations, but on the other hand, lines of inheritance in the human family are rarely consolidated to the extent that an unfavorable genetic factor becomes a Mendelian dominent. Further than this, if a doctor exerts reasonable precaution along the above lines, he is obviously in most cases accomplishing something in eugenic reproduction which is only by chance accomplished under more normal circumstances. When an adequate supply of donors is available, there is indeed a very good chance of selecting a donor with more favorable attributes than those of the husband of the recipient.

It is not possible to anticipate exactly the characteristics of a baby resulting from an artificial insemination, any more than those resulting from a normal insemination. Such matters as the color of the eyes, the color of the hair and of the skin, physiognomy and general body conformation tend to dominate if the same characteristics are present in the parents and the grandparents. If, however, these characteristics of the donor have been diluted by intermarriage between unlike parents, the donor is apt to reproduce any of the various diverse characteristics of his antecedents. Thus, the progeny of a male with black hair and brown eyes may be of blond hair and blue eyes if these other traits are present in his immediate ancestors. On the other hand, the characteristics of the offspring may be determined quite as much by its mother as by genes carried by the sperm. In the background of the wife, there may exist diverse transmissible hereditary characteristics which although not apparent in the mother may nevertheless determine the character of the offspring in spite of the character of the donor which is selected. This should be understood by the husband since it is not possible for a doctor to guarantee that characteristics of the unborn child shall be similar to those of the husband when so many diluting genetic factors are caused to operate by the marriage of unrelated persons having strikingly different characteristics. The prediction of the results of mating in the human race is quite unlike that in some lower animals where the characteristics are established by inbreeding and where cross-breeding may bring out certain characteristics in the offspring with almost mathematical precision.

What is here said relates principally to characteristics in a given race, but it must be recognized that race characteristics are invariably dominant. Under no circumstances should a mixing of races in artificial insemination be permitted, since its product in our modern civilization would almost inevitably invite disaster.

## VIII. Resume of therapy

Ethical therapy of male infertility is based upon a general knowledge of the various etiologic factors. both somatic and those which relate to the health of the gametes. Actually most cases of male infertility are predicated by azoospermia or by faulty sperm populations which because of their genetic origin are not amenable to therapy. Therapy for sterility which is due to faulty spermiogenesis applies principally to the borderline cases but it is always a possibility that a conception may occur if any apparently normal, highly motile spermia are present in the ejaculate. Many cases of male infertility cannot be successfully treated because of their refractory nature. Thus comprehensive examinations which lead to reliable diagnoses and prognoses are very important as a guide to ethical therapy. The omission of such examinations is very conducive to needless therapy for both the male and female partners. In some instances, proper prophylactic measures may conserve fertility and with others, therapy based on a sound diagnosis will be found highly valuable.

### Bibliography

Austin, C.R.: The function of hyaluronidase in fertilization. Nature (Lond.) 162, 63 (1948). — Bayle, H.: Technique de l'anastomose epididmyo-deferentielle. Soc. d'urologie 1945. — Bayle, H., et C. Gouygou: La sterilite masculine. Ass. Francaise d'Urologie, Paris 1953. — Belonoschkin, Boris: Zeugung beim Menschen. Stockholm: Sjobergs Folag 1949. — Bergman, Per.: Spermigation and its relation to morphology and motility of spermatozoa. Int. J. Fertility 1, 45 (1955). — Bielanski, W.: Characteristics of the semen of stallions. Macroscopic and microscopic investigations with an etsimation of fertility, extrait du memoires de l'academie polonaise des science et des letters, Cacovie, 1951. — Birnberg, C. H., D. L. Sherber and R. L. Kurzrok: Fructose and fructolysis in human semen. Amer. J. Obstet. Gynec. 63, 877 (1952). — Blom, E.: Spontaneous detachment of the galea capitis in spermia of bull and stallion. Skand. Veterin.-T. 35, 779—789 (1945). — Blom, E.: One minute live-dead sperm stain by means of eosin-nigrosin. Fertil. and Steril. 1, 176 (1950). — Boreau, J., P. Hermann et R. Fua: L'epididymographie. Presse méd. 59, 1406 (1951). — Breitschneider, L. H.: An electron-microscopical study of sperm IV. Proc. kon. Ned. Akad. Wet. 12, 526 (1949). — An electron-microscopical study of the bull Sperm III. Proc. kon. ned. Akad. Wet. 12, 301 (1949). — Brochart, M., et S. M. Montrose: Morphologie normale et anormale due spermatozoide de taureau. Rec. Med. vet. 127, 449—475 (1951). — Brodny, M. Leopold: Epididymography, varicocelography and testicular angiography. Fertil. and Steril. 6, 158—168 (1955). — Bunge, R. G., and J. K. Sherman: Frozen human semen. Fertil. and Steril. 5, 193, (1954). — Cary, W. H.: Examination of semen with special reference to its gynecologic aspects. Amer. J. Obstet. Gynec. 74, 615—635 (1916). — Castillo, E. B. del, A. Trabucco and F. A. de la Balze: Syndrome produced by absence of the germinal epithelium without impairment of the Sertoli or Leydig cells. J. clin. Endocr. 7, 493—502 (1947). — Castro, E.: Ocupacion y fertilidad masculina: Re-

lacion de ocupaciones a la fertuluda disminuida y a la infertilidad.   Proc. First World
Congr. on Fertility and Sterility, New York 1953. — COHEN, MELVIN R., and IRVING F.
STEIN: Sperm survival at estimated ovulation time. Fertil. and Steril. 2, 20—28 (1951). —
CONKLIN, R. L.: The relation of sexual health of the domestic cock to fertility and hatchability
of the eggs. Cornell Vet. 19, 25—32 (1929). — DAVIS, M. E., and W. W. McCUNE: Fructolysis
of human spermatozoa. Fertil. and Steril. 1, 363 (1950). — DUNN, H. O.: Personal communication, 1958. — New advances in bovine semen preservation. Int. J. Fertility 3, 332 (1958). —
ECHEANDIA, M. ATEEA and MUNOZ, A. PIEROS: Velocidad de progression del espermio humano
en glucose y levulosa. Arch. Med. exp. (Madr.) 2, 273—299 (1954). — EMMONS, C. W.: The
effect of variation in osmotic pressure and electrolyte concentration on the motility of rabbit
spermatozoa at different hydrogen ion concentrations. J. Physiol. (Lond.) 107, 129 (1948). —
FINCHER, M. G., and J. FERGUSON: Sterility in bulls, annual report N. Y. State Vet. College,
1942. — FLECHTER, JOSEPH: Artificial insemination. Fertil. and Steril. 9, 372 (1958). —
FOOTE, R. H., D. C. YOUNG and H. O. DUNN: Fertility of bull semen stored for one and
two days at 5⁰ C. with yolk-citrate, glycine, glucose extenders. J. Dairy Sci. 41, 732 (1958). —
GETZOFF, P. L.: Clinical evaluation of testicular biopsy and the rebound phenomena. Fertil.
and Steril. 6, 465 (1955). — The treatment of male sterility with testosterone. Int. J. Fertility
1, 175 (1956). — The effect of chronic prostatovesiculitis on sperm motility. Int. J. Fertility
3, 316—319 (1958). — Purulent semen and male infertility. Int. J. Fertility 3, 408—412
(1958). — GIAROLA, A.: Biochemical and morphological characters of human semen. Annali,
Milano, 1953. — GREEN, W. W.: The chemistry and cytology of the sperm membrane of
sheep. Anat. Rec. 76, 467 (1940). — HAMAN, JOHN O.: Legal aspects of artificial insemination. Progr. Gynec. 3, 359—373 (1957). — Results in artificial insemination. Trans. Amer.
Urol. Assoc. Aug. 1954. — HAMMEN, R.: Studies on impaired fertility of man with special
reference to the male. Copenhagen: E. Munksgaard 1944. — HAMMOND, J., and S. A. ADSELL:
The vitality of spermatozoa in the male and female reproductive tracts. Brit. J. exp. Biol.
4, 155—185 (1926/27). — HELLINGA, GERHARDUS: Het onderzek nig stoornissen in de
mannelijke. Vruchbaarheld, N. V. Noord-Hollandsche, Uitgevers Mastschappij, 1949. —
HENLEY, HOWARD G.: The surgery of male subinfertility. Ann. roy. Coll. Surg. Engl. 17,
159—183 (1955). — HOYNE, A., J.H. DIAMOND and J. R. CHRISTIAN: Diethylstilbesterol
and prevention of mumps orchitis. J. Amer. med. Ass. 140, 662 (1949). — HUGGINS, C.,
and W. J. NEAL: Coagulation and liquefaction of semen, proteolytic enzymes, and citric
acid in the prostate. J. exp. Med. 76, 527 (1942). — HUGGINS, C. B., W. W. SCOTT and J. H.
HEINEN: Chemical composition of the human semen and of the secretion of the prostate
and seminal vesicles. Amer. J. Physiol. 136, 467 (1942). — HUXLEY, H. E.: Muscular contraction. Endeavour 15, 177—188 (1956). — KLINEFELTER, H. F., E. C. REIFENSTEIN and
F. ALBRIGHT: Syndrome characterized by gynemastia, aspermatogenesis without a-leydigism
and increased secretion of follicle-stimulating hormone. J. clin. Endocr. 2, 615 (1942). —
KNUDSEN, O.: Cytomorphological investigations into the spermocytogenesis of bulls with
normal fertility and bulls with acquired disturbances in spermiogenesis. Acta path. microbiol. scand. Suppl. 100, 1 (1954). — Studies on spermatocytogenesis of bulls. Int. J. Fertility
3, 389—403 (1958). — LAGERLÖF, NILS: Investigations on sterility in swedish bulls during,
the period 1928—1949. Vlaams diergeneesk. T. 19, 285—294 (1950). — Biologic aspects
of infertility of male domestic animals. Int. J. Fertility 2, 99 (1957). — LANE-ROBERTS,
CEDRIC et al.: Sterility and impaired fertility. Hamish Hamilton Med. Books, p. 15. 1948. —
LUNDQUIST, F.: Studies on biochemistry of human semen; amio acids and proteolytic.
enzymes. Acta physiol. scand. 25, 178 (1952). — MACLEOD, J.: The metabolism of human
spermatozoa. Amer. J. Physiol. 132, 193 (1941). — MACLEOD, J., and R. Z. GOLD: The
male factor in fertility and infertility. Fertil. and Steril. 8, 36—49 (1957). — MANN, T.:
Studies in metabolism of semen. Biochem. J. 39, 451 (1945). — Studies in metabolism of
semen, glycolosis in spermatozoa. Biochem. J. 39, 458 (1945). — Studies on the metabolism
of semen. Biochem. J. 40, 481 (1946). — The biochemistry of semen. New York: Wiley
1954. — MARKUS, H.: Über die Struktur der menschlichen Spermien. Arch. Zellforsch.
15, 445—448 (1919/21). — McENTEE, K., and P. OLAFSON: Reproductive trat pathology
in hyperkeratosis of cattle and sheep. Fertil. and Steril. 4, 128—136 (1953). — McKENSIE,
F. F., and V. BERLINER: The reproductive capacity of rams. Missouri Agr. Exp. St. Res.
Bul. No. 265, 1937. — MICHELSON, LEWIS: Treatment of azoospermia by vasoepididymal
anastomosis. Trans. Amer. Soc. Study Sterility 150 (1946). — MICHELSON, LEWIS: Vasoepididymal anastomosis. Surg. Gynec. Obstet. 82, 327 (1946). — MOELLER, A. M., and
N. L. VAN DEMARK: In-vitro speeds of bovine spermatozoa. Fertil. and Steril. 6, 506—512
(1955). — MOENCH, G. L., and H. HOLT: Sperm morphology in relation to fertility. Amer.
J. Obstet. Gynec. 22, 199—210 (1931). — NELSON, W. O.: The physiologic basis of hyper-
gonadism. Med. Clin. N. Amer. 32, 97—110 (1948). — NORDLANDER, E.: The influence of
orchitis parotidea on spermatogneesis. Proc. First World Congr. on Fertility and Sterility,
1953. — PALMER, RAOUL: La sterilite involuntaire. Paris: Masson & Cie. 1950. — PERLOFF,

W. H., and B. J. CHANNICK: Infertility due to large semen volume. Fertil. and Steril. **9**, 171 (1958). — PIUS XII.: Address by His Holiness Second World Congr. on Fertility and Sterility. Int. J. Fertility **2**, 1 (1957). — POLGE, C., and L. E. A. ROWSON: Fertilizing capacity of bull spermatozoa after freezing at —79°C. Nature (Lond.) **169**, 626 (1952). — RAO, B. KRISHNA: Male infertility. Med. Dig. (New Delhi) **23**, 890 (1955). — RISMAN, G. G.: Effect of cortisone in orchitis of epidemic parotitis. J. Amer. med. Ass. **62**, 875 (1956). — REIFENSTEIN, EDWARD C.: The relation of the adrenal cortes to gynecology. Progress in Gynecology. p. 270—283. J. Meigs & S. Sturgis. Grune & Stratton 1950. — SAVAGE, A., W. L. W·LLIAMS and N. M. FOWLER: A study of the head length variability of equine spermatozoa. Cand. J. Res. **3**, 327—355 (1930). — SAVAGE, A., W. W. WILLIAMS and N. M. FOWLER: A statistical study of head length variability of bovine spermatozoa and its application to the determination of fertility. Trans. roy. Soc. Can., Sect. V, **21**, 425 (1927). — SAVIN, J.: Diethylstilbesterolin in prevention of mumps orchitis. Rhode Island Med. J. **29**, 662 (1946). — SCHALL, M. D.: Electromicroscopic study of human spermatozoa. Fertil. and Steril. **3**, 62—82 (1952). — Quoted by Buxton, Artificial insemination. Fertil. and Steril. **9**, 368 (1958). — SCHULTZ-LARSEN, J.: The morphology of the human sperm, Villars. Copenhagen: Lunn 1958. — SEYMOUR, F., C. DUFFY and A. KOERNER: A case of authenticated fertility in a man aged 94. J. Amer. med. Ass. **105**, 1423 (1935). — SIMMONET, H., and M. BRUNAUD: Remarques sur le metabilosme et las motilite du spermatozoide. Atti 1. Congr. Fisiopath. Animal, Milan, 1948. — SORENSEN, ED.: The dehydrogenization power of sperm cells as a mesurea of fertility. Skand. Veter. **32**, 358—373 (1942). — SZENT-GYORGY, A.: Nature of life. New York: Academic Press 1948. — WALTON, A., and W. URUSKI: The effect of low atmospheric pressure of fertility of the male rabbit. J. exp. Biol. **23**, 71—76 (1946). — WEISMAN, ABNER: A technique for aspirating viable spermatozoa from the cavity of the uterus. Amer. J. Obstet. Gynec. **39**, 475 (1940). — Spermatozoa and sterility, p. 129. New York: Hoeber 1941. — WILLIAMS, W. L.: Disease of the genital organs of domestic animals. Ithaca (N.Y.) 1943. — WILLIAMS, W. W.: Spermatic abnormalities. New Engl. J. Med. **217**, 945—951 (1937). — The germ plasm factor in sterility. Urol. cutan. Rev. **43**, 587 (1939). — The routine order of examinations for the diagnosis of sterility. Amer. J. Obstet. Gynec. **47**, 537 (1944). — Mitochondrial and centrosomic disease of spermatozoa. J. Urol. (Baltimore) **64**, 614—617 (1950). — Sterility, the diagnostic survey of the infertility. Int. J. Fertility **1**, 155—169 (1956). — WILLIAMS, W. W., and O. J. POLLAK: Study of sperm vitality with the aid of eosin-nigrosin stain. Fert. and Steril. **1**, 178 (1950). — WILLIAMS, W. W., and A. SAVAGE: Observations on seminal micropathology of bulls. Cornell Vet. **15**, 353 (1925). — WILLIAMS, W. W., and F. A. SIMMONS, The clinical approach to the diagnosis of sterility. Urol. cutan. Rev. **46**, 558—570 (1942). — WILLIAMS, W. W.: Biochemistry of semen. Int. J. Fertility **4**, 29—37 (1959). — YERUSHALMY, G.: Age of father and survival of offspring. Hum. Biol. **2**, 342—356 (1939).

# Namenverzeichnis — Author Index

Mombaerts, J. 3, *56*
Monrad-Krohn, G. H. 87, *110*
Montassut, M., L. Chertok u. P. Aboulker *56*
Montrose, S. M. s. Brochart, M. *294*
More, R. H., u. D. Waugh 120, *169*
Morel, A. s. Leriche, R. *57*
Mosse, W. H. s. Payne, W. W. 159, *169*
Mosso, A., u. P. Pellacani 7, 11, *56*
Mowrer 32
— O. H., u. W. M. Mowrer 32, *57*
— W. M. s. Mowrer, O. H. 32, *57*
Munoz s. Echeandia *295*
Munro, D. 39, 68, 76, 78, 79, 83, 92, 93, *110*
— H. W. Horne jr. u. D. P. Paull *57*
— s. Horne, H. W. 104, *111*
Munter 155
Murnaghan, G. F. 64, *109*

Nachmansohn, D. 116, *169*
Nash, D. F. E. 23, 28, *57*
Nathan, P. W. 85, *110*
Neal, W. J. s. Huggins, C. *295*
Neander, D. G. s. Harrison, F. G. 153, *168*
Nelson, W. O. 217, *295*
Nesbit, R. M., u. J. Lapides 73, *109*
Nichols, L. A. 30, *57*
Nickel, E. s. Hinman jr., F. 94, *110*
Nickels, T. T. s. Kindall, L. 140, 148, *168*
Nissen, K. *201*
Nordlander, E. 206, *295*
Nunez, M. (M. Fernan-Nunez) *169*

Oberman, J. s. Lange, K. 121, *168*
O'Connor jr., V. J. *57*
— V. J. 62
Ogur, G. s. Lange, K. 121, *168*
Olafson, P. s. McEntee, K. 212, *295*
Oldham, J. B. 59, 60, 62, 63, *108*
Ottinger, B. s. Germuth jr., F. G. *168*
Oyma, J. s. Germuth jr., F. G. *168*

Page, J. H. s. Fouts, P. J. *122, 168*
Palmer, Raoul 252, *295*
Pantek, H. s. Schneider, R. C. 77, *110*

Papin, E. 62, *108*
— u. L. Ambard 63, *108*
Parade, G. W. *201*
Paull, D. P. s. Horne, H. W. 104, *111*
— s. Munro, D. *57*
— s. Talbot, H. S. *111*
Payne, W. W., W. H. Mosse u. S. L. Raines 159, *169*
Pearson, G. H. s. English, O. S. 34, *57*
Pellacani, P. s. Mosso, A. 7, 11, *56*
Pendergrass, E. P., G. W. Chamberlin u. E. W. Godfrey u. E. D. Berdick 158, *169*
Perlman 272
Perloff, W. H., u. B. J. Channick *295, 296*
Petersén, I. u. C. Franksson 66, *109*
— s. Franksson, C. 64, 71, *108*, *109*
Pfeiffer, E. F., u. H. E. Bruch 123, *169*
Pflaumer, E. 187, 195, *201*
Pieros, A. s. Echeandia *295*
Pinck s. Anderson 21, 26
— B. D. 23, 26, 28, *57*
Pirquet, C. v. 113, *169*
Pius XII. 290, *296*
Polge 251
— C., u. L. E. A. Rowson *296*
Pollack, O. J. s. Williams, W. W. 263, *296*
Pomeroy,W. B. s. Kinsey, A. C. *57*
Ponsold, A. s. Holtz, F. *201*
— W. s. Quandt, J. 172, 177, 181, 193, 196, *201*
Poole-Wilson, D. S. 64, 66, *109*
Powell, E. B. s. Powell, N. B. 149, *169*
— N. B., u. E. B. Powell 149, *169*
Prather, G. C. 68, 70, 78, 98, *109, 110*
— F. H. Mayfield *111*
Prausnitz, C., u. H. Küstner 118, 141, *169*
Pressman, D. 122, 123, *169*
— H. N. Eisen, M. Siegel, P. J. Fitzgerald, B. Sherman u. A. Siverstein *169*
— L. Korngold u. W. Heyman *169*
Preziozi, P. 123, *169*
Purves-Stewart, J. 87, *110*

Quandt, J. *201*
— u. W. Ponsold 172, 177, 181, 193, 196, *201*

Raffel, S. 125, *169*
— u. J. E. Forney *169*
Raines, S. L. s. Payne, W. W. 159, *169*
Randolph, T. G., J. P. Rollins u. Clyde K. Walter 149, *169*
Rao, B. Krishna *296*
Rattner, H. 152, *169*
Read, G. R. s. Talbot, H. S. *111*
Recklinghausen, v. 175, 180
Reifenstein, Edward C. 266,*296*
— s. Klinefelter 211, *295*
Reingold, I. M. 103, *111*
— s. Bors, E. 87, 94, 105, *109*
Reiter 152
Rhodes, J. 144, *169*
Ribeiro, C. s. Criep, L. H. 160, *167*
Rich, A. R. 119, 120, 121, 123, 127, 129, *169*
— M. Berthrong u. I. L. Bennett jr. 120, *170*
— u. J. E. Gregory 120, *170*
Riches, E. W. 79, *108, 110*
Richet jr., C., A. Tzanck u. A. Couder 145, *170*
Riddoch, G. s. Head, H. 105, *111*
Riethmüller, H. U. s. Heni, F. 185, 186, 187, 190, *201*
Riml, O., u. E. Tscherne 192, *201*
Rinkel, H. J. 141, *170*
— s. Balyeat, R. M. 162, *167*
Ripley, H. S. s. Straub, L. R. 7, 8, 9, 10, 11, *56*
Risak, E. 183, *201*
Risman, G. G. 206, *296*
Robb, W. A. T. s. Milton, G. W. 64, 65, 66, *109*
Robertson, E. G. s. Denny-Brown, D. 66, *109*
Robins, S. A. s. Brodney, M. L. *56*
Robinson s. Guttmann 104
— M. W. 151, *170*
— R. *111*
Roepke, M. H. s. Henderson, V. E. *57*
Rollinghoff, W. 159, *170*
Rollins, J. P. s. Randolph, T. G. 149, *169*
Rolnick u. G. U. Baumrucker 126, *170*
Rose, D. K. s. Meirowsky, A. M. *110*
— S. S. 41, *57*
Rosenblueth, A. 116, *170*
Rosenson, W., u. R. Liswood 32, *57*
Rosenthal 159
Ross, J. Cosbie 71, 86, *109, 110*
— u. M. Damanski 73, 84, 86, 87, *109*

# Sachverzeichnis — Subject Index

REPRINT FROM

# HANDBUCH DER UROLOGIE
# ENCYCLOPEDIA OF UROLOGY
# ENCYCLOPÉDIE D'UROLOGIE

EDITED BY

C. E. ALKEN · V. W. DIX · H. M. WEYRAUCH · E. WILDBOLZ

VOLUME XII

SPRINGER-VERLAG / BERLIN · GÖTTINGEN · HEIDELBERG 1960

(PRINTED IN GERMANY)

# FUNCTIONAL DISEASES

BY

DONALD R. SMITH AND ALFRED AUERBACK

REPRINT FROM

# HANDBUCH DER UROLOGIE
# ENCYCLOPEDIA OF UROLOGY
# ENCYCLOPÉDIE D'UROLOGIE

EDITED BY

C. E. ALKEN · V. W. DIX · H. M. WEYRAUCH · E. WILDBOLZ

VOLUME XII

SPRINGER-VERLAG/BERLIN · GÖTTINGEN · HEIDELBERG 1960
(PRINTED IN GERMANY)

# NEUROMUSCULAR DYSFUNCTION AND PARAPLEGIA

BY

J. COSBIE ROSS

REPRINT FROM

# HANDBUCH DER UROLOGIE
# ENCYCLOPEDIA OF UROLOGY
# ENCYCLOPÉDIE D'UROLOGIE

EDITED BY

C. E. ALKEN · V. W. DIX · H. M. WEYRAUCH · E. WILDBOLZ

VOLUME XII

SPRINGER-VERLAG / BERLIN · GÖTTINGEN · HEIDELBERG 1960
(PRINTED IN GERMANY)

# UROGENITAL ALLERGY

BY

CARL E. BURKLAND

SONDERDRUCK AUS

# HANDBUCH DER UROLOGIE
# ENCYCLOPEDIA OF UROLOGY
# ENCYCLOPÉDIE D'UROLOGIE

HERAUSGEGEBEN VON

C. E. ALKEN · V. W. DIX · H. M. WEYRAUCH · E. WILDBOLZ

BAND XII

SPRINGER-VERLAG / BERLIN · GÖTTINGEN · HEIDELBERG 1960
(PRINTED IN GERMANY)

# TETANIE

VON

G. W. PARADE

REPRINT FROM

# HANDBUCH DER UROLOGIE
# ENCYCLOPEDIA OF UROLOGY
# ENCYCLOPÉDIE D'UROLOGIE

EDITED BY

## C.E. ALKEN · V.W. DIX · H.M. WEYRAUCH · E. WILDBOLZ

VOLUME XII

SPRINGER-VERLAG / BERLIN · GÖTTINGEN · HEIDELBERG 1960
(PRINTED IN GERMANY)

# MALE STERILITY

BY

WALTER W. WILLIAMS